Comprehensive Manuals of Surgical Specialties

Richard H. Egdahl, editor

Robert E. Hermann

Manual of Surgery of the Gallbladder, Bile Ducts, and Exocrine Pancreas

With contributions by Avram M. Cooperman, Caldwell B. Esselstyn, Jr., Ezra Steiger, and R. Thomas Holzbach

Includes 197 color illustrations and 123 illustrations in black and white

Springer-Verlag
New York   Heidelberg   Berlin

Comprehensive Manuals of Surgical Specialties, Volume 3

SERIES EDITOR

Richard H. Egdahl M.D., Ph.D., Professor of Surgery, Boston University Medical Center, Boston, Massachusetts 02118

AUTHOR

Robert E. Hermann M.D., Head, Department of General Surgery, The Cleveland Clinic Foundation, Cleveland, Ohio 44106

CONTRIBUTORS

Avram M. Cooperman M.D., Caldwell B. Esselstyn, Jr., M.D., Ezra Steiger M.D., Department of General Surgery, The Cleveland Clinic Foundation, Cleveland, Ohio 44106

R. Thomas Holzbach M.D., Gastrointestinal Research Unit, Department of Gastroenterology, The Cleveland Clinic Foundation, Cleveland, Ohio 44106

MEDICAL ILLUSTRATOR

Robert M. Reed A.M.I., Head, Department of Medical Illustrations, The Cleveland Clinic Foundation, Cleveland, Ohio 44106

Library of Congress Cataloging in Publication Data

Hermann, Robert E.
    Manual of surgery of the gallbladder, bile ducts,
and exocrine pancreas.

    (Comprehensive manuals of surgical specialties ; v. 3)
    Includes index.
    1. Gall-bladder—Surgery—Handbooks, manuals, etc.
2. Bile-ducts—Surgery—Handbooks, manuals, etc.
3. Pancreas—Surgery—Handbooks, manuals, etc.
I. Cooperman, Avram M. II. Title. [DNLM: 1. Gallbladder—Surgery. 2. Bile ducts—Surgery. 3. Pancreas
—Surgery. WI750 H552m]
RD546.H36   617′.556   78-23697

Printed in the United States of America.

9 8 7 6 5 4 3 2 1

ISBN 0-387-90351-8   Springer-Verlag   New York   Heidelberg   Berlin
ISBN 3-540-90351-8   Springer-Verlag   Berlin   Heidelberg   New York

To all those who have taught me surgery,
especially,

Ewald E. Hermann, M.D.
Carl A. Moyer, M.D.
William D. Holden, M.D.
George Crile, Jr., M.D.
Stanley O. Hoerr, M.D.

Editor's Note

Comprehensive Manuals of Surgical Specialties is a series of surgical manuals designed to present current operative techniques and to explore various aspects of diagnosis and treatment. The series features a unique format with emphasis on large, detailed, full-color illustrations, schematic charts and photographs to demonstrate integral steps in surgical procedures.

Each manual focuses on a specific region or topic and describes surgical anatomy, physiology, pathology, diagnosis and operative treatment. Operative techniques and stratagems for dealing with surgically correctable disorders are described in detail. Illustrations are primarily depicted from the surgeon's viewpoint to enhance clarity and comprehension.

Other volumes in preparation:

Manual of Gynecologic Surgery
Manual of Lower Gastrointestinal Surgery
Manual of Urologic Surgery
Manual of Vascular Surgery
Manual of Cardiac Surgery
Manual of Liver Surgery
Manual of Soft Tissue Tumor Surgery
Manual of Orthopaedic Surgery
Manual of Upper Gastrointestinal Surgery
Manual of Plastic Surgery
Manual of Ambulatory Surgery

Richard H. Egdahl

Foreword

It is appropriate that a surgical teacher, Robert E. Hermann, M.D., with a large experience in a specialized field should author the beautifully illustrated *Manual of Surgery of the Gallbladder, Bile Ducts, and Exocrine Pancreas*. This manual, which takes its place in the distinguished series sponsored by Richard H. Egdahl, M.D., is designed for the working surgeon, resident or practitioner, who wishes to refresh his memory or to bring himself abreast of current thinking and technics. The carefully planned format and the elegant color illustrations of Mr. Robert Reed permit this with the expenditure of a minimum of time and effort, and surgeons who must operate on the organs and structures it covers will wish to have it available for reference.

Stanley O. Hoerr, M.D.
former Chairman, Division of Surgery
Cleveland Clinic

Chairman, Department of Surgery
Fairview General Hospital
Cleveland, Ohio

Preface

Operations on the gallbladder and bile ducts are among the surgical procedures most commonly performed by general surgeons. In most hospitals, cholecystectomy is the most frequently performed operation within the abdomen; approximately 600,000 are performed each year in the United States. In addition, an estimated 120,000 bile duct operations are performed yearly.

Pancreatic surgery is less frequent, but because of the close relation between the biliary system and the pancreas, knowledge of pancreatic problems is equally essential to the surgeon. Acute and chronic pancreatitis and cancer of the pancreas are often encountered by surgeons, with apparently increasing frequency; their treatment remains difficult and perplexing. This book correlates the association between the biliary system and pancreas in a way not done by previous books.

For the gallbladder, bile ducts, and exocrine pancreas, this manual provides an understanding of their anatomy and physiology, their diseases, and most important, methods of operative management. It is written from a personal viewpoint, emphasizing my practice and that of my associates in the operative principles and technics presented.

As in previous manuals in this series, every effort has been made to orient the illustrations to the operative field as seen by the surgeon. We are especially pleased with the many full-color illustrations prepared by Mr. Robert M. Reed and with the publisher's cooperation in the production of this volume.

Robert E. Hermann

Acknowledgments

In the creation of any book, many people contribute to the development of the final manuscript and the illustrations. I would like to especially thank Miss Mary Rita Feran, M.S., Head of the Department of Scientific Publications at the Cleveland Clinic Foundation, for her help in reviewing and editing the manuscript and for checking on innumerable references; Mrs. Margot Lacy and Mrs. Shirley Prokuski of the Department of Word Processing for typing and processing the text; Mr. James T. Suchy and Mr. Jeffrey J. Loerch of the Department of Medical Illustrations for providing additional art work and illustrations for Mr. Robert M. Reed, A.M.I., the principal artist; and to the members of the Department of Medical Photography at the Cleveland Clinic for their help in providing full color photographs and high quality reproductions of roentgenograms.

Robert E. Hermann

Contents

II   Exocrine Pancreas

7   General Introduction 155

8   Congenital Anomalies 167

9   Inflammatory Disease 177

Gallbladder and Bile Ducts

I

General Introduction

1

Surgical Anatomy

The biliary system can be divided into four anatomical areas: (1) intrahepatic bile ducts, (2) common hepatic and common bile ducts, (3) gallbladder and cystic duct, and (4) intrapancreatic (distal) common bile duct and ampullary region (Figure 1-1).

Bile Ducts

The bile ducts are formed in the liver from multiple bile canaliculi that collect the bile excreted by liver cells; these ducts then gather like the branches of a tree into larger ducts to drain the bile from each of the major hepatic segments[1] (Figures 1-2 and 1-3). The segmental ducts then unite into two large hepatic ducts draining both right and left hepatic lobes. A common anomaly is an accessory right hepatic duct, making a total of three main hepatic ducts (Figure 1-4). The right and left hepatic ducts appear to be of generally equal size. In the patient with chronic, obstructive biliary disease, however, the left main hepatic duct frequently becomes much larger than the right hepatic duct (Figure 1-5). The reasons for this developmental finding are unclear.

The common hepatic duct is formed by the junction of the right and left hepatic ducts, proximal to the junction of the cystic duct. After being joined by the cystic duct from the gallbladder, the common hepatic duct becomes the common bile duct.[2,8] The common hepatic duct is 2 to 4 cm in length, the junction with the cystic duct being quite variable; the common bile duct is 6 to 10 cm in length. The diameters of the common hepatic and common bile ducts vary from 4 to 8 mm. After cholecystectomy, they often measure 8 mm to 1.2 cm, undergoing moderate dilatation probably as a response to the loss of the gallbladder as a storage organ or the derangement of the normal choledochal sphincter mechanism at the ampulla of Vater.

The extrahepatic bile duct (the common hepatic and common bile duct) in the hepatoduodenal ligament lies anterior to the portal vein and lateral to (to the right of) the hepatic artery (Figure 1-6). The bile duct is surrounded by a rich plexus of lymphatics and small veins.

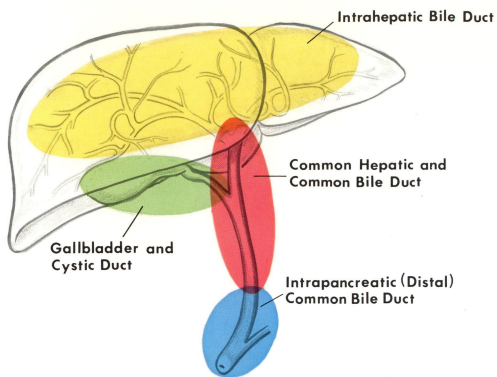

FIGURE 1-1. Four surgical anatomical components of the biliary system: intrahepatic bile ducts (yellow), common hepatic and common bile ducts (pink), gallbladder and cystic duct (green), intrapancreatic (distal) common bile duct and ampullary region (blue).

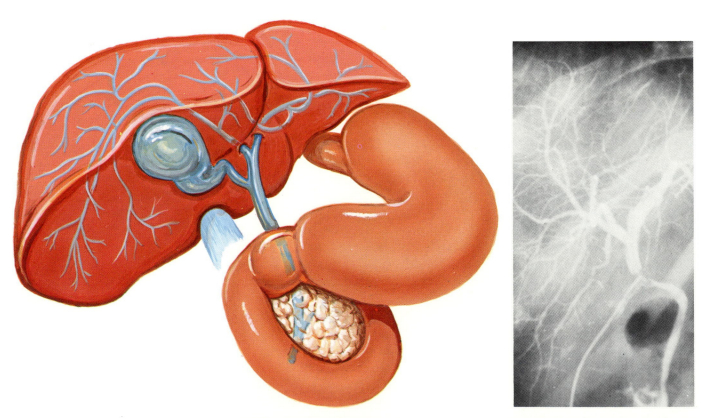

FIGURE 1-2. Intrahepatic bile ducts join to form progressively larger ducts, eventually forming main left and right hepatic ducts. The T-tube cholangiogram shows the intrahepatic bile ducts unusually well as they join to form the main right and left hepatic ducts.

4

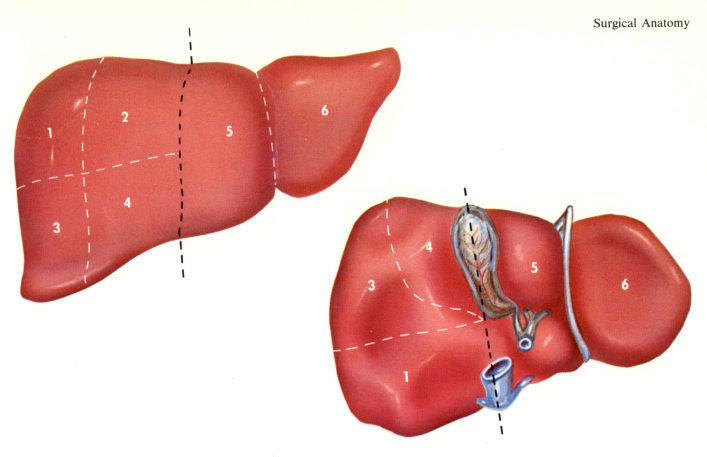

FIGURE 1-3. Major hepatic segments are each drained by segmental, intrahepatic bile ducts. This drawing shows the four major segments of the right hepatic lobe (1 through 4) and the two major surgical divisions of the left hepatic lobe (5 and 6).

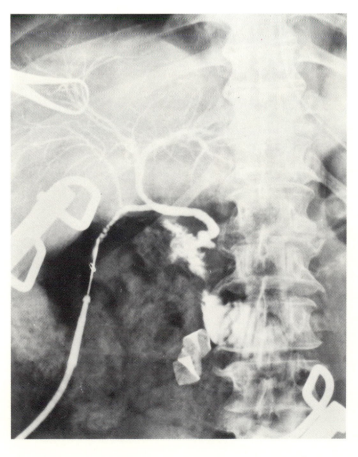

FIGURE 1-4. Operative cholangiogram showing a common anomaly, an accessory right hepatic duct joined by the cystic duct.

5

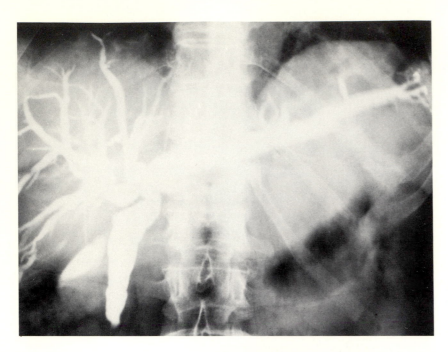

FIGURE 1-5. Left main hepatic duct has become larger than right hepatic duct, as shown on this percutaneous transhepatic cholangiogram in a patient with carcinoma of the pancreas.

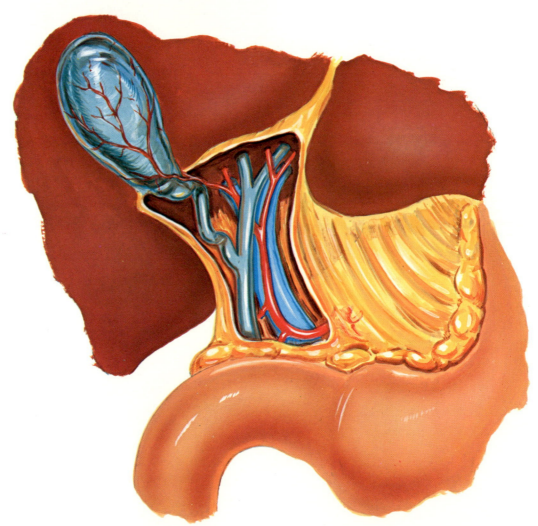

FIGURE 1-6. Bile duct lies anterior and to the right of other structures in the hepatoduodenal ligament. The common hepatic artery lies anterior and to the left, and the portal vein lies behind. The right hepatic artery and cystic artery usually cross behind the common hepatic duct. Anomalies of these arteries are common.

Gallbladder and Cystic Duct

The gallbladder is a pear-shaped organ whose sole purpose is the temporary storage of bile. It lies in a depression on the undersurface of the liver at the anatomical junction of the right and left hepatic lobes. Its size varies from 8 to 12 cm in length and from 4 to 6 cm in greatest diameter. It has a distinctive blue color, is covered by a serosal lining, and consists of a thin layer of smooth muscle and fibrous tissue with an inner lining epithelium of columnar epithelium and mucous-secreting cells. Its average capacity is 30 to 50 ml of bile, although when distended it will stretch to a capacity of 200 ml or more.

The gallbladder may be divided anatomically into a fundus, the main body, an infundibular portion or ampulla, and a neck. The fundus, or rounded end, will occasionally fold on itself and form a "phrygian cap," as shown by cholecystography (Figure 1-7); this has no clinical significance. The body is the main storage portion. The ampulla and neck join with the cystic duct. The cystic duct varies in length from 2 to 4 cm with a diameter of 1 to 1.5 mm. At its distal end a series of valves, the spiral valves of Heister, regulate the flow of bile into and out of the gallbladder. Occasionally the cystic duct is absent or dilated beyond recognition by gallstones, so that the gallbladder empties directly into the common duct, a potentially treacherous anomaly for the unwary surgeon.

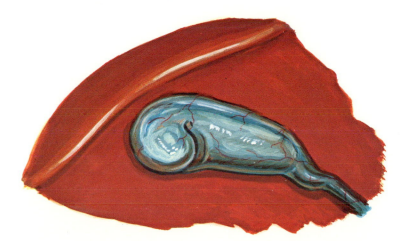

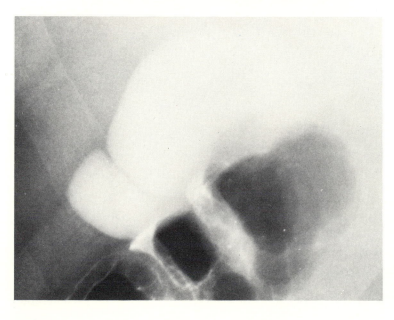

FIGURE 1-7. A "phrygian cap" formed by the fundus of the gallbladder is depicted in this drawing and shown on the oral cholecystogram.

The gallbladder and cystic duct join the common hepatic duct to form the common bile duct in the upper third or central portion of the hepato-duodenal ligament. This junction is variable in its location and type; it may be a 90-degree angle, it may join and run parallel to the common duct, or it may cross behind the common duct and enter medially and low (Figure 1-8). A common anatomical variation (potentially dangerous for the surgeon) is for the cystic duct to insert into or join an accessory right hepatic duct; both ducts then join the common hepatic to form a common bile duct (Figure 1-9).

The triangle of Calot is the anatomical site where the cystic artery can be most readily identified. It is the space bounded by the common hepatic duct medially, the cystic duct inferiorly, and the undersurface of the liver superiorly[2–4] (Figure 1-10). In addition to the cystic artery, an enlarged lymph node, the cystic duct node, is frequently found in this space.

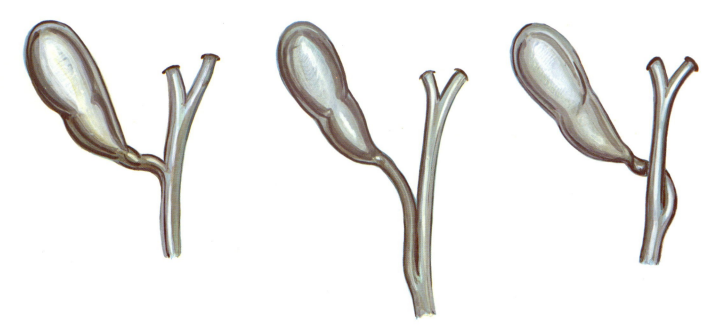

FIGURE 1-8. Three variations of the cystic duct joining the common hepatic duct to form the common bile duct.

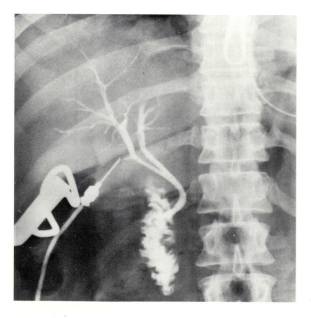

FIGURE 1-9. Operative cholangiogram illustrating the cystic duct inserting into the right main hepatic duct.

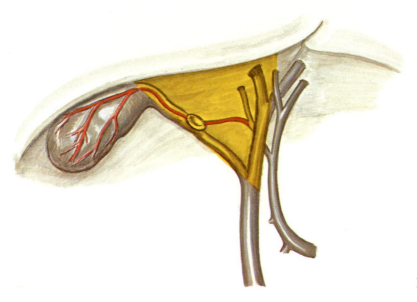

FIGURE 1-10.   Triangle of Calot (yellow).

Distal Common Bile Duct

The terminal or distal common bile duct passes through or behind the head of the pancreas, gradually turning to the right to enter the duodenum at an oblique 45-degree angle. At its point of entry into the duodenum, it joins with the distal pancreatic duct, in a variable pattern, to form the ampulla of Vater.[2,5,6] Both ducts then enter the duodenum, usually (90% of the time) through the papilla of Vater. The anatomy of the ampulla of Vater is variable (Figure 1-11). The terminal common bile duct and major pancreatic duct (duct of Wirsung) may join immediately prior to entry into the duodenum. This is the most common pattern. However, they may open separately side by side or may join at a higher level and enter the duodenum together. In the latter case, there is a possible "common channel" relationship.

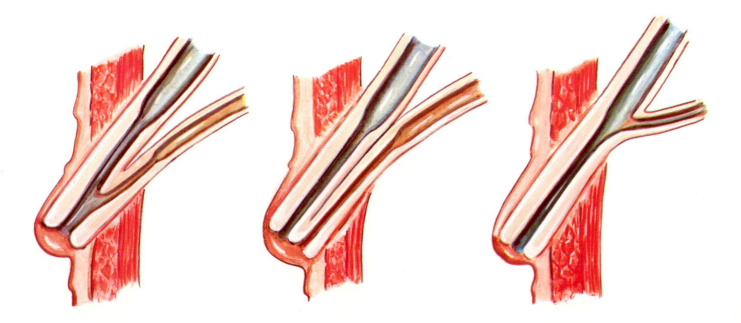

FIGURE 1-11.   Variable anatomy of the ampulla of Vater and the three most common anatomical patterns.

Surrounding the ampulla of Vater is the sphincter of Oddi, an anatomically separate, smooth muscle sphincter distinct from the intrinsic musculature of the duodenal wall. The sphincter of Oddi has three parts: the distal or papillary sphincter, the choledochal sphincter, and the pancreatic sphincter[2] (Figure 1-12). This sphincter complex is the principal regulator of bile flow into the duodenum, pressures within the biliary system, and filling and storage of bile in the gallbladder.[4,7]

The location of the ampulla of Vater along the descending duodenum is also variable.[6] In about 60% of patients, it is located along the medial wall of the duodenum, about midway or two-thirds of the way down the second part of the duodenum. In about 30% of patients it is more distal, at the junction of the second and third part of the duodenum, or in the distal or transverse duodenum (Figure 1-13). In about 10% of patients, the papilla of Vater may be located in the proximal duodenum, rarely as close to the pylorus as 2 or 3 cm.

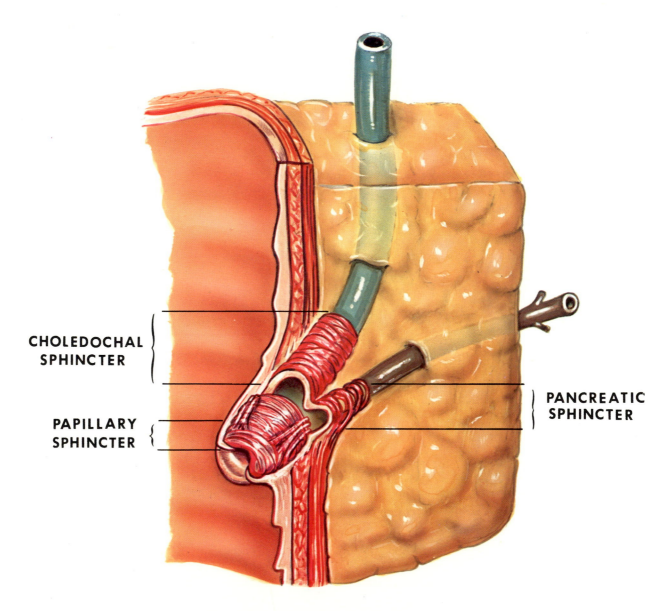

CHOLEDOCHAL SPHINCTER

PAPILLARY SPHINCTER

PANCREATIC SPHINCTER

FIGURE 1-12.   Anatomical relationships of the sphincter of Oddi complex: the choledochal, papillary, and pancreatic sphincters.

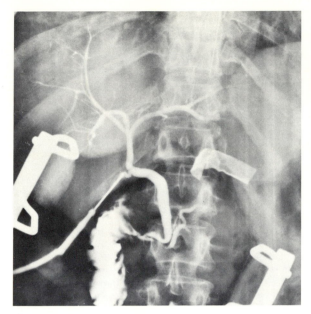

A

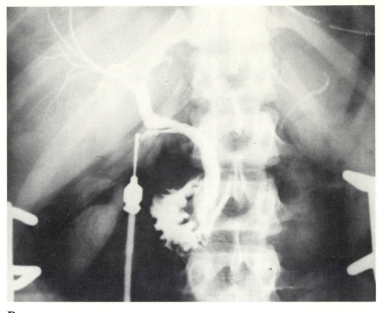

B

FIGURE 1-13. Operative cholangiograms showing the variable location of the papilla of Vater: **(A)** in the mid-duodenum, the most common location; **(B)** in the distal duodenum; **(C)** in the transverse duodenum.

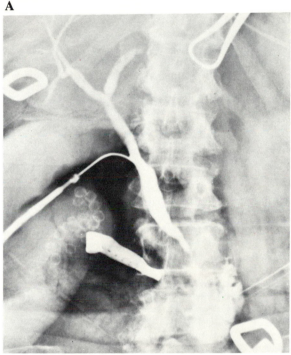

C

Hepatic and Cystic Arteries

The anatomical variations of arterial supply to the liver and biliary system have been known for many years.[8] However, with the frequent use of selective celiac angiography in recent years, the true incidence of great variation in these arteries has only now been appreciated. No single pattern can be said to be normal. The common patterns of the hepatic arteries and cystic artery are depicted in Figures 1-14 and 1-15.

Knowledge of these variations is of major importance to surgeons. In addition, a tortuous hepatic artery that crosses over and lies anterior to the common bile duct may easily be injured during exploration of the common bile duct (Figure 1-16). Such a tortuous hepatic artery is more common in the elderly.

11

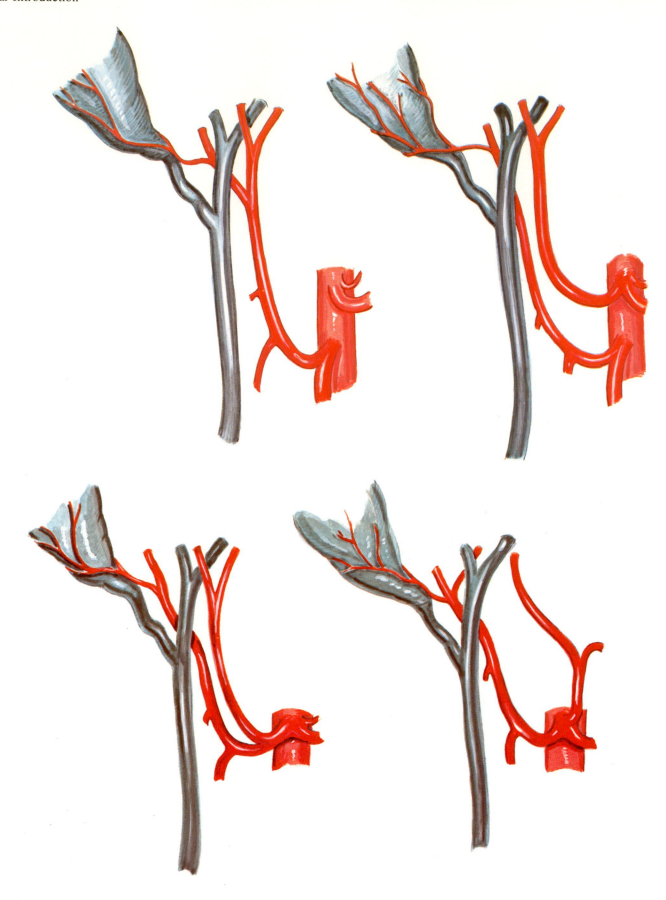

FIGURE 1-14.   Variable anatomy and relationships of the hepatic arteries and cystic artery. A dual hepatic blood supply is more common (15%) than previously suspected.

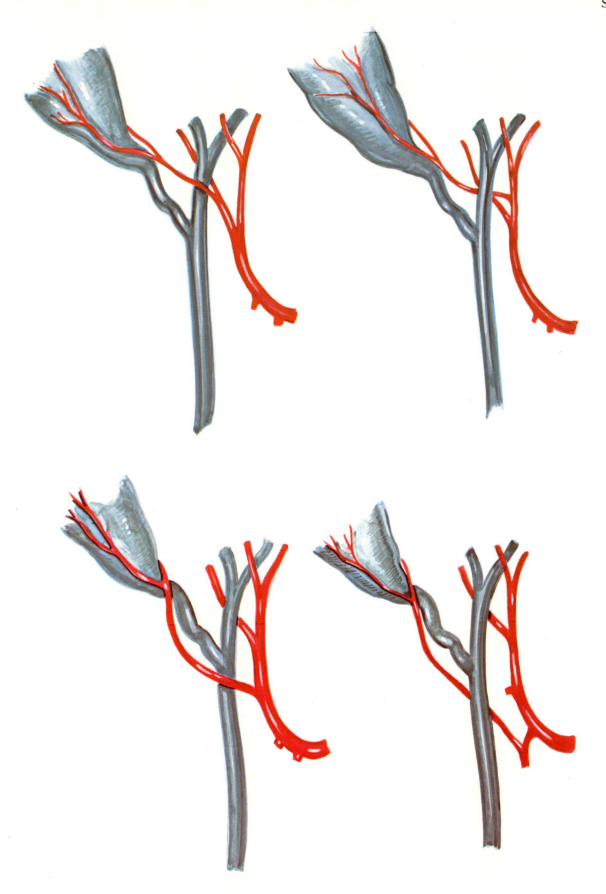

FIGURE 1-15.   Variable origin of the cystic artery. It may arise from the right or left hepatic, common hepatic, or an accessory artery from the superior mesenteric. It may cross the common bile duct anteriorly or occasionally join the gallbladder below the cystic duct.

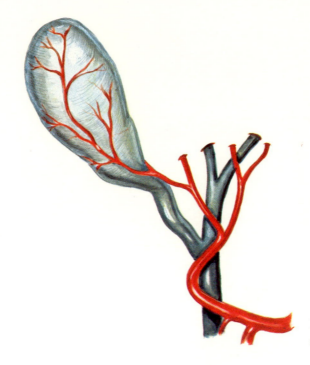

FIGURE 1-16. Tortuous hepatic artery.

Portal Vein

The portal vein is formed by the junction of the splenic and superior mesenteric veins and their tributary mesenteric veins (Figure 1-17). As indicated previously, it lies behind and slightly medially to the common bile duct in the hepatoduodenal ligament (Figure 1-6). The venous drainage of the bile ducts and gallbladder empty directly into the portal venous system in the hilus of the liver.

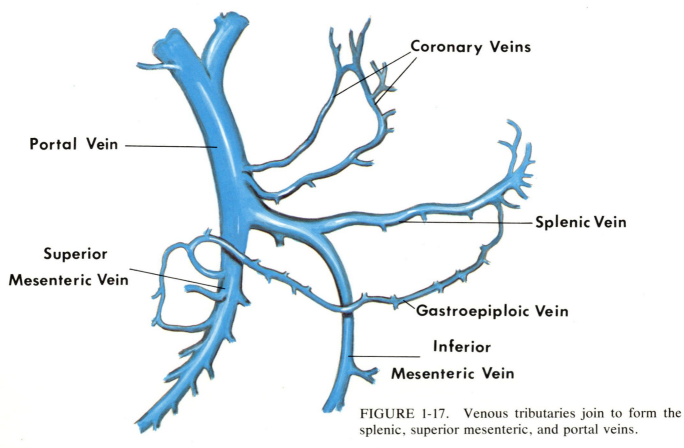

Coronary Veins

Portal Vein

Splenic Vein

Superior Mesenteric Vein

Gastroepiploic Vein

Inferior Mesenteric Vein

FIGURE 1-17. Venous tributaries join to form the splenic, superior mesenteric, and portal veins.

Biliary Lymphatics

The biliary system has a rich lymphatic plexus that drains into lymph nodes in the hepatoduodenal ligament and thence to the celiac nodes (Figure 1-18).

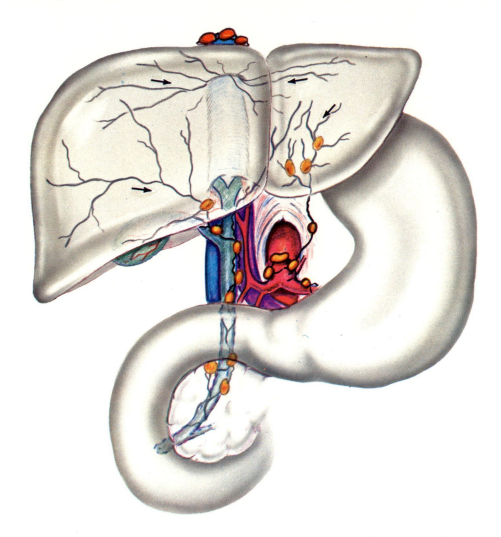

FIGURE 1-18. Principal lymphatics of the biliary system drain into lymph nodes (yellow) in the hepatoduodenal ligament, subpancreatic and common bile duct nodes, and nodes of the celiac axis.

Physiology of Bile Production and Storage
R. Thomas Holzbach

The amount of bile produced each day is estimated to vary from 500 to over 1,200 ml, depending on the method of collection, amount and type of diet, state of hydration, and influence of other stimuli such as vagal stimulation, secretin, and the reabsorption of acids. Normal hepatic bile is approximately 97% water, 1% bile salts, phospholipids, and varying but small amounts of cholesterol, mucin, bilirubin, lipids, electrolytes, vitamins, and enzymes.[9] The pH of bile is usually alkaline, varying between 6.0 and 8.5; its specific gravity is approximately 1.040.

Interdigestive Phase

In the interdigestive phase, the choledochal sphincter slows the rate of bile excretion into the duodenum, intrabiliary pressure rises in the common duct (from 10 to 30 cm H_2O), and bile flows into the gallbladder for storage. The gallbladder concentrates bile 6- to 10-fold by water absorption and secretes mucin into the bile (approximately 20 ml/day). With ingestion of food, especially a fatty meal, the gallbladder contracts, intracholecystic pressure rises (from 20 to 30 cm H_2O), the choledochal sphincter relaxes, and bile flows out of the gallbladder into the common duct and into the duodenum.[9,10] Stimulation of the gallbladder to contract is predominantly under hormonal control, the major stimulus being that of cholecystokinin released by the duodenal cells when fatty or amino acids are present in the duodenum.[11,12] Although vagal stimulation can cause weak contractions of the gallbladder, it cannot induce emptying of the gallbladder. The lack of vagal innervation, as after vagotomy, causes a moderate decrease in overall tonicity and pressures in the biliary system, with some dilatation of the gallbladder seen on cholecystograms. However, emptying of the gallbladder under the influence of cholecystokinin is essentially normal, with only some delay in complete emptying and in peristaltic contractions.[10]

Formation and Excretion of Bile

Bile is excreted into the bile duct canaliculi following formation within parenchymal liver cells. The liver is central to the synthesis of a variety of specific body proteins and lipids and plays a key role in the intermediary metabolism of carbohydrates and fatty acids. Among its many functions are the detoxification and conjugation of bile acids and other substances for excretion into the intestinal tract and removal from the body.

A variety of endogenously synthesized and exogenous materials are excreted in bile unchanged or as metabolites, including bilirubin, fatty acids, cholesterol, bile acids, various drugs, radiocontrast materials, and alcohol. Bilirubin is produced in the reticuloendothelial system of the body as a hemoglobin breakdown product, and it is excreted by the liver cell. In certain hemolytic states, excessive hepatic excretion can result in the formation of bile pigment gallstones. Bile acids, in contrast, are produced within the liver from the catabolism of cholesterol. The uptake of materials by the liver cell in most cases appears to be an active, energy-requiring process involving several mechanisms. Upon entering the hepatocyte, chemical substances undergo metabolic alteration to produce catabolites, or are conjugated: for example, bilirubin is conjugated primarily to glucuronic acid; bile acids are conjugated with one of two amino acids (glycine or taurine); and hormones commonly undergo sulfation or other conjugate formation. The net effect of these forms of conjugation is to convert

16

lipid-soluble materials to make them soluble in cell water and in bile, a solution system based on water. Excretion of catabolites occurs across the bile canalicular wall, the microvillous surface which is the boundary between the liver cell and the smallest intrahepatic tributaries of the biliary collecting system.

Figure 1-19 depicts an overall view of the anatomical arrangements between venous and arterial blood supply and the bile-collecting system in juxtaposition to hepatic cells.

Independent, carrier-mediated, active transport mechanisms also exist for bile acids, cations and anions such as sodium, potassium, chloride, and bicarbonate, and for certain neutral compounds. The prevailing view regarding the formation of bile is that active solute transport leads to local osmotic flow in the biliary canaliculi, which begin as fine channels between adjacent hepatocytes (Figure 1-20). The entire process is best explained by the "standing gradient" hypothesis proposed by Diamond and Bossert.[13] Bile acids comprise the major portion of actively transported anions, and their excretion rate is one of the major determinants of the rate of bile production. This has come to be designated as the *bile acid–dependent* component of bile flow.[14]

Canalicular bile production cannot be solely attributed to bile acid secretion, however, and a number of recent studies have probed the magnitude of bile acid–independent canalicular bile production.[15,16] There are a number of other interacting contributions to bile flow, such as that resulting from bile duct activity which is responsive to various stimuli, e.g., the secretin effect. Figure 1-21 portrays a number of the complex factors involved in the generation and secretion of bile.[17]

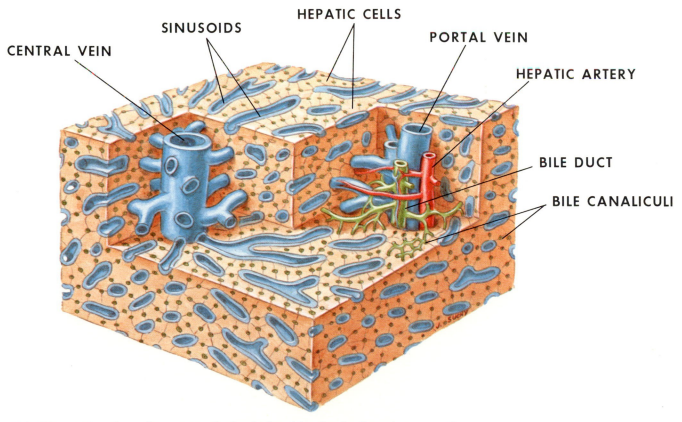

FIGURE 1-19.   Complex anatomical relationships in the liver between the venous and arterial blood supply to the hepatic cells, intrahepatic sinusoids, and central collecting veins of the liver. Interspersed between the hepatic cells are the bile duct canaliculi, which unite to form intrahepatic bile ducts.

17

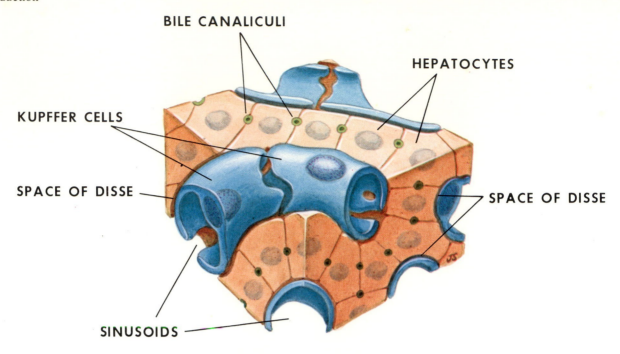

FIGURE 1-20.   Relationship between individual hepatic cells, intrahepatic sinusoids, space of Disse, and bile duct canaliculi.

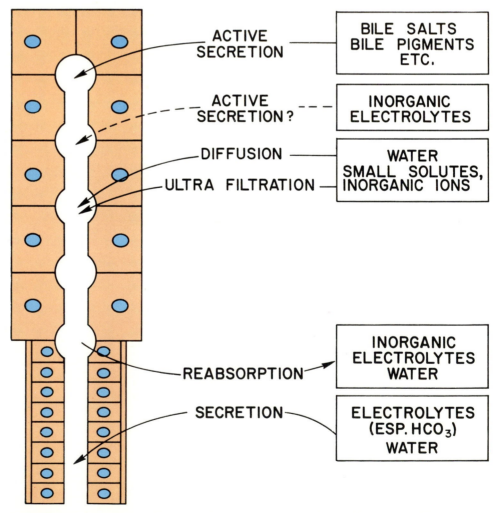

FIGURE 1-21.   Some of the mechanisms involved in bile formation. From H. O. Wheeler. In L. Schiff (ed.): *Diseases of the Liver*, 4th ed., 1975. Courtesy of Lippincott.

The rate of bile flow is primarily influenced by its aqueous component and by the flux of bile acids through the liver. When the solute composition of bile is examined it is found that lipids comprise about 75% of its total mass; the greater portion of this is in the form of bile acids. In addition, significant concentrations of phospholipid (lecithin) and cholesterol are found. All three substances are synthesized by enzymes in the liver cells; the liver is the largest single organ source for cholesterol synthesis in the body. There are apparently two separate hepatic pools of cholesterol: one is partially esterified within the liver and secreted into the serum as a lipoprotein, the other is excreted in bile without esterification and is in the free form.[18]

Some microsomal cholesterol also undergoes catabolism to form the two primary bile acids, cholic and chenodeoxycholic acids. Following conjugation with glycine or taurine, these acids are secreted (along with lecithin and free cholesterol) into bile. Although bile acids differ only slightly in structure from cholesterol, these structural differences permit their aggregation into groups of similar molecules termed *micelles*. Micelles have the property of aggregating into sphere-like particles and incorporating the other primary lipids, lecithin and cholesterol. The molecules in watery solution orient themselves so that the charged portions, which have an affinity for water, face the exterior; the non-water-soluble portions comprise the core[19] (Figure 1-22). This aggregation also confers an additional benefit: it explains the isotonicity of bile with plasma. If the number of bile acid molecules normally present in bile acted osmotically as separate entities, bile would be hypertonic and physiological problems in the biliary tract would ensue. As a result of micellar aggregation, each polymolecular aggregate exerts the same osmotic force as that which would result from a single molecule. A final advantage to this arrangement is that the hydrophobic core of the micellar bile salt aggregate is able to incorporate lecithin as an expander, swelling its interior. This permits a considerable incorporation of free cholesterol into the micellar structure and permits cholesterol to be dissolved in bile.

Enterohepatic Circulation

A schematic representation of the enterohepatic circulation (EHC) is shown in Figure 1-23. This drawing depicts the gastrointestinal tract in man following ingestion of a meal containing common nutritional fat in the form of triglycerides. Emulsification of the cleavage products from triglyceride hydrolysis by pancreatic lipase results in the incorporation of fat into micelles with a structure similar to that described. Absorption of fat takes place primarily in the upper intestine, whereas bile acids undergo little absorption until the lower third of the small intestine is reached. In the ileum there are specific high-affinity binding sites for the active absorption of bile acids. Due to the efficiency of this absorptive process, less than 5% the excreted daily bile acids reach the colon. Upon absorption, bile acids enter the portal vein and return to the liver. As the bile acids re-enter the liver at the sinusoidal membrane (Figure 1-20), they again encounter an avid, high-affinity binding process, so that these conjugated bile acids are almost entirely cleared on a single pass through the hepatic circulation.[20]

The efficiency of this hepatic removal process for bile acids accounts for the extremely low peripheral blood levels normally found. This 95% return rate of bile acids to the liver has two consequences. First, most of the bile acids excreted in bile are actually recycled rather than newly synthesized. Second, bile acids exert a feedback inhibition that regulates their

19

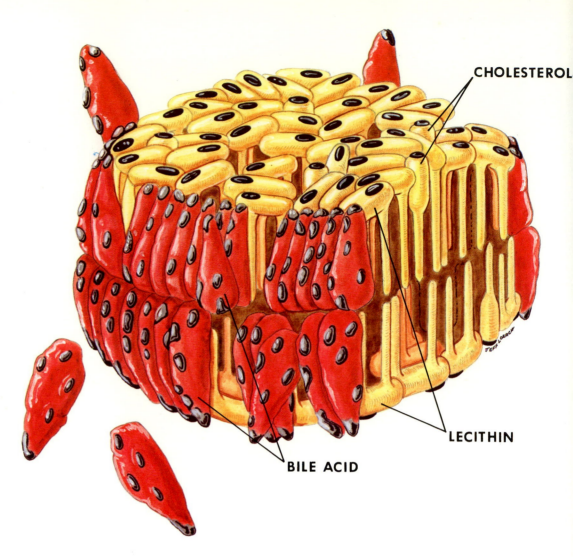

CHOLESTEROL

LECITHIN

BILE ACID

FIGURE 1-22. Most probable structure of a biliary micelle, a polymolecular aggregate of molecules into sphere-like particles containing bile acids, cholesterol, and lecithin. A vertical section has been cut away to enable visualization of the micelle core. Recent evidence indicates that the particle is probably a sphere having a different internal structure than the conventional ringed bilayer model represented here (K. Müller, Personal communication).

rate of synthesis. Because of the abundance of recycled bile acids in the liver, the normal synthesis rate is low, although the liver has a large reserve capacity to increase synthesis in the event of increased intestinal losses.

Many other substances, such as steroids, estrogens, cholesterol, fat-soluble vitamins, radiographic dyes such as iopanoic acid (Telepaque), and digitalis preparations, also cycle in lesser magnitude, but in a manner similar to that described for bile acids. These materials all share a feature in common with bile acids—i.e., their insolubility in water.

Storage of Bile

When bile is secreted by the liver in the fasting state, most of the hepatic bile is carried through the cystic duct into the gallbladder and stored. From radioisotope measurements, it has been estimated that after an overnight fast about 70% of the total-body bile acid pool confined to the EHC has become localized within the gallbladder[20] (Figure 1-24). During storage

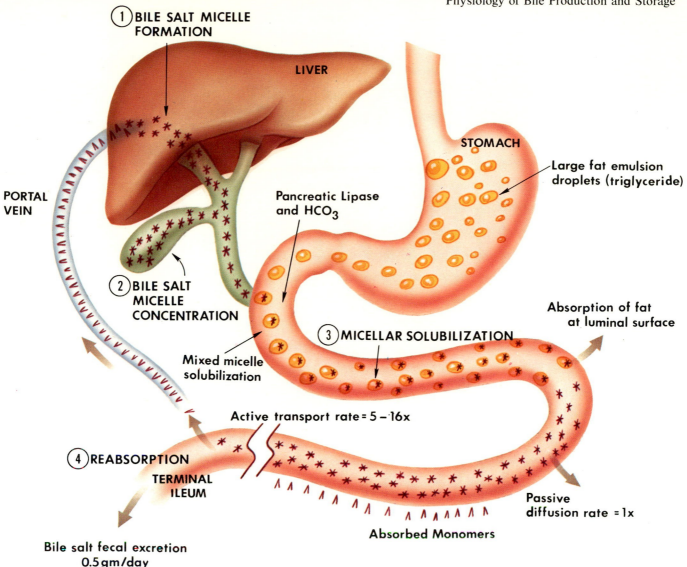

1 BILE SALT MICELLE FORMATION

LIVER

STOMACH

Large fat emulsion droplets (triglyceride)

PORTAL VEIN

Pancreatic Lipase and HCO₃

2 BILE SALT MICELLE CONCENTRATION

3 MICELLAR SOLUBILIZATION

Absorption of fat at luminal surface

Mixed micelle solubilization

Active transport rate = 5 – 16x

4 REABSORPTION
TERMINAL ILEUM

Absorbed Monomers

Passive diffusion rate = 1x

Bile salt fecal excretion 0.5 gm/day

FIGURE 1-23.   Gastrointestinal tract following ingestion of a meal containing fat illustrating enterohepatic circulation (EHC). Fat is incorporated into micelles and absorbed; bile acids are reabsorbed into the portal venous system, returned to the liver, and re-excreted through the bile canaliculi.

within the gallbladder, water and electrolytes are actively reabsorbed, concentrating the solute fraction 6 to 10 times. Bile in the gallbladder, however, remains isotonic because the fluid removed during concentration is isotonic, and the nonabsorbed lipids, though more concentrated, are in micellar structure. With storage of bile within the gallbladder, the rate of bile flow from the liver during fasting decreases.

Upon ingestion of a meal, especially one containing fats or essential amino acids,[11,12] cholecystokinin is released into the circulation from the duodenum. This hormone causes vigorous contraction of the gallbladder and relaxation of the sphincter of Oddi, resulting in release of concentrated bile into the intestine to aid in fat absorption (Figure 1-25). Once bile acids have been released into the small intestine they rapidly pass downstream, the rate of enterohepatic cycling is increased, and the flow rate of bile from the liver is again increased.

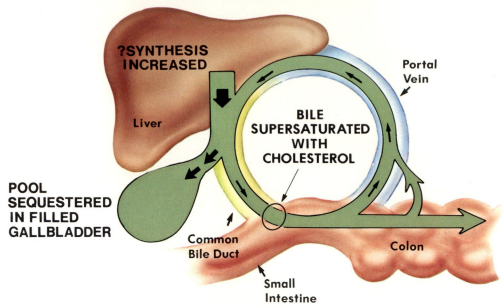

FIGURE 1-24. Functional interruption of the EHC during fasting. Adapted with permission from Dr. Martin C. Carey and Milner-Fenwick, Inc., Baltimore.

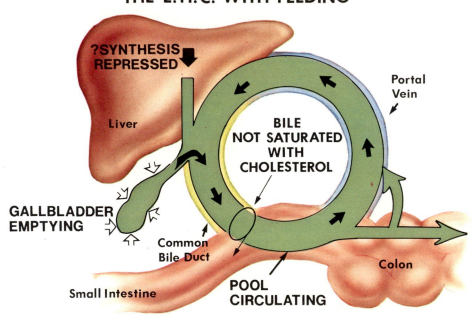

FIGURE 1-25. Restored physiological status of the EHC after a meal. Adapted with permission from Dr. Martin C. Carey and Milner-Fenwick Inc., Baltimore.

Disturbances of Enterohepatic Circulation

The most important way in which the recycling of bile acids becomes disordered is through the loss of function of the ileum in the conservation of bile from excretory losses. For example, this mechanism can be disrupted or bypassed under the following conditions: (1) the development of an external bile fistula, (2) severe inflammatory bowel disease of the ileum or resection of the ileum, and (3) oral administration of a chelating substance, e.g., cholestyramine, which is not absorbed and binds bile acids within the intestinal lumen, increasing fecal bile acid excretion. In each of these three situations, there results a broken EHC with marked depletion of the bile acid pool. Bile acid losses may exceed the capacity of new bile synthesis by the liver. The bile acid pool becomes depleted, and the net effect is a decrease in the flow rate of hepatic bile, 95% of which normally comes from recirculation of the EHC of bile acids.

Formation of Gallstones

Man is the only known animal species that forms cholesterol gallstones. Recent studies have shown that the bile salt–lecithin micelle is not only responsible for cholesterol solubilization in bile, but that this structure also has a limitation of saturation. It is possible to represent this saturation limit for cholesterol on a tricoordinate graph.[21] When the amount of cholesterol in bile exceeds the saturation limit, bile is supersaturated with cholesterol. In earlier terminology this bile was called *lithogenic*.[22] We now know that the concept of lithogenic bile is not this simple. It is clear that biliary cholesterol supersaturation occurs frequently in man without cholelithiasis, as indicated by data from a U. S. population (Figure 1-26). On the other hand, it is true that there is, in general, a parallelism between the degree of supersaturation and the incidence of cholesterol gallstones. One example is the high incidence of this disease in some population groups, such as in Sweden, where high levels of biliary cholesterol supersaturation are reported[23] (Figure 1-27). At the other extreme is the Masai tribe of Africa, which has the lowest incidence of cholelithiasis known and the lowest published figures for biliary cholesterol saturation. Furthermore, a comparison of human bile with that obtained from the gallbladder of other mammalian species in whom gallstones never occur shows that the latter are characterized by low levels of biliary cholesterol saturation.[21] Gallstones occur more frequently in obese patients, a group known to have high levels of biliary cholesterol secretion and cholesterol supersaturation.[24] The female to male ratio for incidence of gallstones is in the range of 3:1. Recent studies have suggested that this female propensity to cholesterol gallstone formation has a hormonal basis.[25]

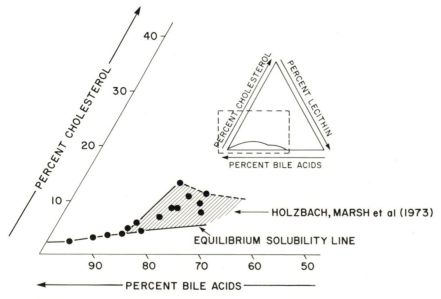

FIGURE 1-26. Frequency of biliary cholesterol supersaturation in healthy persons in a U. S. population. Adapted from R. T. Holzbach et al.: *J. Clin. Invest.*, **52**, 1467–1479, 1973.

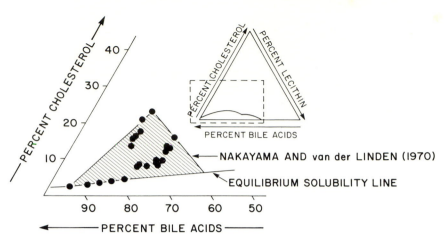

FIGURE 1-27. Frequency of biliary cholesterol supersaturation in healthy persons in a Swedish population. Adapted from F. Nakayana and W. Van der Linden: *Acta Chir. Scand.*, **136**, 605, 1970.

All evidence indicates that biliary cholesterol supersaturation is a necessary condition for gallstone formation. This is not a totally sufficient explanation, however, as indicated by the observation that gallbladder bile in fasting, healthy man is supersaturated, often to a striking degree. Recent studies have shown that this high degree of biliary cholesterol supersaturation is a function of the bile flow rate related to fasting[26] (Figure 1-28). These studies indicate that although the secretion rates of both phospholipids and cholesterol parallel those of bile acids during fasting,[27] the secretion rate of cholesterol decreases less than that of bile acids and phospholipids; with eating, flow rates of bile acids and phospholipids increase markedly in association with a much more modest rise in cholesterol output.[28] Thus bile becomes supersaturated in the fasting state.

Physiological Effects of Cholecystectomy

Most studies of patients with cholesterol gallstones have shown, for unexplained reasons, that these patients have a low bile acid pool as measured by isotope dilution methods.[24,29] Previously, this was felt to be an important factor in the lithogenic process. Recent studies have shown that when the bile acid pool is diminished in humans, the 24-hr outputs of bile acids, phospholipids, and cholesterol from the liver are not significantly different from similar measurements in patients with normal bile acid pool sizes.[28] The most likely explanation for these observations lies in the fact that patients with smaller bile acid pools experience greater recycling rates through the EHC to maintain normal levels of bile secretory output. When the gallbladder is removed, the physiological effect of normal gallbladder function is also removed. The result is a dampening of the intermittency pattern or a decrease in the fluctuation rate of bile flow and an increase in the net overall flow rate. Such an effect tends to reduce the frequency and duration of bile cholesterol supersaturation,[24] which, in turn, reduces the rate of recurrent cholelithiasis.

Current Status of Oral Gallstone Dissolution Therapy

Some patients, because of comparatively poor health or unwillingness to undergo surgery, are potential candidates for medical therapy aimed at gallstone dissolution. Oral chenic (chenodeoxycholic) acid therapy has been shown to reduce cholesterol supersaturation in bile.[30] Although

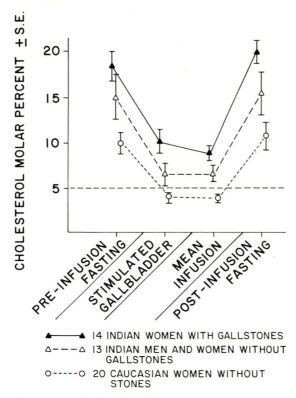

FIGURE 1-28. Diurnal variation in biliary cholesterol saturation with fasting and feeding. Mean (±SE) molar percentage of cholesterol (which reflects degree of cholesterol saturation) in bile from three groups of subjects: 14 Indian women with gallstones (closed triangles), 13 Indian men and women without gallstones (open triangles), and 20 white women without stones (open circle). The dashed horizontal line approximates the limit of cholesterol solubility.[21] A diurnal variation in molar percentage of cholesterol was found in all groups, and the mean fasting bile was supersaturated with cholesterol in every group, including white women without stones.[15] Adapted from A. L. Metzger et al.: *N. Engl. J Med.,* **288,** 333, 1973.

chenic acid is hepatotoxic in most animals, studies during the past 7 years indicate no substantial evidence of toxicity in man. Recently obtained data can explain this on the basis of a difference in metabolism.[31] There are several shortcomings to this compound, which is still unavailable for general use and is restricted to experimental studies. First, the success rate in achieving dissolution is less than 60% of treated patients.[32] The failure rate of more than 40%, could be due in part to the patient having pigment, rather than cholesterol, gallstones or a layer of calcification surrounding the gallstone. A second liability is its required duration of administration. Although small stones may dissolve in 1 year, total dissolution of most stones takes, on the average, about 2 years. Finally, once the stones have been dissolved and the patient ceases taking medication, the stones often recur within 1 or 2 years. Thus, patients offered this treatment in its present form will apparently require medication on a regular or intermittent basis for the rest of their lives. Because the drug has these limitations, its importance at the moment is more symbolic than practical. An analogy might be drawn between the use of this compound and the introduction of the first sulfonamide in 1935.

A new bile acid compound, ursodeoxycholic acid, and several other new chemotherapeutic compounds are receiving investigative attention at present. In a few years, perhaps, an even more effective chemotherapeutic agent may be available as a practical alternative to cholecystectomy. Such treatment, however, is never likely to assume predominance because of two limitations already known to exist from the trials with chenic acid. First, if the patient has symptomatic disease, cholecystectomy will afford more rapid relief and the development of complications will be less likely. Second, with or without symptoms, if the gallbladder fails to visualize roentgenographically, it seems improbable that orally administered medications will successfully enter the gallbladder to dissolve the stones contained therein. In such a circumstance it would also be impossible to monitor the effects of the medication (i.e., dissolution of the gallstones).

References

Surgical Anatomy
1. Healey, J. E., Jr., and Schroy, P. C.: Anatomy of the biliary ducts within the human liver. *Arch. Surg.*, **66,** 599, 1953
2. Anson, B. J., and McVay, C. B.: *Surgical Anatomy*, 2 vols., 2nd ed. Philadelphia, Saunders, 1971.
3. Hess, W.: *Surgery of the Biliary Passages and the Pancreas*. Princeton, N.J., Van Nostrand, 1965, p. 638.
4. Orloff, M. J.: The biliary system. In, D. C. Saliston, Jr. (ed.): *Davis-Christopher Textbook of Surgery*, 11th ed. Philadelphia, Saunders, 1977.
5. Lindner, H. H., Pena, V. A., and Ruggeri, R. A.: A clinical and anatomical study of anomalous terminations of the common bile duct into the duodenum. *Ann. Surg.*, **184,** 626, 1976.
6. Wood, M.: Anomalous location of the papilla of Vater. *Am. J. Surg.*, **111,** 265, 1966.
7. Schwartz, S. I.: Gallbladder and extrahepatic biliary system. In, S. I. Schwartz, R. C. Lillehei, G. T. Shires, et al. (eds.): *Principles of Surgery*, 2nd ed. New York, McGraw-Hill, 1974, pp. 1221–1254.

Physiology of Bile Production and Storage
8. Puestow, C. B.: *Surgery of the Biliary Tract, Pancreas, and Spleen*, 4th ed. Chicago, Year Book, 1970, p. 388.
9. Schwartz, S. I.: Gallbladder and extrahepatic biliary system. In, S. I. Schwartz (ed.): *Principles of Surgery*, 2nd ed. New York, McGraw-Hill, 1974, pp. 1077.
10. Watts, J. M., and Dunphy, J. E.: The role of the common bile duct in biliary dynamics. *Surg. Gynecol. Obstet.*, **122,** 1207, 1966.
11. Malagelada, J. R., DiMagno, E. P., Summerskill, W. H., et al.: Regulation of pancreatic and gallbladder functions by intraluminal fatty acids and bile acids in man. *J. Clin. Invest.* **58,** 493, 1976.
12. Malagelada, J. R., Go, V. L. W., DiMagno, E. P., et al.: Interactions between intraluminal bile acids and digestive products on pancreatic and gallbladder function. *J. Clin. Invest.*, **52,** 2160, 1973.
13. Diamond, J. M., and Bossert, W. H.: Standing-gradient osmotic flow. A mechanism for coupling of water and solute transport in epithelia. *J. Gen. Physiol.*, **50,** 2061, 1967.
14. Forker, E. L.: Mechanisms of hepatic bile formation. *Annu. Rev. Physiol.*, **39,** 323, 1977.
15. Berthelot, P. Erlinger, S., Dhumeaux, D., et al.: Mechanism of phenobarbital-induced hypercholeresis in the rat. *Am. J. Physiol.*, **219,** 809, 1970.
16. Erlinger, S., Dhumeaux, D., Berthelot, P., et al.: Effect of inhibitors of sodium transport on bile formation in the rabbit. *Am. J. Physiol.*, **219,** 416, 1970.
17. Wheeler, H. O.: Secretion of bile. In, L. Schiff (ed.): *Diseases of the Liver*, 4th ed. Philadelphia, Lippincott, 1975, pp. 87–110.

18. Gregory, D. H., Vlahcevic, Z. R., Schatzski, P., et al: Mechanism of secretion of biliary lipids. I. Role of bile canalicular and microsomal membranes in the synthesis and transport of biliary lecithin and cholesterol. *J. Clin. Invest.*, **55**, 105, 1975.

19. Oh, S. Y., McDonnell, M. E., Holzbach, R. T., et al.: Diffusion coefficients of single bile salt and bile salt–mixed lipid micelles in aqueous solution measured by quasielastic laser light scattering. *Biochem. Biophys. Acta*, **488**, 25, 1977.

20. Hofmann, A. F.: The enterohepatic circulation of bile acids in man. *Adv. Intern. Med.*, **21**, 501, 1976.

21. Holzbach, R. T., Marsh, M., Olszewski, M., et al.: Cholesterol solubility in bile: evidence that supersaturated bile is frequent in healthy man. *J. Clin. Invest.*, **52**, 1467–1479, 1973.

22. Tompkins, R. K.: Current status of investigations into the etiology of gallstones. *Am. J. Surg.*, **122**, 1, 1971.

23. Nakayama, F., and Van der Linden, W.: Bile from gallbladder harbouring gallstone: can it indicate stone formation? *Acta Chir. Scand.*, **136**, 605, 1970.

24. Shaffer, E. A., and Small, D. M.: Biliary lipid secretion in cholesterol gallstone disease. The effect of cholecystectomy and obesity. *J. Clin. Invest.*, **59**, 828, 1977.

25. Bennion, L. J., Ginsberg, R. L., Garnick, M. B., et al.: Effects of oral contraceptives on the gallbladder bile of normal women. *N. Engl. J. Med.*, **294**, 189–192, 1976.

26. Metzger, A. L., Adler, R., Heymsfield, S., et al.: Diurnal variation in biliary lipid composition: possible role in cholesterol gallstone formation. *N. Engl. J. Med.*, **288**, 333, 1973.

27. Nilsson, S., and Schersten, T.: Importance of bile acids for phospholipid secretion into human hepatic bile. *Gastroenterology*, **57**, 525, 1969.

28. Northfield, T. C., Hofmann, A. F.: Biliary lipid output during three meals and an overnight fast. I. Relationship to bile acid pool size and cholesterol saturation of bile in gallstone and control subjects. *Gut*, **16**, 1, 1975.

29. Almond, H. R., Vlahcevic, Z. R., Bell, C. C., Jr., et al.: Bile acid pools, kinetics and biliary lipid composition before and after cholecystectomy. *N. Engl. J. Med.* **289**, 1213, 1973.

30. LaRusso, N. F., Hoffman, N. E., Hofmann, A. F., Northfield, T. C., and Thistle, J. L.: Effect of primary bile acid ingestion on bile acid metabolism and biliary lipid secretion in gallstone patients. *Gastroenterology*, **69**, 1301, 1975.

31. Cowen, A. E., Korman, M. G., Hofmann, A. F., et al.: Metabolism of lithocholate in healthy man. II. Enterohepatic circulation. *Gastroenterology*, **69**, 67, 1975.

32. Iser, J. H., Dowling, H., Mok, H. Y., et al.: Chenodeoxycholic acid treatment of gallstones: a follow-up report and analysis of factors influencing response to therapy. *N. Engl. J. Med.*, **293**, 378, 1975.

Congenital Anomalies

2

Introduction

The biliary system develops from the embryonic hepatic diverticulum during the fourth to sixth week of fetal development. Anomalies in the development of the gallbladder or bile ducts probably occur as a result of failure of growth or differentiation. Canalization of the bile ducts from a solid cord of cells appears to begin in the 6th week and continues until the 12th week of intrauterine life.[1]

A variety of anomalies of the biliary system have been recognized in approximately 15% of individuals. Some anomalies are more common, such as variations in the number or arrangement of the hepatic ducts, variations in the length or junction of the cystic duct with the hepatic ducts, and variations in the insertion of the distal common bile duct into the duodenum or its junction with the pancreatic duct. These anomalies, all of which permit unimpeded bile flow from the liver to the duodenum, are important to surgeons only because they are potentially dangerous at operation and injury to an important structure must be avoided (Figure 2-1).

Other anomalies, such as atresia or duplication of the gallbladder or bile ducts, absence of the gallbladder, intrahepatic gallbladder, and cystic dilatation of the common bile duct, are rare (Figure 2-2). For some unexplained reason, the incidence of these anomalies appears to be higher in Japan than in other areas of the world.[2] The presence of patent extrahepatic bile ducts is not essential to intrauterine life and development, but it is critical to growth and development after birth. Without normal bile flow, obstructive jaundice, biliary cirrhosis, liver failure, and death are the expected sequence of events, with survival of most children limited to 14 months to 2 years of life.[3,4]

The two types of congenital anomalies of greatest importance to surgeons are biliary atresia and choledochal cysts. These will be discussed in detail.

Biliary Atresia

The incidence of biliary atresia in the United States has been estimated to be from 1/5,000 to 1/20,000 births.[1] As noted, the incidence appears to be higher in Japan.

29

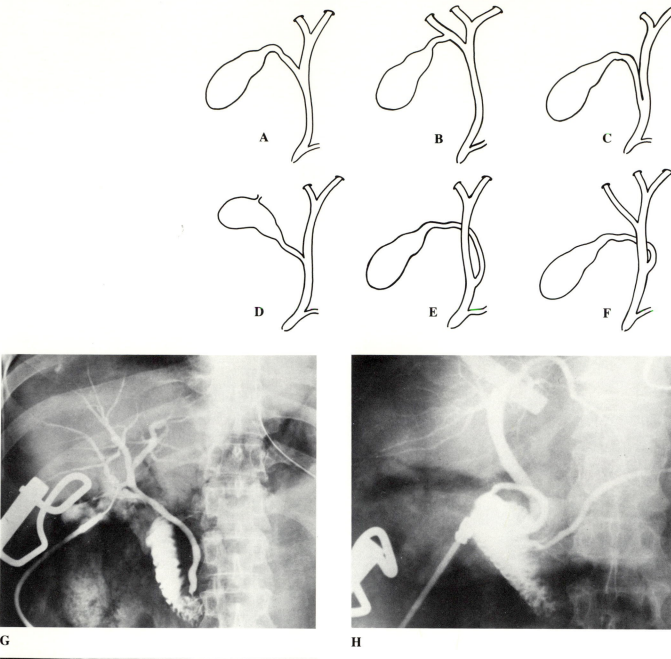

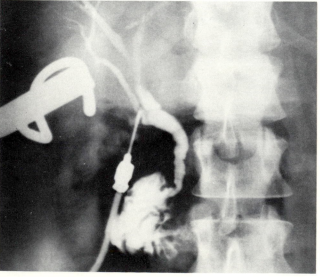

FIGURE 2-1. Variations in cystic and common hepatic duct anatomy. Some of these variations or anomalies, especially those of (**B**) and (**E**), are potentially dangerous if the surgeon fails to identify a duct structure adequately before dividing or ligating it. The operative cholangiograms (**G-I**) depict several of these anomalies.

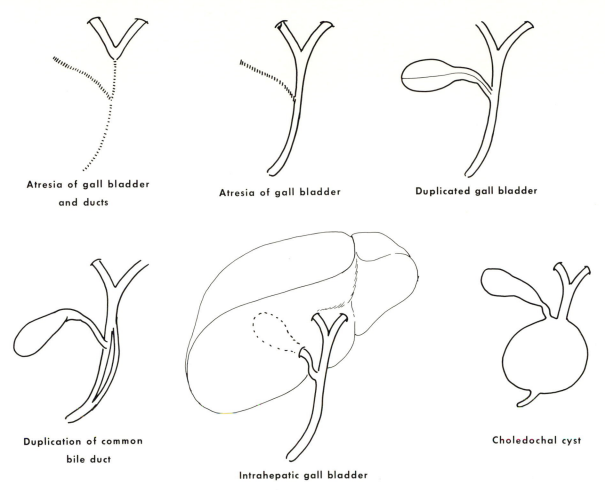

Atresia of gall bladder
and ducts

Atresia of gall bladder

Duplicated gall bladder

Duplication of common
bile duct

Intrahepatic gall bladder

Choledochal cyst

FIGURE 2-2.   Less common, major anomalies of the biliary system.

Pathology

Atresia of the bile ducts may be segmental, extrahepatic, intrahepatic, or complete.[5] The various anatomical types are depicted in Figure 2-3. From reports of several series, it is estimated that approximately 85% to 90% of cases are "uncorrectable" by surgery; only 10% to 15% of patients have a surgically "correctable" type of atresia.[1,4-8]

The histological findings at surgery, if the bile ducts can be identified or located, show fibrous and small cord-like duct structures (Figure 2-4). The histological findings on biopsy of the liver in patients with biliary atresia are remarkably similar to those in patients with neonatal hepatitis (Figure 2-5). Bile canaliculi and intrahepatic bile ducts may or may not be seen, depending on the severity and extent of the atretic process.

Whether biliary atresia is actually a failure of canalization of the bile ducts in intrauterine life or whether it is an acquired process from a perinatal viral infection, with development of sclerosing cholangitis related in some way to neonatal hepatitis, has not been definitely determined. Because there are many similarities between patients with biliary atresia and neonatal hepatitis, recent studies are progressively indicating that biliary atresia is a result of an acquired, ongoing prenatal or perinatal infection. Bill and Koop, in discussions of the ongoing cirrhosis after portoenterostomy reported by Altman and associates,[9] both believe that biliary atresia is an acquired condition due to a viral infection, a progressive sclerosing cholangitis of the entire biliary system. Hays[10] has recently discussed this controversy in an excellent review article.

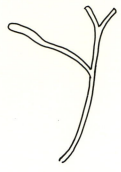

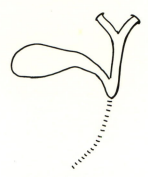

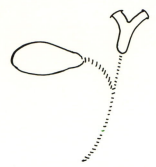

Hypoplasia of ducts

Hepatic duct, cystic duct
and gall bladder patent

Hepatic duct patent, G.B. normal,
all other ducts atretic

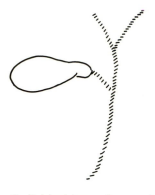

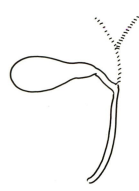

Gall bladder only, no ducts

Gall bladder and distal ducts only

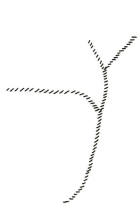

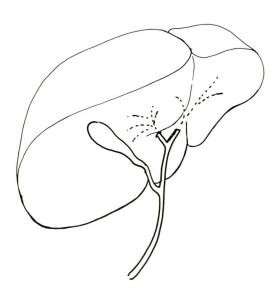

Total atresia

No intrahepatic ducts

FIGURE 2-3. Various types of biliary atresia and hypoplasia. Those depicted in the top row, found in 10% to 15% of infants, are all potentially correctable lesions. Those depicted in the bottom two rows, found in 85% to 90% of infants, are considered "uncorrectable" by surgery.

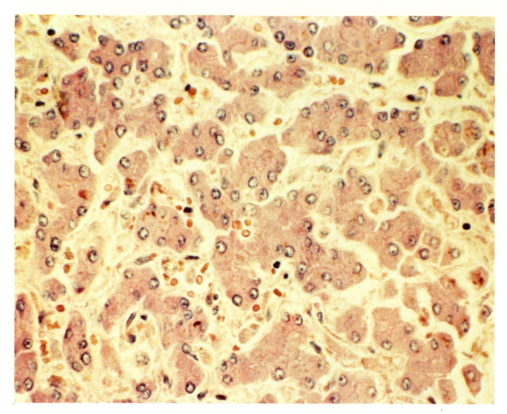

FIGURE 2-4. Photomicrograph showing the micro histology of biliary atresia—atretic or absent bile ducts with swollen liver cells and fibrosis.

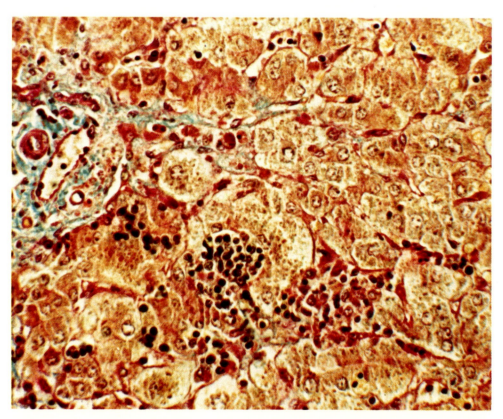

FIGURE 2-5. Photomicrograph of neonatal hepatitis. The histological findings can be remarkably similar to those of patients with biliary atresia. Bile ducts are seen here.

Diagnosis

Clinical Features. The newborn infant with biliary atresia usually has little or no jaundice at birth. During the first 2 weeks of life, progressive jaundice becomes apparent and worsens. Approximately 70% of neonates with jaundice persisting beyond the second week of life have atresia of the bile ducts, about 20% have neonatal hepatitis, and 10% have jaundice from a variety of other causes (physiological jaundice, "inspissated" bile, choledochal cyst, biliary hypoplasia, hemolytic anemia, cytomegalic inclusion disease, sepsis, Crigler-Najjar syndrome, or toxoplasmosis).[1]

The infant's stools are noted to be light in color and frequently large and bulky; the urine becomes dark. Although the parents and pediatricians observing the child may occasionally note some fluctuation in the jaundice, bilirubin levels progressively increase, usually to the range of 15 to 20 mg/dl. The child usually appears healthy and gains weight normally (Figure 2-6).

Laboratory Studies. Laboratory studies show a high level of bilirubin in the serum with high levels of conjugated bilirubin levels. Bilirubin is noted in the urine, there is an absence of urobilinogen in the stool and urine, and the serum alkaline phosphatase levels are elevated.[11,12] Serum transaminase levels may be mildly elevated.

The ^{131}I rose bengal excretion test has been helpful in diagnosing biliary atresia in many instances.[4,10,13,14] Less than 2% to 4% of injected radioactive dye is excreted in the stool of patients with biliary atresia (Figure 2-7).

A Coombs' test, serology, urine studies for cytomegalic inclusion bodies and for galactose, and blood cultures should be negative. The challenge in diagnosis is to distinguish between biliary atresia, neonatal hepatitis, and choledochal cyst, all of which give the clinical and laboratory picture of obstructive jaundice. In neonatal hepatitis and choledochal cyst, the obstruction may not be as complete and there may be more fluctuation in the levels of jaundice. The infant with neonatal hepatitis usually appears sicker and gains little weight. The child with choledochal cyst usually has onset of jaundice at a later age, frequently after the first weeks or months

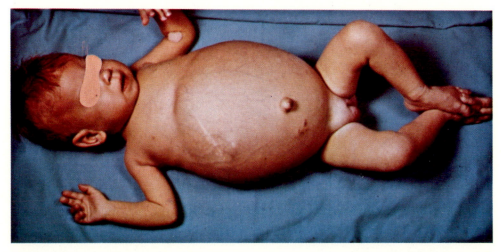

FIGURE 2-6. Child with biliary atresia at age 14 months. She appears well nourished, although she has obvious ascites. She subsequently had a liver transplant at age 16 months in an unsuccessful attempt to correct the biliary atresia.

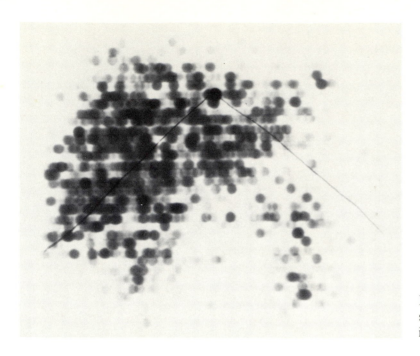

FIGURE 2-7. ^{131}I rose bengal scan at 12 h shows most radioactivity is in the liver, some is in the kidneys, and none is in the intestine.

of life. However, all clinical and laboratory studies may be remarkably similar in these three conditions. The most accurate diagnostic test is operative exploration of the liver and bile ducts, open-liver biopsy, and operative cholangiography.

Treatment

Any infant who has had persistent jaundice beyond 4 to 6 weeks of age, especially if the jaundice has been progressive and the ^{131}I rose bengal excretion tests have shown minimal amounts of radioactivity in the intestine or stool, should have operative exploration of the liver and bile ducts, open-liver biopsy, and operative cholangiography.[7,13-15]

Operative Strategy. At operation, the initial procedures should be diagnostic: (1) adequate exposure of the liver, (2) liver biopsy and frozen section, (3) exposure of the gallbladder and porta hepatis to look for bile ducts, and (4) operative cholangiography through the gallbladder, if present. If the gallbladder cannot be identified, the incision should be enlarged for better exposure of the undersurface of the liver and porta hepatis to aid identification of the extrahepatic bile ducts.[6-8,10,13,15,16] If bile ducts can be found, operative cholangiography with a small 23-gauge needle should be performed.

Occasionally, by operative cholangiography, hypoplasia of the bile ducts may be found and small but patent bile ducts may be present (Figure 2-8).[17] Infrequently, inspissated bile in the ducts or the "bile-plug" syndrome has also been found. The possibility of this syndrome as a cause of jaundice has been questioned. After cholangiography has shown that the ducts are patent, irrigation of the ducts with saline may improve the flow of bile.

If, on operative cholangiography through the gallbladder, all dye goes distally into the duodenum and no dye goes proximally up into the hepatic ducts, a small bulldog vascular clamp is placed across the distal bile ducts to occlude them and another cholangiogram is performed (Figures 2-9 and 2-10). If a patent biliary system is found the operation is terminated.

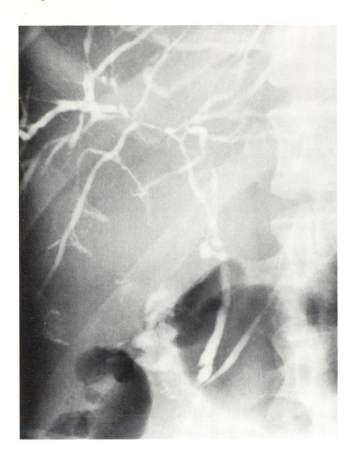

FIGURE 2-8. Operative cholangiogram showing hypoplasia of the bile ducts throughout the liver and extrahepatic biliary system.

Operative procedures for Biliary Atresia. If the gallbladder is absent, a careful exploration of the porta hepatis and hilar area of the liver should be undertaken. If patent upper bile ducts can be found, they are anastomosed to a Roux-Y jejunal segment (a choledochojejunostomy). From 10% to 15% of patients have such a potentially correctable lesion (Figure 2-3).

If no extrahepatic bile ducts can be found, the hilar area of the liver at the point where the right and left hepatic ducts should join is exposed and entered, and about 2 cm of liver tissue is removed, including any occluded or nonpatent ducts. A Roux-Y jejunal segment is then sewn to this area (a portoenterostomy). This procedure was described and popularized by Kasai et al,[8] Suruga et al,[18] and Lilly and Altman[19] have modified this procedure by dividing the Roux-Y jejunal segment, thereby creating an isolated upper segment with a double-barreled jejunostomy stoma to prevent ascending cholangitis. (see Chapter 6).

Results. The results of surgical treatment of biliary atresia are disappointing and controversial. In patients with uncorrectable atresia, the average length of survival is approximately 19 months. Early reports of the results of the Kasai procedure indicated a significant improvement in these survival statistics.[8,20,21] Recent long-term follow-up reports, especially those from the United States, have again shown discouraging results to be prevalent.[2,9,10,18,19,22,23] In several series, although jaundice may have been corrected in up to 45% of patients, evidence of biliary cirrhosis, cholangitis, and portal hypertension continued and long-term survival was limited.

At present, although the prognosis for long-term survival in patients with "correctable" lesions after choledochojejunostomy is improving, cholangitis, stricturing of the anastomosis, and the development of biliary cirrhosis seem to be a problem in 50% of patients. In patients with uncor-

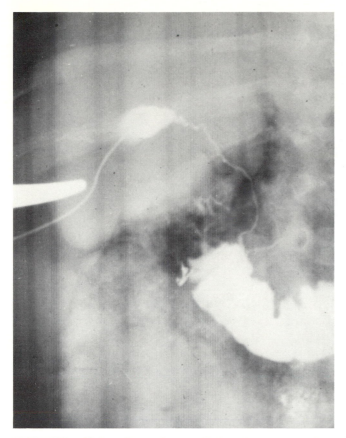

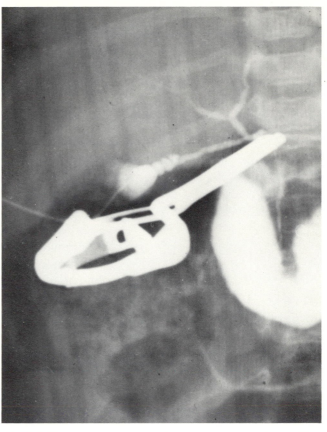

FIGURE 2-9. Operative cholangiogram taken through the gallbladder showing a patent gallbladder and distal bile duct; no proximal bile duct can be seen.

FIGURE 2-10. Second cholangiogram taken after placement of a small bulldog vascular clamp across the distal bile duct seen in Figure 2-9 to occlude it. This cholangiogram shows a patent common hepatic and proximal bile duct.

rectable lesions, the initial enthusiastic reports after portoenterostomy are now being tempered and the long-term results appear to be that at least 85% of patients develop biliary cirrhosis and portal hypertension. Of all patients with biliary atresia, probably no more than 5% to 10% will be cured by operation and live to adulthood.

Choledochal Cyst

Choledochal cyst is a less common congenital anomaly of the biliary system than is biliary atresia. Its incidence is estimated by Tsardakas and Robnett[24] to be approximately 1/200,000 infant hospital admissions. The incidence of this anomaly, like that of biliary atresia, is higher in the Japanese; almost one-third of reported patients have been Japanese children.[25–27] More than 600 cases have now been reported in the English literature. The defect appears to be more common in females than in males (7:2).[24,25,28–32]

Pathology

Choledochal cysts may be found in various forms (Figure 2-11). The most common form, type A, is a congenital cystic dilatation of the extrahepatic common bile duct with stenosis of the distal bile duct, but a normal intrahepatic ductal system. Type B, a cystic diverticulum arising from an otherwise normal or slightly dilated common bile duct, is rare. Type C, a choledochocele dilatation limited to the distal or intraduodenal portion of the common bile duct, is also rare.[33] Occasionally, multiple cysts are found[34] or the intrahepatic bile ducts may also be dilated.[35]

A variation of choledochal cyst may be the lesion originally described by Caroli, now termed Caroli's disease.[36] This lesion, a congenital cystic dilatation of the intrahepatic bile ducts, is seen most often in young women (Figure 2-12). Intrahepatic bile duct stones frequently form as a complication of this problem.[37] Cystic dilatation of the intrahepatic bile ducts may be seen alone, without extrahepatic bile duct anomalies, or in association with dilatation of the extrahepatic bile ducts.[38–40]

The cause of choledochal cyst formation is unknown. Many possible causes have been considered in the past.[24,25,29,32] Pickett[41] has suggested that the lesion may be a variant of biliary atresia; stenosis of the common bile duct occurs with cystic dilatation of the duct behind the stenotic segment. Others have emphasized abnormal epithelial cell proliferation as an obstructing factor, with congenital weakness of the bile duct walls as

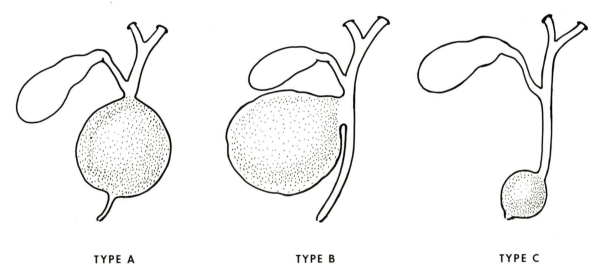

TYPE A   TYPE B   TYPE C

FIGURE 2-11.   Three major types of choledochal cysts. Type A, the most common, is a congenital cystic dilatation of the common bile duct. Type B is a cystic diverticulum arising from an otherwise normal or slightly dilated common bile duct. Type C is a choledochocele limited to the distal common bile duct.

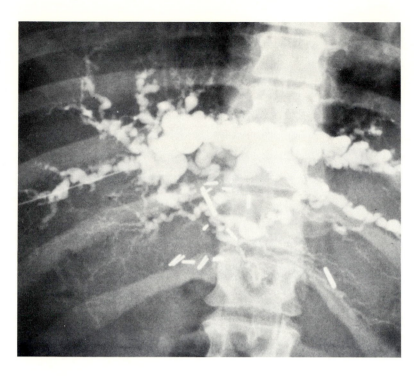

FIGURE 2-12. Percutaneous transhepatic cholangiogram of a patient with Caroli's disease.

a secondary feature. Weakening and thinning of the wall of the bile duct might occur during the stage of canalization of the solid bile duct between the 6th and 12th weeks of intrauterine life.

The cysts may vary in size from 3 to 25 cm. They may contain up to several liters of bile, depending on their size. The wall of the cyst usually is composed of columnar epithelium. Bile duct stones are occasionally found in older patients. Infection is rare.

Diagnosis

Clinical Features. Symptoms of choledochal cyst are jaundice, colicky right upper abdominal pain, and a palpable abdominal mass. Symptoms may occur from several weeks of age to adulthood. Symptoms begin in infancy or childhood in approximately 50% of patients. By age 30, more than 80% of patients with choledochal cysts have had the onset of symptoms; 20% of patients are over 30 years of age when symptoms begin.[24,25,32]

Thus, choledochal cyst, unlike biliary atresia, is not always seen in the infant during the first few weeks of life. Obviously, the greater the degree of stenosis or biliary obstruction, the greater the likelihood that symptoms will occur in the young patient. Several patients have been found to have cirrhosis of the liver with portal hypertension and bleeding esophagogastric varices at the time of diagnosis; all these findings are secondary to a previously unrecognized choledochal cyst[42]

The abdominal mass may fluctuate in size to some extent and may be cystic to palpation. The differential diagnosis of a multicystic or polycystic kidney, hepatoblastoma, or cirrhosis of the liver (etiology unknown) may be considered.

Laboratory Studies. Laboratory studies and liver function tests usually indicate the presence of obstructive jaundice. Dark urine and light-colored stool are commonly found.

An intravenous urogram, intravenous cholangiogram, and barium contrast upper gastrointestinal roentgenogram series may be helpful. The

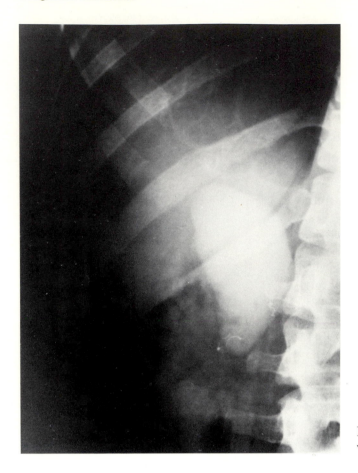

FIGURE 2-13. Type A choledochal cyst seen on intravenous cholangiography in an adult.

urogram excludes renal lesions; the intravenous cholangiogram, if it visualizes, may identify cystic dilatation of the common bile duct (Figure 2-13); barium studies of the stomach may show displacement of the antrum of the stomach or duodenum. In addition, an ultrasonic scan or computed tomography (CT) may identify the presence of a cystic mass beneath the liver. In the teenage or adult patient, selective celiac and superior mesenteric arteriograms may help determine the site and size of the mass and its relation to the liver.

A diagnostic laparotomy with operative cholangiography should be performed in any child or adult with unexplained jaundice, especially if abdominal pain or an abdominal mass is part of the clinical picture.

Treatment

Operative Strategy. At operative exploration, the recognition of a choledochal cyst may occasionally be a problem because of the rarity of these lesions. The size, configuration, and attachments of the cystic mass should be thoroughly and carefully explored and identified. The presence of the gallbladder and its relationship to the cyst should be noted (Figure 2-14). An operative cholangiogram can be obtained simply by needle aspiration of the cystic mass, removal of 10 to 250 ml (more if necessary) of bile, and instillation of 10 to 50 ml of Renografin-60 solution or another water-soluble dye. Operative cholangiography is essential to appreciate fully the size of the cyst and the type of lesion (Figure 2-15).

Operative Procedures. TYPE A. Treatment of most choledochal cysts (type A deformity, congenital cystic dilatation of the common bile duct), is effectively obtained by anastomosing the cyst to the duodenum or to a Roux-Y jejunal segment for internal biliary–intestinal drainage. For the

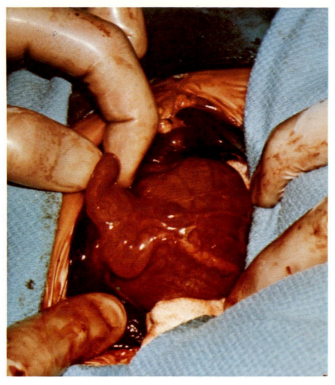

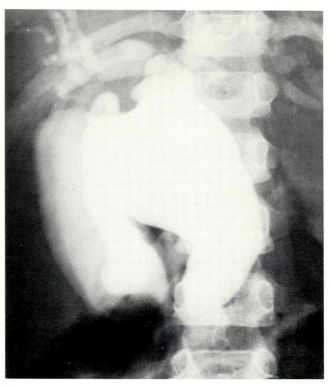

FIGURE 2-14. Choledochal cyst seen at operation in a child. A small, atrophic gallbladder is held in the surgeon's hand.

FIGURE 2-15. Operative cholangiogram demonstrating a large choledochal cyst in another child. The gallbladder is also greatly dilated.

newborn or infant, choledochocystoduodenostomy may be the most expeditious procedure, the treatment of choice.[25,26,28,29,37,43,44] For the older child or adult, choledochocystojejunostomy with a Roux-Y jejunal segment probably is a superior diversionary procedure with better long-term results.[33,40]

Trout and Longmire[44] have reported a significant number of late complications (recurrent jaundice, cholangitis, and stricture of the biliary–intestinal anastomosis) associated with choledochocystoduodenostomy in patients followed for longer than 5 years. In addition, they and others have recommended the addition of cholecystectomy as a concomitant procedure, whenever possible, in patients operated upon for choledochal cyst to prevent the later development of cholelithiasis and cholecystitis. In my opinion, cholecystectomy should not be performed in the infant or very young child, especially if it is hazardous or likely to prolong unduly the operative procedure. Excision of the choledochal cyst is not recommended because it would require resection of the entire common bile duct.

TYPE B.   For cystic diverticula (type B anomalies), excision of the cyst may be considered. Excision of the cyst should only be performed in the patient with type B deformity; in patients with type A or type C deformity the operation is hazardous and has been associated with a high mortality rate.[25,44] If excision is not possible, a choledochocystojejunostomy to a Roux-Y jejunal segment is the procedure of choice.

TYPE C.   For patients with a choledochocele (type C deformity), transduodenal exposure of the cyst with excision of the duodenal–cyst wall (opening the cyst into the duodenum) should be performed. This creates a wide choledochocystoduodenal opening for biliary decompression.

CAROLI'S DISEASE. If multiple cystic dilatations of the intrahepatic bile ducts are found, drainage by means of a hepatojejunostomy with a Roux-Y jejunal segment is the procedure of choice. This may be performed in the hilum of the liver or it may be done by partially transecting the left hepatic lobe (Longmire procedure). Occasionally resection of a segment of the liver is necessary.[37]

Results. Operative mortality rates reported for the surgical treatment of choledochal cyst range from 5% to 10% if it is diagnosed promptly, before the onset of multiple biliary stones, biliary cirrhosis, portal hypertension, or other complications.[24,25,30,32,38–40,44] Long-term survival results are also good, especially in patients treated by choledochocystojejunostomy to a Roux-Y segment. Patients treated by choledochocystoduodenostomy, in the experience of Trout and Longmire[44] and others, have had a somewhat greater incidence of late complications requiring secondary reconstructive biliary operations at a later time.

References

Biliary Atresia
1. Gray, S. W., and Skandalakis, J. E.: Extrahepatic biliary ducts and the gallbladder. In, Embryology for Surgeons. Philadelphia, Saunders, 1972.
2. Campbell, D. P., Smith, E. I., Bhati, M., et al.: Hepatic portoenterostomy: an assessment of its value in the treatment of biliary atresia. *Ann. Surg.* **181,** 591, 1975.
3. Hays, D. M., and Snyder, W. H., Jr.: Life-span in untreated biliary atresia. *Surgery,* **54,** 373, 1963.
4. Holder, T. M.: Atresia of the extrahepatic bile duct. *Am. J. Surg.* **107,** 458, 1964.
5. Stowens, D.: *Pediatric Pathology,* 2nd ed. Baltimore, Williams & Wilkins, 1966.
6. Arima, E., Fonkalsrud, E. W., and Neerhout, R. C.: Experiences in the management of surgically correctable biliary atresia. *Surgery,* **75,** 228, 1974.
7. Izant, R. J., Akers, D. R., Hays, D. M., McParland, F. A., and Wrenn, E. L., Jr.: *Biliary Atresia Survey.* Section on Surgery, American Academy of Pediatrics, 1965.
8. Kasai, M. Kimura, S., Asakura, Y., et al.: Surgical treatment of biliary atresia. *J. Pediatr. Surg.,* **3,** 665, 1968.
9. Altman, R. P., Chandra, R., and Lilly, J. R.: Ongoing cirrhosis after successful porticoenterostomy in infants with biliary atresia. *J. Pediatr. Surg.* **10,** 685, 1975.
10. Hays, D. M.: Biliary atresia: the current state of confusion. *Surg. Clin. North Am.,* **53,** 1257, 1973.
11. Thaler, M. M.: Jaundice in the newborn. *J.A.M.A.,* **237,** 58, 1977.
12. Thaler, M. M., and Gellis, S. S.: Studies in neonatal hepatitis and biliary atresia. IV. Diagnosis. *Am. J. Dis. Child.,* **116,** 280, 1968.
13. Hays, D. M., Wooley, M. M., Snyder, W. H., et al.: Diagnosis of biliary atresia: relative accuracy of percutaneous liver biopsy, open liver biopsy, and operative cholangiography. *J. Pediatr. Surg.* **71,** 598, 1967.
14. Miller, S., Fonkalsrud, E. W., and Longmire, W. P., Jr.: Current concepts in the management of congenital biliary atresia. *Arch. Surg.,* **92,** 813, 1966.
15. Mason, G. R., Northway, W., and Cohn, R. B.: Difficulties in the operative diagnosis of congenital atresia of the biliary duct system. *Am. J. Surg.,* **112,** 183, 1966.

16. Altman, R. P., and Lilly, J. R.: Technical details in the surgical correction of extrahepatic biliary atresia. *Surg. Gynecol. Obstet.,* **140,** 952, 1975.
17. Porter, S. D., Soper, R. T., Tidrick, R. T.: Biliary hypoplasia. *Ann. Surg.,* **167,** 602, 1968.
18. Suruga, K., Nagashima, K., Kohno, S., et al.: A clinical and pathological study of congenital biliary atresia. *J. Pediatr. Surg.,* **7,** 655, 1972.
19. Lilly, J. R., and Altman, R. P.: Hepatic portoenterostomy (the Kasai operation) for biliary atresia. *Surgery,* **78,** 76, 1975.
20. Kasai, M., Watanabe, I., and Ohi, R.: Follow-up studies of long-term survivors after hepatic portoenterostomy for "non-correctable" biliary atresia. *J. Pediatr. Surg.,* **10,** 173, 1975.
21. Miyata, M., Satani, M., Ueda, T., et al.: Long-term results of hepatic portoenterostomy for biliary atresia: special reference to postoperative portal hypertension. *Surgery,* **76,** 234, 1974.
22. Lilly, J. R.: The Japanese operation for biliary atresia: remedy or mischief? *Pediatrics,* **55,** 12, 1975.
23. Lilly, J. R., and Javitt, N. B.: Biliary lipid excretion after hepatic portoenterostomy. *Ann. Surg.,* **184,** 369, 1976.

Choledochal Cyst
24. Tsardakas, E., and Robnett, A. H.: Congenital cystic dilatation of the common bile duct. *Arch. Surg.,* **72,** 211, 1956.
25. Alonso-Lej, F., Rever, W. B., Jr., and Pessagno, D.J.: Congenital choledochal cyst with a report of 2, and an analysis of 94 cases. *Int. Abstr. Surg.,* **108,** 1, 1959.
26. Mahour, G. H., and Lynn, H. B.: Choledochal cyst in children. *Surgery,* **65,** 967, 1969.
27. Tsuchiya, R., Nishimura, R., and Toshiya, I.: Congenital cystic dilatation of the bile duct associated with Laurence-Moon-Biedel-Bardet syndrome. *Arch. Surg.* **112,** 82, 1977.
28. Fonkalsrud, E. W., and Boles, E. T., Jr.: Choledochal cysts in infancy and childhood. *Surg. Gynecol. Obstet.* **121,** 733, 1965.
29. Gross, R. E.: Idiopathic dilatation of the common bile duct in children. *J. Pediatr.* **3,** 730, 1933.
30. Hays, D. M., Goodman, G. N., Snyder, W. H., Jr., et al.: Congenital cystic dilatation of the common bile duct. *Arch. Surg.* **98,** 457, 1969.
31. Muakkasah, K., Obeid, S., and Shin, M.: Congenital choledochal cysts. *Arch. Surg.* **111,** 1112, 1976.
32. Ravitch, M. M., and Snyder, G. B.: Congenital cystic dilatation of the common bile duct. *Surgery,* **44,** 752, 1958.
33. Reinus, F. Z., and Weingarten, G.: Choledochocele of the common bile duct. *Am. J. Surg.,* **132,** 646, 1976.
34. Engle, J., and Salmon, P.: Multiple choledochal cysts. *Arch. Surg.,* **88,** 345, 1964.
35. Loubeau, J. M., and Steichen, F. M.: Dilatation of intrahepatic bile ducts in choledochal cyst. *Arch. Surg.* **111,** 1384, 1976.
36. Caroli, J., and Covinaud, C.: Une affection nouvelle, sans doute congenitales des voies biliares: la dilatation kystique unilobaire des canaux hepatiques. *Sem. Hôp. Paris,* **34,** 136, 1958.
37. Pridgen, J. E., Jr., Aust, J. B., McInnis, W. D.: Primary intrahepatic gallstones. *Arch. Surg.,* **112,** 1037, 1977.
38. Glenn, F., and McSherry, C. K.: Congenital segmental cystic dilatation of the biliary ductal system. *Ann. Surg.,* **177,** 705, 1973.
39. Hadad, A. R., Westbrook, K. C., Campbell, G. S., et al.: Congenital dilatation of the bile ducts. *Am. J. Surg.,* **132,** 799, 1976.
40. Lorenzo, G. A., Seed, R. W., and Beal, J. W.: Congenital dilatation of the biliary tract. *Am. J. Surg.,* **121,** 510, 1971.
41. Pickett, L. K.: Liver and biliary tract. In, C. D. Benson et al. (eds.): *Pediatric Surgery.* Chicago, Year Book, 1962, p. 618.

42. Gillis, D. A., and Sergeant, C. K.: Prolonged biliary obstruction and massive gastrointestinal bleeding secondary to choledochal cyst. *Pediatr. Surg.*, **52,** 391, 1962.
43. Gross, R. E.: *The Surgery of Infancy and Childhood*. Philadelphia, Saunders, 1953.
44. Trout, H. H., III, and Longmire, W. P., Jr.: Long-term follow-up study of patients with congenital cystic dilatation of the common bile duct. *Am. J. Surg.*, **121,** 68, 1971.

Inflammatory Disease

3

Cholecystitis and Cholangitis

It has been estimated from autopsy studies and clinical investigations in defined populations that gallstones develop in 15% to 20% of all adults. The incidence of gallstones is increased in certain countries (notably the Scandinavian countries), in women (twice the incidence of men), and in older age groups.[1-4] From approximately age 35 the incidence increases so that at age 75 about one of every three persons has cholelithiasis.

Studies from Denmark, Sweden, and the United States have shown that 40% to 60% of patients with cholelithiasis are asymptomatic.[2-4] Among asymptomatic patients with gallstones who were followed for 5 to 20 years without operation, cholecystitis eventually developed in 50% to 60%; complications (acute gangrenous cholecystitis, jaundice, cholangitis, or pancreatitis) developed in approximately 20%.[2] It can be said that the longer gallstones are present and the older the patient, the greater the incidence of symptomatic cholecystitis.

Of all symptomatic patients, about one-fifth have vague, mild symptoms, about two-fifths have typical chronic cholecystitis and one-fifth have acute cholecystitis, and about one-fifth have jaundice, cholangitis, pancreatitis, or other complications related to cholecystitis.[3]

Approximately 600,000 cholecystectomies are performed annually in the United States. Cholecystectomy is the abdominal operation most frequently performed.[5]

Pathology

The earliest change of acute or chronic cholecystitis is usually the precipitation or formation of gallstones in the gallbladder. These stones may then cause temporary obstruction of the cystic duct, with edema and thickening of the wall of the gallbladder (Figure 3-1). If infection supervenes in the obstructed system, inflammatory changes increase and there is a loss of the normal mucosal lining, vascularity increases in the wall of the inflamed organ, and hemorrhagic necrosis of the mucosa and, eventually, gangrenous changes in the gallbladder wall occur (Figures 3-2 and 3-3). In some patients, probably no more than 3% to 5%, loss of normal gallbladder function occurs without the presence of stones in the gallbladder. Dilatation of

45

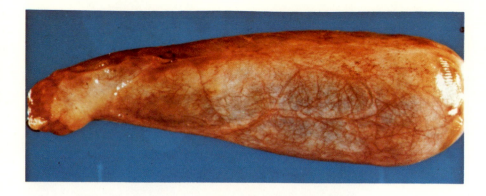

FIGURE 3-1. Operative specimen with edematous cholecystitis removed 36 to 48 h after the onset of acute cholecystitis.

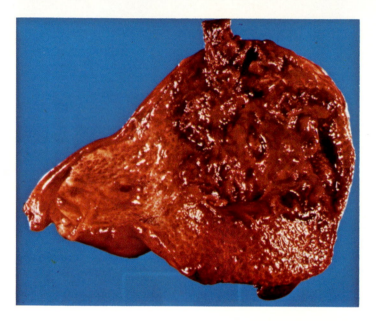

FIGURE 3-2. Operative specimen of a gallbladder with hemorrhagic necrosis of the mucosa.

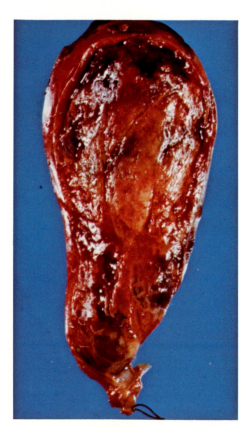

FIGURE 3-3. Operative specimen of a gallbladder with gangrenous changes in the wall.

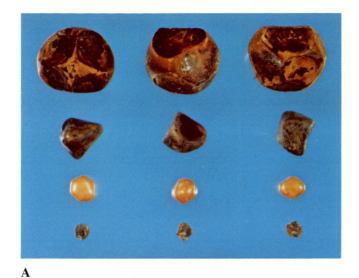

A

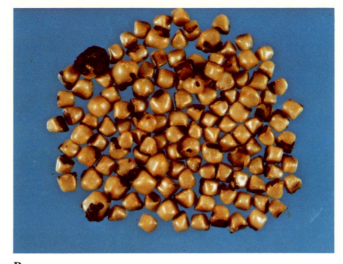

B

FIGURE 3-4. Common types of gallstones recovered at surgery. Primary bile duct stones are shown in (C).

C

the gallbladder and secondary infection may occur as a metabolic process resulting from decreased vascular perfusion, dehydration, or other systemic diseases.

Most stones in the biliary system form in the gallbladder; approximately 12% to 18% pass into the bile ducts.[6,7] In less than 5% of patients with bile duct stones, no stones are found in the gallbladder. In some patients, the stones in the bile duct were formed there, as *primary* duct stones.[8] The incidence of primary bile duct stones is greater with advancing age, as is the incidence of all bile duct stones in patients with cholelithiasis[6] (Table 3-1).

Careful studies of stool specimens in patients with cholecystitis by Kelly[9] and others have shown that, although small stones apparently pass spontaneously through the papilla of Vater into the duodenum in only 11% of patients with uncomplicated cholecystitis, this incidence is increased to 80% in patients with pancreatitis secondary to cholecystitis.

Types of Stones. Three general types of gallstones have been identified: pure or laminated cholesterol stones, bile pigment stones, and mixed cholesterol–bile pigment–calcium stones (Figure 3-4). Mixed stones are by far the most common. The structure of gallstones has been of interest to many surgeons;[10] most gallstones form around a central nidus of cholesterol, mucous, mucopolysaccharide, cellular debris, or mixtures of all of these with calcium bilirubinate. The stones gradually become larger by accretion, accumulation of more debris, or precipitation on the surface of the stone.

47

TABLE 3-1 Relationship of age to incidence
of stones in the bile ducts in 437 patients
with cholecystitis

Age (yr)	No. of patients with cholecystitis/no. of patients with bile duct stones	Incidence of bile duct stones (%)
10–20	7/1	14
21–30	26/3	11.5
31–40	64/6	9.4
41–50	92/8	8.7
51–60	134/19	14.2
61–70	78/24	31
71–80	33/16	48.5
81–90	3/3	100
Total	437/80	18.3

SOURCE Data from Hermann and Martin.[6]

Bacteriology of Bile. Bile in normal patients is sterile. Once gallstones have developed, obstruction has occurred, or inflammation has begun, the incidence of bacterial infection in bile steadily increases. A variety of bacterial organisms have been cultured from bile in 5% to 40% of patients with chronic cholecystitis, in about 75% of patients with acute cholecystitis, and in up to 90% of patients with common duct stones or cholangitis. The most common organisms found are listed in Table 3-2.[11–18] Obviously, in treating patients with cholecystitis or cholangitis it is important to choose a broad-spectrum antibiotic that covers the gram-negative group of organisms as well as some gram-positive organisms and clostridia. In addition, the antibiotic chosen should be excreted by the liver into bile in reasonably high concentrations.[17]

Diagnosis
Symptoms. The typical symptoms of cholecystitis are right upper quadrant abdominal pain that is colicky at first and then becomes constant with colicky exacerbations. The pain radiates to the back or parascapular area and is often accompanied by a feeling of upper abdominal distention, bloating, nausea, and vomiting. Pain is characteristically brought on or precipitated by a heavy meal, fried or fatty foods, or certain vegetables such as cabbage, onions, or cucumbers. Many patients have atypical symptoms. Sometimes back pain is more pronounced or severe than anterior abdominal pain. Frequently, the abdominal pain or discomfort is epigastric, not right upper quadrant; rarely, it may appear to be in the left upper quadrant. Sometimes a vague feeling of general upper abdominal heaviness or bloating is the only discomfort experienced. There may be no relationship to fatty foods or, in some patients, all foods may seem to cause discomfort. Some patients have no pain or discomfort but have episodes of fever with or without chills or malaise.

When stones have passed into the common bile duct, episodes of biliary colic may be more severe and jaundice may be apparent. If pancreatitis occurs secondary to biliary disease, the pain may be band-like, encircling the entire upper or central abdomen or radiating to the midback. When the gallbladder becomes acutely obstructed due to a stone or inflammatory obstruction of the cystic duct, hydrops of the gallbladder occurs, the pain becomes steady and constant, and a globular, tender right upper quadrant mass can be palpated.

48

TABLE 3-2   Bacteria cultured from bile in patients
with cholecystitis and/or cholangitis

Bacteria	Incidence[a] (percent of positive cultures)
Escherichia coli	30
Enterococcus } Staphylococci }	25
Klebsiella pneumonia } *Enterobacter* }	20
Diphtheroids	15
Clostridium perfringens	10
Alpha streptococci	5
Proteus } *Bacteroides* } *Pseudomonas* } Others }	<5

[a] Incidence equals greater than 100%. Most patients have multiple organisms.
SOURCE   Data from selected reports.[11-18]

Physical Findings.   The patient with acute or chronic cholecystitis rarely has pain as well localized to the area of inflammation as does a patient with appendicitis. However, a definite area of increased or severe tenderness is noted in the right upper abdomen over the gallbladder or edge of the liver. A hydrops of the gallbladder can be palpated in about 10% of patients. Jaundice may be apparent in approximately 10% of patients. In the elderly, occasionally jaundice may be the first or sometimes the only evidence of biliary tract disease.

Differential Diagnosis.   This should include acute appendicitis, pancreatitis without cholecystitis, acute or chronic duodenal ulcer, acute pyelonephritis, diverticulitis of the right colon, pneumonia of the right lower lung, perforating carcinoma of the right colon, hepatitis, and carcinoma of the pancreas or bile ducts (when jaundice is the principal finding.)

Laboratory Studies.   Routine blood counts, urinalysis, a chest x-ray, and a plain roentgenogram of the abdomen should always be obtained. Liver function tests, serum amylase, blood urea nitrogen (BUN), serum creatinine, blood glucose levels, and an electrocardiogram should be ordered as soon as feasible after admission to the hospital to assess other organ systems and the risks of possible surgery.

Roentgenographic Studies.   INDIRECT CHOLANGIOGRAPHY.   If previous roentgenographic studies have not shown gallstones, or if they are not apparent on plain roentgenograms of the abdomen (Figure 3-5), an oral cholecystogram or intravenous cholangiogram (if the patient is vomiting or has a nasogastric tube in place) should be ordered to confirm or rule out the tentative diagnosis of cholecystitis (Figure 3-6). The demonstration of stones in these studies or of nonvisualization of the gallbladder, along with the clinical picture and laboratory findings, supports the diagnosis of cholecystitis. It should be remembered, however, that nonvisualization of the gallbladder during oral or intravenous cholecystography may be due to liver disease. The accuracy of cholecystography, at best, is about 95%.[19-21] Neither oral nor intravenous cholecystography should be utilized in patients with clinical jaundice or bilirubin levels above 2.5 or 3.0 mg/dl; nonvisualization of the biliary system is to be expected in this situation.

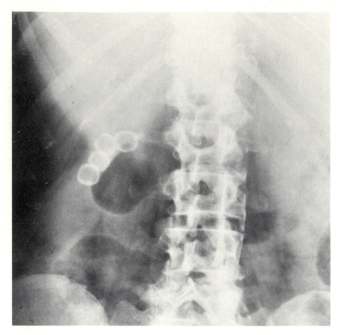

FIGURE 3-5. Plain roentgenogram of the abdomen showing gallstones in the right upper quadrant.

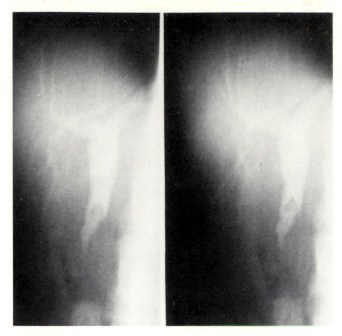

FIGURE 3-6. Intravenous cholangiograms showing non-visualization of the gallbladder, moderate dilatation of the biliary system, and radiolucent common bile duct stones.

ULTRASONOGRAPHY, RADIOISOTOPE SCANS. Recently, ultrasound (echograms), using gray-scale scanners, and radioisotope scans of the biliary system after the injection of ^{99m}Tc-pyridoxylidene glutamate have been introduced.[22–26] These technics are being studied and have additional value in confirming the diagnosis of inflammatory disease of the gallbladder and bile ducts. Ultrasound can identify a dilated gallbladder or bile ducts, and stones in the biliary system may be detected (Figure 3-7).

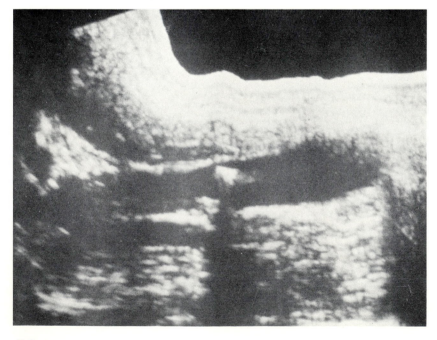

FIGURE 3-7. Ultrasound study showing a dilated gallbladder containing a stone.

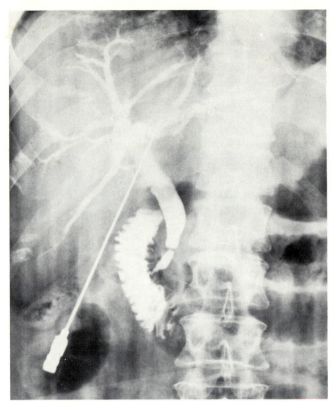

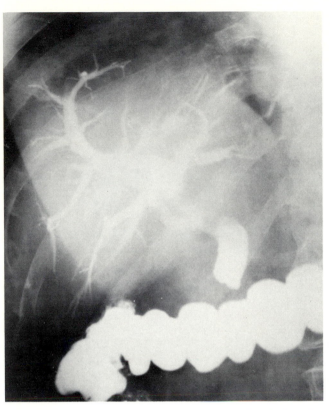

FIGURE 3-8. Percutaneous transhepatic cholangiogram showing a stricture of the distal bile duct, dilatation of the biliary system, and several radiolucent filling defects that were primary duct stones.

FIGURE 3-9. Percutaneous transhepatic cholangiogram showing recurrent stones in the common bile duct. Barium is seen in the colon.

DIRECT CHOLANGIOGRAPHY. Percutaneous transhepatic cholangiography, the direct needling of the intrahepatic bile ducts with instillation of dye into the biliary system, is a valuable method of direct cholangiography in patients who are jaundiced or who have had repeated episodes of jaundice (Figures 3-8 and 3-9).[12,27,28] In such patients, the biliary system is dilated and easier to enter with a needle. A success rate of 80% to 85% in entering and visualizing the dilated biliary system can be expected. Among jaundiced patients with a nondilated biliary system, such as those with chronic hepatitis, normal or small biliary ducts in the liver are successfully demonstrated in a much lower percentage, probably in the range of 20% to 30%. With the use of a Chiba "skinny" needle and small injections of dye into the liver parenchyma under the fluoroscope, some radiologists have demonstrated the normal biliary system in up to 50% of patients.[27]

Endoscopic retrograde cholangiography has recently been introduced in many major medical centers as an additional method of direct cholangiography. A flexible fiberoptic duodenoscope is passed, the ampulla of Vater is visualized, and a small catheter is passed retrograde into the common bile duct. This technic of visualization of the biliary system has been of great value in ruling out obstructive jaundice in patients with hepatitis or unexplained jaundice (Figures 3-10 and 3-11). It is hazardous in the patient with active inflammatory disease; in the acute situation, cholangitis and septicemia may result. Endoscopic retrograde cholangiography has its greatest value in patients with chronic or episodic problems.

Operative cholangiography is of enormous value to the surgeon during the operative procedure.[29] It should be used routinely as an expected

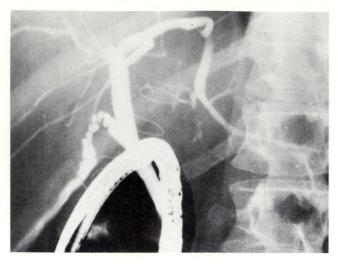

FIGURE 3-10.   ERC showing a normal biliary system in a patient with hepatitis.

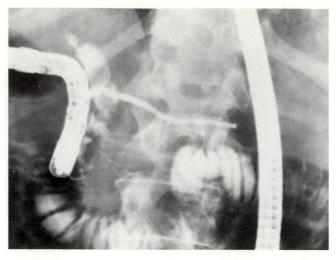

FIGURE 3-11.   ERC showing recurrent common bile duct stones. The pancreatic duct is visualized and appears normal.

part of all biliary procedures.[30] It identifies the presence of ductal anomalies and is of great importance in identifying unsuspected bile duct stones in 7% to 8% of patients (Figure 3-12). It provides complete visualization of the entire biliary system from the hepatic radicles to the duodenum and, if used routinely, adds less than 10 min to the operating time. An abnormal cholangiogram is the best indication of the need to explore the common bile duct.

Post-operative T-tube cholangiography should be performed after all bile duct explorations (1) immediately after completion of the bile duct exploration and placing a T-tube, prior to closing the abdomen, and (2) 8 to 10 days post-operatively, before removing the T-tube.

Treatment

Asymptomatic Patient.   Since symptoms will develop in approximately 50% of all asymptomatic patients with gallstones if they are not operated on over a 10-year period, I advise elective cholecystectomy to all patients younger than 60 years old and otherwise healthy; in older patients the operative risk is greater.[31,32] For patients with diabetes, angina pectoris that is not progressive, or small stones in the gallbladder, I advise elective cholecystectomy even more strongly. These three groups of patients have a greater risk of complications developing with cholecystitis: the diabetic because of the increased incidence of gangrene or perforation of the gallbladder; the patient with angina because of the association of acute myocardial infarction with episodes of acute cholecystitis; and the patient with small stones because of the increased hazard of stones migrating into the common bile duct and causing jaundice or pancreatitis.

For patients of any age with chronic renal disease, advanced cardiac disease, liver failure, or other major health problems, or for elderly patients (older than 65 or 70 years) without symptoms I would not advise cholecystectomy.

In all asymptomatic patients with gallstones, it is important for the surgeon to discuss with the patient and his family the pros and cons of elective cholecystectomy, to consult with the referring physician or family doctor, and to let the patient participate in the decision as to whether cholecystectomy should be performed now or in the future. An elective cholecystectomy is always safer than cholecystectomy during an acute attack.

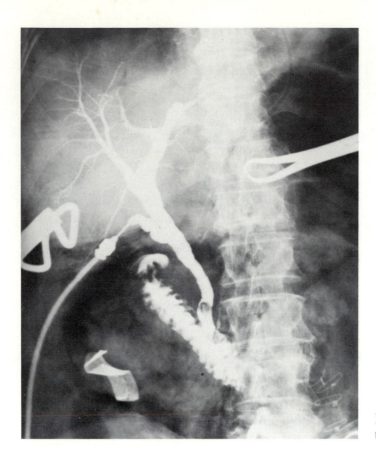

FIGURE 3-12. Operative cholangiogram showing an unsuspected stone in the distal common bile duct.

Acute Cholecystitis. The patient with acute cholecystitis should be hospitalized and treated initially with nasogastric suction, intravenous fluid replacement, and antibiotics (if there is evidence of fever or a significantly elevated white blood cell count). Relief of pain with meperidine hydrochloride (Demerol) or other agents is essential. During the first 12 to 24 hr of hospitalization, a general assessment of the patient's condition and potential risk for surgery should be made, including an evaluation of cardiorespiratory status, liver and renal function tests, and a serum amylase determination to identify pancreatitis. An oral cholecystogram, intravenous cholangiogram, or ultrasound study should be obtained if previous roentgenographic documentation of gallstones or a nonfunctioning gallbladder has not been obtained.

In the past, the controversy of "emergency" cholecystectomy versus "urgent" cholecystectomy versus medical therapy of the acute episode and later "elective" cholecystectomy has been much discussed in the surgical literature.[5,33–36] Although most patients (90%) with acute cholecystitis will recover from the episode with medical therapy alone, the hazards of complications, especially perforation, in the few who do not, the prolonged hospitalization required for some patients, the incidence of recurrent acute episodes, and the economic costs of a second hospitalization for later cholecystectomy have convinced me that the safest, most efficient management of most patients with acute cholecystitis is early, elective cholecystectomy and operative cholangiography 24 to 72 hr after the patient has been hospitalized. By this time, the acute symptoms have usually been aborted or modified by medical therapy, an evaluation of the patient's general health has been accomplished, and elective cholecystectomy can be performed safely and reasonably easily in an edematous dissection plane. If the acute symptoms cannot be controlled medically, if an enlarging hy-

53

drops of the gallbladder is palpated, or if the patient appears to become increasingly febrile or toxic, then an emergency cholecystectomy or cholecystostomy should be performed as soon as possible, even if it must be done under local anesthesia because the patient is too ill to be given a general anesthetic.[37,38]

Conversely, if the patient has another complicating problem, such as severe acute pancreatitis, myocardial infarction, congestive heart failure, renal failure, or severe lung disease, and is recovering from the cholecystitis on medical therapy, then cholecystectomy should be delayed.[39] An elective operation in such a patient can be performed more safely 6 weeks to 3 months or later, depending on symptoms and general recovery.

The worst, most difficult time to perform a cholecystectomy, in my experience, is 10 days to 3 weeks after an acute attack, during the period of resolving inflammation, vascularity, and fibrosis that follows the acute episode.

Perforation of the Gallbladder. Perforation of the gallbladder occurs in 5% to 10% of patients with acute cholecystitis.[40,41] It occurs most frequently in (1) the elderly, (2) patients with diabetes mellitus, (3) patients with generalized arteriosclerosis, (4) patients with hydrops of the gallbladder, and (5) patients with emphysematous cholecystitis (cholecystitis caused by gas-forming organisms). In most patients, the perforation is walled off by omentum or adjacent organs; in less than 5% of patients it is a free perforation into the peritoneal cavity. It rarely occurs sooner than 3 days after the onset of symptomatic acute cholecystitis. Whenever the diagnosis of perforation of the gallbladder is made or strongly suspected because of peritoneal signs or peritonitis, urgent operative exploration for cholecystectomy or cholecystostomy with drainage of the right upper abdomen is indicated.

Chronic Cholecystitis. In the patient with atypical symptoms, the diagnosis of chronic cholecystitis may be difficult. Care must be exercised in the patient who has atypical symptoms, but has gallstones or a non-visualizing gallbladder. Other studies, such as an upper gastrointestinal roentgenogram, barium enema, or intravenous urogram, should be obtained to rule out other problems. If the patient has functional symptoms, such as irritable bowel syndrome, gastritis, or psychosomatic problems, cholecystectomy will give little relief. Such patients make up a large segment of those who have post-cholecystectomy symptoms.

In the patient with typical symptoms of chronic cholecystitis, confirmed by roentgenographic studies, elective cholecystectomy and operative cholangiography is advised. As stated previously, operative cholangiography should be performed routinely with all cholecystectomies to evaluate the entire biliary tract.[30] In addition, a careful intra-abdominal exploration and palpation of other organs should be performed to identify any other organic pathology in the abdomen.

Occasionally, patients have classical symptoms of chronic cholecystitis but normal oral cholecystograms. If symptoms continue after repeated cholecystograms with laminograms of the gallbladder, ultrasonograms, a trial of a low-fat diet and anticholinergics, and a thorough diagnostic effort to identify and correct other causes of the symptoms, then an exploratory laparotomy and probable elective cholecystectomy with operative cholangiograms are indicated. Careful deliberation and discussion with the patient, as well as consultation with another physician, is wise before deciding on cholecystectomy for such patients. In my opinion, cholecystectomy will correct the symptoms in about 50% of such patients.

Bile Duct Stones. As noted earlier, 12% to 18% of patients with cholecystitis have stones in the common bile duct. Approximately one-half of this group of patients have or have had jaundice. An operative cholangiogram performed routinely at all cholecystectomies should identify stones in the common bile duct with an accuracy of about 98%.[29] Studies have shown that in about 6% to 8% of patients with common duct stones, the stones would have been unsuspected or missed at operation if an operative cholangiogram were not performed.

In patients with obstructive jaundice, a pre-operative endoscopic retrograde cholangiogram (ERC) or a percutaneous transhepatic cholangiogram will give important information and frequently shorten the operative time. If a percutaneous transhepatic cholangiogram is done pre-operatively, even with a "skinny" Chiba needle, and biliary obstruction is found, operative exploration and decompression of the obstructed bile ducts should optimally be done the same day. We schedule these studies in the morning and plan the operative procedure to follow. If biliary obstruction is not found to be the cause of the jaundice, the operation can be canceled. At operation, the use of intraoperative choledochoscopy is gaining increasing acceptance as a valuable adjunct to bile duct exploration (Figure 3-13).[42,43]

For most patients with stones in the bile ducts, bile duct exploration, removal of the stones, irrigation of the ducts, and closure with a T-tube (the largest T-tube that comfortably fits the duct should always be used) for post-operative drainage is all that is necessary. For some patients, however, who have stones recurring in the bile ducts after previous bile duct explorations, especially if the stones have recurred a second or third time, a bile duct drainage procedure (choledochoduodenostomy, choledochojejunostomy using a Roux-Y segment, or a sphincteroplasty) should be considered.[44,45]

If, after exploration of the common bile duct and placement of a T-tube, despite a normal closing T-tube cholangiogram, a stone (or stones) is

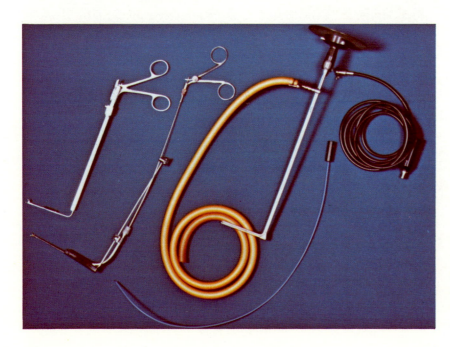

FIGURE 3-13. Storz-Hopkins choledochoscope is a valuable adjunct to bile duct exploration, especially in patients with dilated ducts and recurrent bile duct stones.

55

missed and is retained in the ducts, the T-tube should be left in place with open drainage into a bile bag, or clamped if the patient has no symptoms, for 6 to 8 weeks post-operatively. At that time, the T-tube can be removed and instruments can be passed into the bile duct through the fibrous T-tube tract, in the Department of Radiology, under fluoroscopic control, to retrieve the retained stone.[46] Other methods used to dissolve stones employing instillations of ether, heparin, or chenodeoxycholate have been unsuccessful, time consuming, or uncomfortable for the patient.

Acute Suppurative Cholangitis. Although chills and fever commonly occur along with jaundice in patients who have common bile duct stones, there are some patients who rapidly become septic, often showing signs of shock and extreme toxicity. These patients usually have a completely obstructed common bile duct and have early or obvious jaundice. A gram-negative infection develops in the obstructed biliary system. The syndrome of acute suppurative cholangitis is a surgical emergency.[47-49] Rapid restoration of fluids, the use of whole blood, and the vigorous use of appropriate antibiotics should be followed as rapidly as possible by surgical exploration and drainage of the common bile duct. Cholecystostomy may be used to drain an obstructed gallbladder, but it is not adequate in the treatment of suppurative cholangitis; common bile duct drainage with a T-tube must be employed.[50]

Gallstone Ileus

Occasionally a large gallstone will erode, by pressure or ischemic necrosis, through the wall of the gallbladder into the lumen of an adjacent segment of intestine, usually the duodenum. When such a stone passes down into the lower small intestine, it may obstruct the small intestine by virtue of its size.[51-53] The clinical picture of small bowel obstruction results, with nausea, vomiting, and dehydration, plus the complication (frequently) of biliary infection.

A major clue to the diagnosis of gallstone ileus can be seen on plain roentgenograms of the abdomen, which may show dilated small bowel loops plus air in the biliary system (Figure 3-14).

Treatment is primarily that of the small bowel obstruction: operative exploration, dislodgment of the stone back into a dilated segment of more proximal intestine, and enterostomy to remove the stone (always look for more than one). The management of the biliary problem *at that time* is of secondary importance. Only if the patient is in good condition and is not elderly, and the cholecystoduodenal fistula is not acutely inflamed or surgically hazardous from extensive scarring or the presence of an inflammatory mass, should a cholecystectomy and closure of the duodenal fistula be undertaken. Almost always it is safer to leave the biliary system alone, let the inflammation subside, and return at another elective operative procedure to perform a cholecystectomy and close the duodenal fistula.

Other Internal Biliary Fistulas. Other internal biliary fistulas, which are rarely seen, include the following: cholecystocholedochal fistulas, which occur when a stone erodes from the gallbladder into the common bile duct; cholecystocolic fistulas, which result when a stone erodes into the colon; or choledochoduodenal fistulas, which are usually caused by penetration of a duodenal ulcer into the common bile duct. These types of biliary fistulas rarely cause an emergency problem, as does gallstone ileus. They most frequently cause symptoms of chronic cholecystitis or of chol-

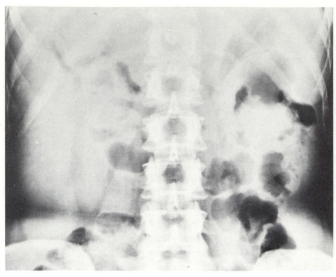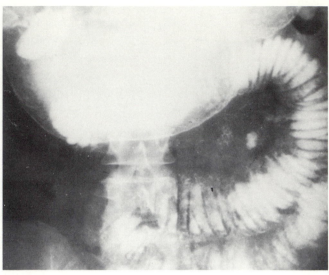

A   B

FIGURE 3-14. (A) Plain abdominal roentgenogram in a patient with gallstone ileus showing air in the biliary system. (B) In later film, barium is seen in the biliary system and in dilated small intestine.

angitis and are discovered by pre-operative studies or at the time of cholecystectomy. Treatment is essentially removal of the gallbladder, exploration of the common bile duct, and repair or closure of the enteric fistula.

Chronic Sclerosing Cholangitis.   Sclerosing cholangitis is an unusual, chronic inflammatory thickening of the extrahepatic bile ducts.[54,55] Its cause is unknown; it is only occasionally associated with gallstones and usually occurs primarily. Etiological factors suspected include bacterial and viral infections, an autoimmune process, or an underlying carcinoma of the bile ducts, with which it is often confused. It has been reported with increasing frequency in association with Crohn's disease of the intestine and with chronic ulcerative colitis.

The walls of the bile ducts are thickened, fibrotic, and chronically inflamed. The mucosa is often destroyed or ulcerated (Figure 3-15). The process is usually diffuse, involving the entire extrahepatic biliary system.

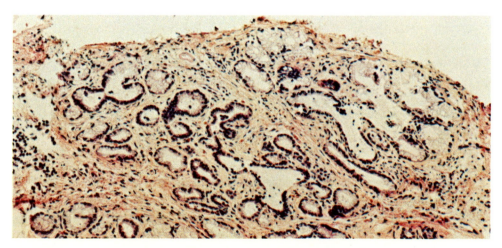

FIGURE 3-15.   Photomicrograph showing diffuse inflammatory changes involving the wall of the bile duct in a patient with sclerosing cholangitis.

58

The lumen of the bile duct is occluded by inspissated cells and debris, or it is narrowed to the point of obstruction by the thickened wall of the duct.

The symptoms are usually those of fluctuating obstructive jaundice, occasionally with pain, but frequently without. Chills and fever are common, as is some degree of nausea, loss of appetite, and weight loss. The differential diagnosis with chronic hepatitis may be difficult.

Percutaneous transhepatic cholangiography is usually not successful. ERC may show the small, abnormally narrowed ducts (Figure 3-16).

Operative exploration should be performed to make the diagnosis or to treat the biliary obstruction. If a thickened, dilated gallbladder is found cholecystectomy is indicated. The common duct should be explored, a biopsy performed to rule out carcinoma, the duct dilated and irrigated to remove all debris, and a T-tube left for post-operative drainage (Figure 3-17). Prolonged (6 months or longer) drainage may be of value. Long-term treatment post-operatively with antibiotics and with steroids has been used with success. However, the prognosis for permanent relief of symptoms and cure of the disease for most patients is poor. The disease frequently recurs or continues and progresses to biliary cirrhosis. In addition, the incidence of later development of carcinoma of the bile ducts is high, making some surgeons suspect that many patients with sclerosing cholangitis may have had bile duct carcinoma all along.

Stenosis of the Sphincter of Oddi. Stenosis of the sphincter of Oddi (stenosing papillitis, odditis) is a result of chronic irritation from bile duct stones in the majority of patients. Rarely, it is a primary entity. Some degree of spasm or fibrosis of the sphincter of Oddi may be seen in most patients with choledocholithiasis and in about 10% of patients with cholecystitis alone.[56] Significant stenosis is rarely suspected pre-operatively. It is usually an operative diagnosis found by palpation of the sphincter of Oddi at the time of cholecystectomy or common bile duct exploration (hypertrophy or thickening is noted), by operative cholangiography (spasm is seen on x-ray) (Figure 3-18), by inability to pass a 3-mm Bake's sound

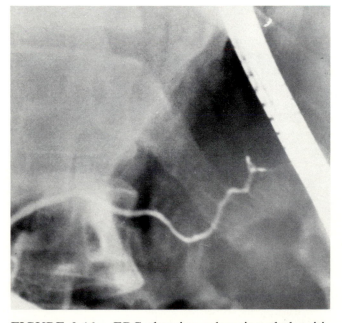

FIGURE 3-16. ERC showing sclerosing cholangitis and a normal pancreatic duct.

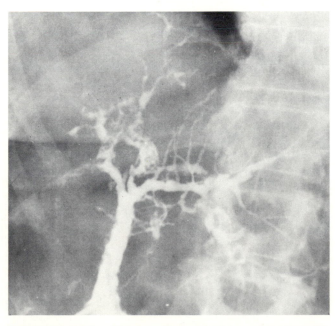

FIGURE 3-17. T-tube cholangiogram showing diffuse inflammatory changes in a patient with sclerosing cholangitis.

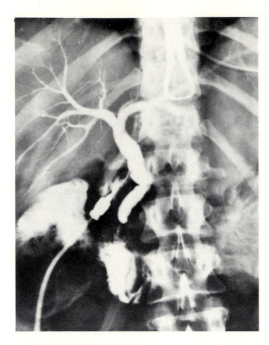

FIGURE 3-18. Operative cholangiogram showing moderate distention of the common bile duct with narrowing of the distal duct. On common bile duct exploration, fibrosis and stenosis of the sphincter of Oddi were found.

through the papilla of Vater (stenosis), or by manometric pressure recordings taken in the common bile duct.

If significant stenosis is present such that a 3-mm Bake's sound will not pass through the sphincter of Oddi, a duodenotomy should be performed and the papilla of Vater exposed. The sphincter should be divided by means of a sphincteroplasty (sphincterotomy) and a biopsy should be taken to confirm the diagnosis of papillary stenosis or hypertrophy and to rule out a carcinoma of the terminal bile duct or ampulla of Vater.[57]

Occasionally, stenosis of the sphincter of Oddi is a cause of post-cholecystectomy symptoms or of recurrent episodes of pancreatitis.[58-61] If it is suspected, cholangiographic studies (an intravenous cholangiogram or an ERC) should be obtained. In addition, an "evocative test" has been described by Nardi[59] that consists of an intramuscular injection of 10 mg morphine sulfate and 1 mg prostigmine. If this test reproduces the episodes of pain and elevates serum amylase to more than twice normal levels, papillary stenosis should be suspected.

Post-Cholecystectomy Syndrome and Biliary Dyskinesia

Avram M. Cooperman

The post-cholecystectomy syndrome (PCS)[51] includes a variety of organic and functional disorders that persist or, less frequently, develop after cholecystectomy.[62-64] It has been difficult to evaluate this syndrome critically because there are predominantly subjective symptoms (pain, bloating, dyspepsia), few objective tests (mostly cholangiography), and a large percentage of abnormal psychometric examinations (as high as 43% in one series).[63] Recently, the application of assays for hepatic lipids has quantitated bile acid abnormalities in some patients with PCS, and perhaps firmer grounds exist for a physiological explanation for some abnormalities.[62,65-67]

Incidence

The frequency or incidence of PCS is unknown because few long-term studies are available for analysis. In an analysis of 36 studies involving 20,000 cholecystectomies followed for up to 32 years, Bodvall[62] concluded that symptomatic cure occurred in 32% to 88% of cases, mild symptoms persisted in 9% to 35%, and severe symptoms (colic or dyspepsia) persisted in 2.6% to 32%. In another study of 1,930 cholecystectomy patients, 60% were symptomatically cured, 11% had dyspepsia, 24% had mild pain (biliary colic of low intensity and short duration), and 5% had severe colic or pain.[68] In both studies PCS was more common in women, especially when the indication for surgery was nonspecific symptoms rather than colic, when no stones were found in the gallbladder at surgery, and in functioning rather than non-functioning gallbladders. It is more common after operations for chronic than for acute cholecystitis.

Pathology

A variety of lesions, both organic and functional, have been associated with PCS. Some of the more common organic lesions include common duct stones, bile duct tumors, cystic duct remnants, stenosis of the sphincter of Oddi, and overlooked carcinoma of the pancreas. Some of the functional causes include motility or sphincter abnormalities (without pathological abnormalities) and abnormalities in bile salt metabolism. The functional causes have been collectively designated *biliary dyskinesia,* a term that awaits accurate pathological definition in most patients.

Diagnosis

A thorough and systematic evaluation is in order for all patients. Careful evaluation of all symptoms prior to cholecystectomy is important to determine if functional abnormalities are likely. A history of jaundice, colic, and known cholelithiasis makes one more optimistic about a good result from cholecystectomy than a pre-operative history of epigastric bloating, fullness, or dyspepsia.

Physical examination should exclude an incisional hernia (not found frequently enough) and local abnormalities such as a chronic stitch abscess. Laboratory studies of liver function should be obtained. An elevated alkaline phosphatase or bilirubin is evidence of recurrent or uncorrected biliary pathology.

A gastrointestinal series using barium will identify ulcer disease, congenital webs, or an annular pancreas. A barium enema should be per-

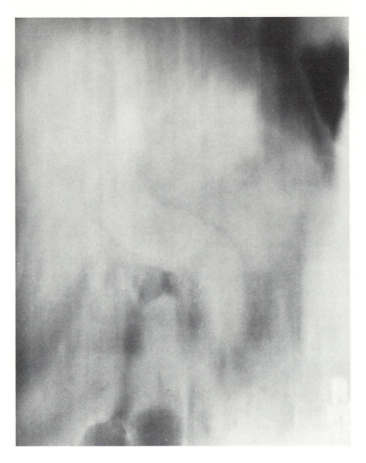

FIGURE 3-19. Intravenous cholangiogram of a dilated common bile duct containing several stones.

formed to exclude colonic disorders such as diverticulosis or the irritable bowel syndrome, a functional disorder which can mimic both upper and lower gastrointestinal organic disease. An intravenous cholangiogram should be obtained to identify the size of the common bile duct as well as to demonstrate any filling defects (Figure 3-19). In some patients, a questionable sensitivity to iodinated dyes precludes this study. For these patients, ultrasound examination or CT scans may show the size and configuration of the duct and the presence of stones if their density is different from the density of bile. Endoscopic examination will exclude ampullary tumors.

If these studies are normal, psychometric examination (we prefer a modification of the Minnesota Multiphasic Personality Examination) may be of value. Additional tests include the morphine transaminase test and cholecystokinin infusion.[69]

The morphine transaminase test was introduced by Sorensen[70] in 1964 and Laursen and Schmidt in 1966.[69] This test is based on the ability of morphine to raise intraductal biliary pressures by contracting the sphincter of Oddi and secondarily increasing the levels of transaminase (both SGOT and SGPT), amylase, and fraction 5 of lactic acid dehydrogenase. Despite these theoretical reasons to support the use of this test, a number of false-negative and false-positive tests have limited its use. In one series of 77 patients with PCS the morphine test was positive in 19%; of 9 patients submitted to sphincterotomy, none improved.[63]

The cholecystokinin infusion test is based on the principle that cholecystokinin will contract the bile duct and may reproduce the pain symptoms. This test has had sporadic application and limited critical analysis. Since the parameters are presently subjective and the availability of cholecystokinin is limited, this test is seldom used.

Common Bile Duct Stones.   If symptoms of biliary colic or obstructive jaundice are present, an overlooked or retained common duct stone should be a strong consideration. This problem should occur less frequently as intraoperative cholangiography becomes routine (Figure 3-20). Bodvall[2] reported and compared two groups of patients who underwent cholecystectomy: Group I comprised 938 patients operated on from 1949 to 1951; group II comprised 992 patients operated on during 1956 and 1957. In the first group cholangiography was performed in 14%, and in the second, in 66%. Common duct stones were found in 7.8% of group I and 14.6% of group II. In group I patients with PCS, 199 intravenous cholangiograms were performed; stones were identified in 12 pre-operatively and in four additional patients at surgery. In group II, in 192 intravenous cholangiograms, no stones were seen. Other studies have confirmed the value of intraoperative cholangiography. To reduce further the incidence of retained stones, intraoperative choledochoscopic examination has now been utilized. I am an enthusiast of this procedure since it provides direct visualization of the bile duct, is easy to use, and adds little time to the operation.

Stenosis of the Sphincter of Oddi.   This is thought to be an uncommon cause of PCS. Inflammation and subsequent scarring of the sphincter of Oddi may be due to the passage of stones or alcoholic pancreatitis. This condition is certainly not common, but it should be suspected when the common duct is dilated and a 3-mm probe cannot be passed into the duodenum through the ampulla. In one study reported by Grage et al.,[71] biopsies were taken from the sphincter in 50 patients with PCS and 50 "normal" autopsies. No pathological lesion was identified in either group. Although this study does not disprove this entity, fibrosis or scarring would be a welcome pathological finding to place this entity on firmer ground. Even then, identification and correction of this abnormality may not provide relief of symptoms. Lehmann[72] reported on a group of patients with stenosis of the ampulla who underwent choledochoduodenostomy to equalize biliary and duodenal pressures; PCS was rarely relieved postoperatively.

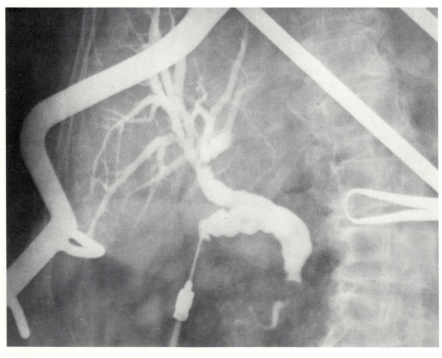

FIGURE 3-20.   Operative cholangiogram showing multiple stones in an enlarged cystic duct stump and a dilated common bile duct.

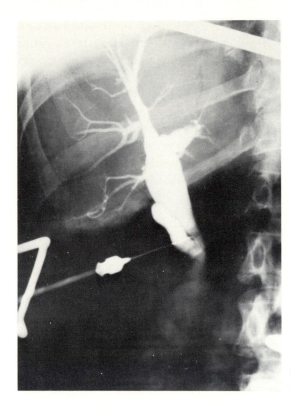

FIGURE 3-21 Operative cholangiogram demonstrating an enlarged cystic duct remnant.

Bile Duct Tumors. Occasionally a sclerosing carcinoma of the proximal bile duct or an ampullary tumor may mimic PCS. The former is almost always accompanied by an elevation in alkaline phosphatase level and 5-nucleotidase or by an abnormal cholangiogram. An ampullary tumor is far less frequent and can be best diagnosed by endoscopy.

Bile Duct Strictures. Although bile duct strictures are not uncommon, they usually occur in the immediate post-operative period and are accompanied by objective findings of jaundice, proximal bile duct dilatation, and elevated alkaline phosphatase levels. They are usually not difficult to differentiate from functional PCS.

Cystic Duct Syndrome. Uncommon causes of PCS are abnormalities due to a long cystic duct remnant or a neuroma that develops subsequent to amputation of the cystic duct[6,73,74] (Figure 3-21).

The frequency of a cystic duct remnant varies. Glenn and Johnson[66] found it in 1% of 3862 cholecystectomies; Bodvall and Overgaard,[68] using radiographic criteria, identified a remnant in 55% of patients. The importance of this anatomical finding as a cause of PCS, in my opinion, has been both overemphasized and underemphasized, depending on the source quoted. In one study of patients without PCS a cystic duct remnant was identified in 43%. It was present in 40% of mild and in 84% of severe PCS[62] patients.

There are a few theoretical reasons why a cystic duct remnant could cause symptoms. Residual or recurring inflammation or a nidus for stone formation are two of the more popular theories. Certainly, if stones or cholangitis are present with a long remnant there is a reason to hope that removal of the remnant will relieve symptoms. Excision of a cystic duct remnant will relieve symptoms in up to 50% of patients if stones or cholangitis are present and much less frequently if nonspecific symptoms are present.

A second pathological abnormality of a cystic duct remnant is an amputation neuroma. Fewer than 20 cases have been described since Florcken's[75] description in 1912. The symptoms that neuromas cause vary from crampy epigastric pain (sympathetic) to dyspepsia and vomiting (parasympathetic), depending on which autonomic nerve endings are stimulated. Even jaundice has been reported by extrinsic compression of the common duct by a neuroma.[73] The diagnosis of a cystic duct neuroma cannot be made pre-operatively and its finding at surgery does not ensure relief of symptoms. In Bodvall's[62] series, 15% of patients with severe epigastric distress of PCS had neuromas of the cystic duct, but none were improved after surgical excision.

Biliary Dyskinesia. In many cases of PCS no organic lesions may be found. They have been classified as *biliary dyskinesia,* implying that motor abnormalities of the common duct or sphincter may be the cause. That this relationship does exist has been corroborated by case reports. For example, Manier et al.[76] reported an unusual instance following cholecystectomy in which biliary colic was reproduced during intravenous cholangiography. The common duct dilated to twice its normal size, the transaminase level increased, and the right upper quadrant pain was reproduced. At subsequent surgery, the duct was normal in size and a probe passed easily into the duodenum through the sphincter. A choledochoduodenostomy was done and there was symptomatic relief.

Other authors, using the morphine provocative test and clinical impressions, have had limited success with sphincteroplasty or choledochoduodenostomy.[62,63] Good results are obtained in less than 30% of cases by most surgeons. To increase good results, manometric tests have been employed to detect increased pressures in the bile duct.[77] When these tests are done at surgery under anesthesia they may not reflect true pressures under basal condition.[64] Despite its popularity abroad, manometry has been of limited use in the United States, and sphincteroplasty is not widely endorsed unless a dilated duct with an abnormal cholangiogram is encountered.

Chemical Abnormalities. Studies of conjugation of 14-C-labeled cholic acid with liver homogenates of glycine and taurine have shown both an increase and decrease in the normal ratio with intrahepatic or extrahepatic diseases. Bodvall[62] and Bodvall and Eckdahl[65] studied both normal patients and those with mild and severe PCS. In some patients, bile aspirated from the common duct showed abnormalities in conjugation ratios and in ratios of bile salts. Bodvall fed a solution of cholic and dehydrocholic acid to some of these patients; 90% of 269 patients with dyspepsia or mild pain became symptom free. This symptom-free period lasted from 1 to 10 years while the patients had bile salt feedings. In patients with severe epigastric distress this treatment was inadequate, but feeding of progestational steroids was of benefit. The reasons for the efficacy of this treatment remain unclear, despite the apparent beneficial results in a small number of patients. This work and its applications have not been adapted in the United States, and most cases of functional PCS remain unsatisfactorily resolved.[62,78]

Treatment

The treatment of PCS will vary depending on the abnormality. For organic causes, especially retained or recurrent bile duct stones, treatment is standard. Removal of these stones by reoperation or a trans-sphincteric endoscopic approach is indicated. For bile duct strictures, reoperation with reanastomosis of the hepatic or common bile duct to the lower duct, jejunum, or duodenum may provide long-lasting relief. These technics are discussed elsewhere.

If a bile duct tumor is the cause of symptoms, operative treatment is dependent on the location of the tumor and the local findings. If stenosis of the sphincter of Oddi is found, a sphincteroplasty or choledochoduodenostomy should be performed. I will speculate that endoscopy-guided transduodenal sphincterotomy may replace the operative approach, particularly since its definition is unclear. A cystic duct remnant with calculi, when identified, should be excised.

For biliary dyskinesia, treatment is more difficult. Medical therapy with antispasmodics has been of some help in selected patients. Avoidance of fatty and spicy foods has helped other patients. The use of bile salts and acids to dissolve gallstones has been limited to a few centers in the United States; their use in biliary dyskinesia has not yet been reported. Thus, a search for other causes of upper gastrointestinal disease and biofeedback may be appropriate until controlled studies evaluate these biochemical modalities.

Biliary Stricture

In most patients, strictures of the bile ducts are the result of an operative injury to the ducts.[79-82] In 90% to 95% of patients the operative injury has occurred during cholecystectomy; in about 5% the injury occurred during common bile duct exploration, gastric resection, or an operation on the pancreas. Infrequently, strictures may occur as a result of progressive stenosis from chronic pancreatitis, injuries to the bile duct from external trauma, erosion of a common bile duct stone, sclerosing cholangitis, or spontaneously from a congenital stenosis that progresses to stricture.

The incidence of injuries to the common bile duct during cholecystectomy or other operative procedures is not known. Since the advent of routine operative cholangiography during cholecystectomy, anomalies of the biliary system are recognized in 10% to 15% of patients. Despite this incidence of anomalies of the ducts, it is estimated that injury to the bile ducts occurs during cholecystectomy in less than 0.5% of patients.[5] Careful operative technic, avoiding the division of any duct stricture until the anatomy is completely clear, and the routine use of operative cholangiography should help to make this complication become even more rare in the future.[83,84]

Pathology

Strictures of the bile duct are located in the hepatic ducts, above the junction with the cystic duct in more than one-half of all patients.[79-82,85,86] Frequently, the area of scarring extends to the bifurcation of the right and left hepatic ducts; less often, the central or distal common bile duct is the site of stricture formation (Table 3-3).

Gross inspection of the area of stricture shows dense scar tissue surrounding the duct, making dissection and exposure of the duct difficult. Proximal to the stricture, the ducts are dilated and their walls thickened.

Histologically, the integrity of the mucosa is lost and is replaced by scar tissue, with complete, or nearly complete, occlusion of the lumen of the duct. The entire wall of the common bile duct may be replaced with scar tissue.

Diagnosis

Clinical Features. Most patients have a history of an operative procedure, usually a cholecystectomy, or have had symptoms of biliary disease or pancreatitis. In some patients, after operative injury of the bile ducts, an external biliary fistula or a subhepatic collection of bile may result. Reoperation to correct the bile leakage may precede the development of a stricture of the bile duct at the point of suture repair of the duct.

TABLE 3-3   Location of strictures of the bile ducts in 100 patients (1951–1971)

Location	No. of Patients
Common hepatic duct or junction of right and left hepatic ducts	54
Central common bile duct	28
Distal common bile duct	18

SOURCE   Data from Hermann.[81]

The classic symptoms of stricture of the bile duct are jaundice if the stricture is complete (as after suture ligation of the bile duct), or intermittent chills, fever, and jaundice if the stricture is incomplete. These symptoms may occur within days after an operative procedure or may occur weeks or months later. They indicate, of course, the presence of cholangitis secondary to the stricture.

The differential diagnosis should include a stone in the common bile duct, sclerosing cholangitis, or hepatitis. If jaundice alone occurs, carcinoma of the bile ducts, ampulla of Vater, or head of the pancreas, missed at the previous operative procedure, may be suspected. However, when chills and fever are present or the jaundice is intermittent, the diagnosis of a malignant lesion is unlikely.

Laboratory Studies. Routine laboratory studies should be obtained, the most important being those of liver function. The serum alkaline phosphatase is significantly elevated; the serum bilirubin is elevated; and the SGOT is only slightly elevated in patients with a biliary stricture. High SGOT levels indicate the possibility of hepatitis.

Roentgenographic Studies. Intravenous cholangiography is of no value in patients with obstructive jaundice. Direct methods of cholangiography are of the utmost importance to visualize the obstructed biliary system, to locate the site of the stricture, and to confirm the diagnosis. Endoscopic retrograde cholangiography may be attempted, but it will only visualize the distal biliary system below the point of obstruction. If the obstruction is incomplete, the stricture may be visualized (Figure 3-22). Percutaneous transhepatic cholangiography will visualize the dilated, proximal biliary system in the liver and will show the point of obstruction (Figure 3-23). For this reason, I have found it an extremely valuable pre-operative study. I usually schedule the percutaneous transhepatic cholangiogram for the morning of the operation. After the study is completed, the patient is sent to the operating room for correction of the stricture, usually within 2 to 4 hr after the diagnostic procedure.

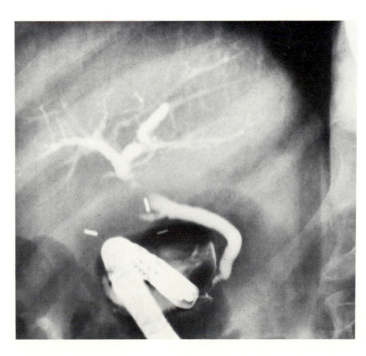

FIGURE 3-22.   ERC showing an incomplete stricture of the upper central bile ducts.

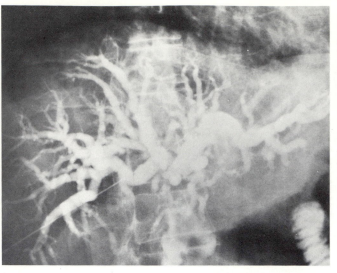
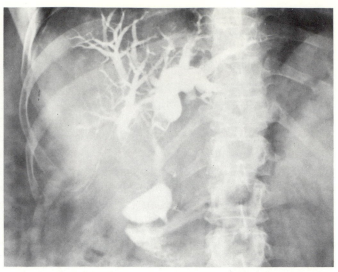

A   B

FIGURE 3-23.   Percutaneous transhepatic cholangiograms showing strictures of the proximal biliary system. One film (**B**) shows hepatic duct stones proximal to a stricture.

Treatment

Operative Strategy.   Antibiotics should be given pre-operatively, prior to endoscopic retrograde cholangiography or percutaneous transhepatic cholangiography, especially in patients who have a history of cholangitis. I select an antibiotic that is excreted in the bile, such as ampicillin or sodium cephalosporin.

The aim of operative treatment of a stricture of the bile ducts is to resect the stricture and all surrounding scar tissue and to reconstruct the biliary system so that unobstructed bile flow is returned to the duodenum or jejunum. The operative procedure can be difficult. It is important to choose an incision that will give good exposure of the subhepatic space; I prefer a right subcostal incision for most patients. The bile ducts must be carefully exposed and identified. The pre-operative cholangiogram is of great help in identifying the site of the stricture and of the intrahepatic anatomy of the biliary system.[81] Frequently, intraoperative needling of the bile ducts or repeat intraoperative cholangiograms are an aid in localizing the ducts (Figure 3-24). All scar tissue should be resected, if possible, back to normal duct strictures. The distal duct should be exposed to see if it might be usable in the reconstruction. Frequently, the distal duct is involved in scar tissue and is so collapsed or small as to be unusable.

Choice of Repair.   The choice of repair includes duct-to-duct repair, plastic revision or dilatation of a partial or incomplete stricture, choledochoduodenostomy, or choledochojejunostomy using a Roux-Y segment or a loop with an enteroenterostomy below. I prefer complete resection of the stricture rather than plastic revision or dilatation for most patients. Duct-to-duct repairs (choledochocholedochostomy) are not often possible because the difference in size between the dilated proximal duct and the small distal duct is too great.[79,85,87] In addition, mobilization of the distal duct to allow an anastomosis without tension is difficult.

I prefer a choledochoduodenostomy or choledochojejunostomy with a Roux-Y segment for most patients. If the duodenum is mobile, I prefer choledochoduodenostomy because this operation is simpler, involves only

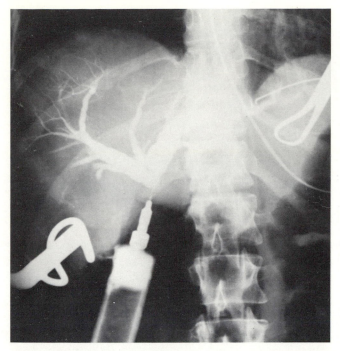

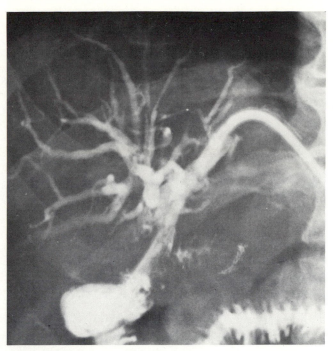

FIGURE 3-24. Operative cholangiogram, obtained by transhepatic needling of the biliary system during the operative procedure, showing total obstruction of the biliary system at a high level.

FIGURE 3-25. Postoperative cholangiogram through an intrahepatic tube after hepatojejunostomy repair of a high biliary stricture.

one anastomosis, and would appear to be more physiological in that bile is returned into the duodenum.[88-91] Many surgeons are afraid of reflux of duodenal contents into the bile ducts and ascending cholangitis, but this is seldom seen. It does occur if the anastomosis is too small or becomes strictured. If a choledochoduodenostomy cannot be performed because of duodenal scarring, or if a previous choledochoduodenostomy has failed, then a choledochojejunostomy is performed. The hepatojejunostomy technic of Wexler and Smith,[92] using a jejunal mucosal graft, is an excellent method for the repair of high bile duct strictures in which all scar tissue cannot be resected (Figure 3-25). These technics are illustrated in Chapter 6.

Use of Tubes. The use of a T-tube, Y-tube, or straight catheter stents for bile duct repairs and the length of time such tubes should be left in place is controversial.[86,93] When greatly dilated and thickened ducts are found at surgery and a satisfactory, two-layer anastomosis can be achieved, I frequently do not use any tube to stent or splint the anastomosis. We have had excellent long-term results in those patients in whom no tubes were used. In most patients, however, a T-tube or Y-tube splint is left in place to protect the anastomosis for 6 weeks and is then removed in the office. When all scar tissue has been removed, reasonably "normal" bile ducts are available for the anastomosis, and the anastomosis has gone well, I believe that the continuing presence of a tube in the bile duct is an irritant to the anastomosis and a foreign body that collects bile sludge that may lead to further stricture formation[94] (Figure 3-26). I therefore remove the tube about 6 weeks postoperatively.

In some patients, however, scar tissue cannot be completely removed at the site of stricture repair, especially when the stricture is high in the liver or when several previous repairs have failed and the stricture has recurred. In such patients, I agree with those who advocate leaving the T-

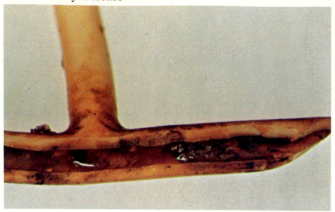 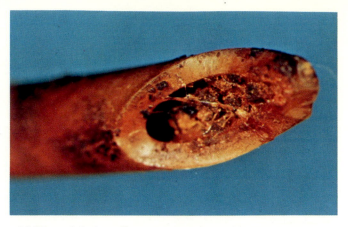

FIGURE 3-26. Sludge and biliary debris collects on T-tubes; these T-tubes were removed at 6 weeks.

tube or Y-tube splint in for much longer periods of time—up to 1 or 2 years after operation.[86] Occasionally, a U-tube may be used and left in place for 6 to 9 months.[87,95] At this time, a previously matched tube is tied and fitted to one end of the tube, the first tube is removed, and the second tube is passed into its place (Figure 3-27). Each 6 to 9 months, a new tube is thus positioned through the area of the biliary intestinal anastomosis.

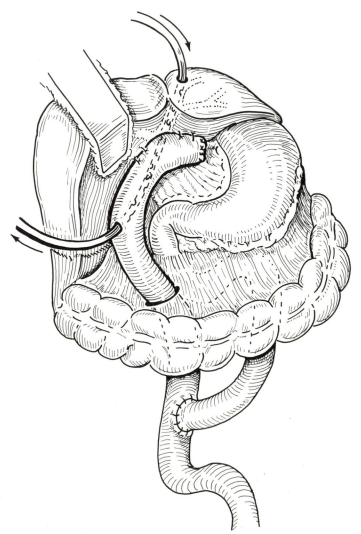

FIGURE 3-27. Straight catheter splint placed through a hepatojejunostomy anastomosis in the U-tube technic. This catheter is removed in the direction of the arrows for replacement with a matched catheter each 6 to 9 months.

TABLE 3-4 Results of repair of strictures of bile duct in 100 patients (1951–1971)

Procedure	Excellent/Good		Poor	
	No.	%	No.	%
Choledochoduodenostomy	53	90	6	10
Choledochocholedochostomy	8	73	3	27
Choledochojejunostomy, Roux-Y	7	78	2	22
Plastic revision of stricture	5	71	2	29
Dilatation of stricture	11	78	3	22
All procedures	84	84	16	16

Results. Our operative mortality for repair of strictures of the bile duct has been approximately 3%.[81] The operative mortality reported by other groups for stricture repair has ranged from 2% to 5%.

Long-term success with excellent or good results are now being reported in 65% to 85% of patients after repair of strictures of the bile ducts.[80,81,85,87,92–96] At the Cleveland Clinic, in 100 patients operated upon between 1951 and 1971 with a follow-up of 2 to 20 years, we have had good or excellent results in 84% of the patients (Table 3-4). In this group of patients, some of the best results were achieved after choledochoduodenostomy. Sixteen patients who did poorly after repair of the stricture have required an additional 22 operative procedures to reconstruct the bile ducts. The success with repair of a biliary stricture is related to the length of follow-up, the number of previous repairs that have failed, the delay in repairing a stricture that has occurred (or recurred), and the presence of coexisting (secondary) biliary cirrhosis.

References

Cholecystitis and Cholangitis
1. Hermann, R. E.: Cholelithiasis and cholecystitis. In, H. F. Conn (ed.): *Current Therapy*. Philadelphia, Saunders, 1971, p. 278.
2. Lund, J.: Surgical indications in cholelithiasis: prophylactic cholecystectomy elucidated on the basis of long-term followup on 526 nonoperated cases. *Ann. Surg., 151,* 153, 1960.
3. Wenckert, A., and Robertson, B.: The natural course of gallstone disease. Eleven-year review of 781 nonoperated cases. *Gastroenterology, 50,* 376, 1966.
4. Wilbur, R. S., and Bolt, R. J.: Incidence of gallbladder disease in normal men. *Gastroenterology, 36,* 251, 1959.
5. Glenn, F.: Trends in surgical treatment of calculous disease of the biliary tract. *Surg. Gynecol. Obstet, 140,* 877, 1975.
6. Hermann, R. E., and Martin, J. C.: Biliary disease and advancing age. *Geriatrics 24,* 139, 1969.
7. Saypol, G. M.: Indications for choledochostomy in operations for cholelithiasis. Analysis of 525 cases. *Ann. Surg., 153,* 567, 1961.
8. Madden, J. L., Vanderheyden, L., and Kandalaft, S.: The nature and surgical significance of common duct stones. *Surg. Gynecol. Obstet., 126,* 3, 1968.
9. Kelly, T. R.: Gallstone pancreatitis: pathophysiology. *Surgery, 80,* 488, 1976.

10. Womack, N. A., Zeppa, R., and Irvin, G. L., III: The anatomy of gallstones. *Ann. Surg.* **157,** 670, 1963.
11. Chetlin, S. H., and Elliott, D. W.: Biliary bacteremia. *Arch. Surg.,* **102,** 303, 1971.
12. Flemma, R. J., Flint, L. M., Osterhout, S., et al.: Bacteriologic studies of biliary tract infection. *Ann. Surg.,* **166,** 563, 1967.
13. Fukunaga, F. H.: Gallbladder bacteriology, histology, and gallstones; study of unselected cholecystectomy specimens in Honolulu. *Arch. Surg.,* **106,** 169, 1973.
14. Goswitz, J. T.: Bacteria and biliary tract disease. *Am. J. Surg.,* **128,** 644, 1974.
15. Keighley, M. R. B., McLeish, A. R., Bishop, H. M., et al.: Identification of the presence and type of biliary microflora by immediate gram stains. *Surgery,* **81,** 469, 1977.
16. Pyrtek, L. J., and Bartus, S. A.: An evaluation of antibiotics in biliary tract surgery. *Surg. Gynecol. Obstet.,* **125,** 101, 1967.
17. Schoenfield, L. J.: Editorial. Biliary excretion of antibiotics. *N. Engl. J. Med.,* **284,** 1213, 1971.
18. Stefanini, P., Carboni, M., Patrassi, N., et al.: Factors influencing the long-term results of cholecystectomy. *Surg. Gynecol. Obstet.,* **139,** 734, 1974.
19. Fiegenschuh, W. H., and Loughry, C. W.: The false-normal oral cholecystogram. *Surgery,* **81,** 239, 1977.
20. Freedman, J. N.: X-ray evaluation of patients with gallbladder disease. *Contemp. Surg.,* **8,** 53, 1976.
21. Wise, R. E.: Roentgenology of the liver and biliary tract. *Gastroenterology,* **45,** 644, 1963.
22. Bartrum, R. J., Jr., Crow, H. C., and Foote, S. R.: Ultrasound examination of the gallbladder as alternative to "double-dose" oral cholecystography. *J.A.M.A.,* **236,** 1147, 1976.
23. Berger, M., Smith, E., Holm, H. H., and Mascatello, V.: Utility of ultrasound in the differential diagnosis of acute cholecystitis. *Arch. Surg.,* **112,** 273, 1977.
24. Isikoff, M. B., and Diaconis, J. N.: Ultrasound. A new diagnostic approach to the jaundiced patient. *J.A.M.A.* **238,** 221, 1977.
25. Matolo, N. M., Stadalnik, R. C., and Wolfman, E. F., Jr.: Hepatobiliary scanning using ^{99m}-Tc-pyridoxylideneglutamate. *Am. J. Surg,* **133,** 116, 1977.
26. Williams, J. A. R., Baker, R. J., Walsh, J. F., et al.: The role of biliary scanning in the investigation of the surgically jaundiced patient. *Surg. Gynecol. Obstet.,* **144,** 525, 1977.
27. Elias, E., Hamlyn, A. N., Jain, S., Long, R. G., Summerfield, J. A., Dick, R., and Sherlock, S.: Liver physiology and disease. A randomized trial of percutaneous transhepatic cholangiography with the chiba needle versus endoscopic retrograde cholangiography for bile duct visualization in jaundice. *Gastroenterology,* **71,** 439, 1976.
28. Flemma, R. J., and Shingleton, W. W.: Clinic experience with percutaneous transhepatic cholangiography. Experience with 107 cases. *Am. J. Surg.,* **111,** 13, 1966.
29. McCormick, J. S., Bremner, D. N., Thomson, J. W. W., and Philp, T.: The operative cholangiogram: its interpretation, accuracy, and value in association with cholecystectomy. *Ann. Surg.,* **180,** 902, 1974.
30. Hermann, R. E., and Hoerr, S. O.: The value of the routine use of operative cholangiography. *Surg., Gynecol. Obstet.,* **121,** 1015, 1965.
31. Glenn, F., and Hays, D. M.: The age factor in the mortality rate of patients undergoing surgery of the biliary tract. *Surg. Gynecol. Obstet,* **100,** 11, 1955.
32. Seltzer, M. H., Steiger, E., and Rosato, F. E.: Mortality following cholecystectomy. *Surg. Gynecol. Obstet.,* **130,** 64, 1970.
33. Gagic, N., Frey, C. F., and Gaines, R.: Acute cholecystitis. *Surg. Gynecol. Obstet.,* **140,** 868, 1975.
34. Haff, R. C., Butcher, H. R., Jr., and Ballinger, W. F.: Factors influencing morbidity in biliary tract operations. *Surg. Gynecol. Obstet.,* **132,** 195, 1971.

35. Hermann, R. E.: Acute cholecystitis. *J.A.M.A.*, **234**, 1261, 1975.
36. Wright, H. K., and Holden, W. D.: The risks of emergency surgery for acute cholecystitis. *Arch. Surg.*, **81**, 341, 1960.
37. Gagic, N., and Frey, C. F.: The results of cholecystostomy for the treatment of acute cholecystitis. *Surg. Gynecol. Obstet.*, **140**, 255, 1975.
38. Gingrich, R. A., Awe, W. C., Boyden, A. M., and Peterson, C. G.: Cholecystostomy in acute cholecystitis. Factors influencing morbidity and mortality. *Am. J. Surg.*, **116**, 310, 1968.
39. Hermann, R. E., and Hertzer, N. R.: Time of biliary surgery after acute pancreatitis due to biliary disease. Report of six illustrative cases. *Arch. Surg.*, **100**, 71, 1970.
40. MacDonald, J. A.: Perforation of the gallbladder associated with acute cholecystitis: 8-year review of 20 cases. *Ann. Surg.*, **164**, 849, 1966.
41. McEachern, C. G., and Sullivan, R. E.: Perforation of the gallbladder. Analysis of 21 cases. *Arch. Surg.*, **87**, 489, 1963.
42. Nora, P. F., Berci, G., and Dorazio, R. A.: Operative choledochoscopy. Results of a prospective study in several institutions. *Am. J. Surg.*, **133**, 105, 1977.
43. Shore, J. M., Berci, G., and Morgenstern, L.: The value of biliary endoscopy. *Surg. Gynecol. Obstet.*, **140**, 601, 1975.
44. Glenn, F.: Post-cholecystectomy choledocholithiasis. *Surg. Gynecol. Obstet.*, **134**, 249, 1972.
45. Madden, J. L., Chun, J. Y., Kandalaft, S., et al.: Choledochoduodenostomy. An unjustly maligned surgical procedure? *Am. J. Surg.*, **119**, 45, 1970.
46. Burhenne, H. J., Richards, V., Mathewson, C., Jr., et al.: Nonoperative extraction of retained biliary tract stones requiring multiple sessions. *Am. J. Surg.*, **128**, 288, 1974.
47. Dow, R. W., and Lindenauer, S. M.: Acute obstructive suppurative cholangitis. *Ann. Surg.*, **169**, 272, 1969.
48. Haupert, A. P., Carey, L., Evans, W. E., et al.: Acute suppurative cholangitis. Experience with 15 consecutive cases. *Arch. Surg.*, **94**, 460, 1967.
49. Hinchey, E. J., and Couper, C. E.: Acute obstructive suppurative cholangitis. *Am. J. Surg.*, **117**, 62, 1969.
50. Saik, R. P., Greenburg, A. G., and Peskin, G. W.: Cholecystostomy hazard in acute cholangitis. *J.A.M.A.*, **235**, 2412, 1976.
51. Cooperman, A. M., Dickson, E. R., and ReMine, W. H.: Changing concepts in the surgical treatment of gallstone ileus: a review of 15 cases with emphasis on diagnosis and treatment. *Ann. Surg.*, **167**, 377, 1968.
52. Day, E. A., and Marks, C.: Gallstone ileus. Review of the literature and presentation of thirty-four new cases. *Am. J. Surg.*, **129**, 552, 1975.
53. Hudspeth, A. S., and McGuirt, W. F.: Gallstone ileus. A continuing surgical problem. *Arch. Surg.*, **100**, 668, 1970.
54. Glenn, F., and Whitsell, J. C., II: Primary sclerosing cholangitis. *Surg. Gynecol. Obstet.*, **123**, 1037, 1966.
55. Perry, A. W., Djang, E., Kafrouni, G., and Ludington, L. G.: Primary sclerosing cholangitis. *Am. J. Surg.*, **121**, 743, 1971.
56. Shingleton, W. W., and Gamburg, D.: Stenosis of sphincter of Oddi. *Am. J. Surg.* **119**, 35, 1970.
57. Jones, S. A., Steedman, R. A., Keller, T. B., et al.: Transduodenal sphincteroplasty (not sphincterotomy) for biliary and pancreatic disease. Indications, contraindications and results. *Am. J. Surg.*, **118**, 292, 1969.
58. Acosta, J. M., Civantos, F., Nardi, G. L., et al: Fibrosis of the papilla of Vater. *Surg. Gynecol. Obstet.*, **124**, 787, 1967.
59. Nardi, G. L.: Papillitis and stenosis of the sphincter of Oddi. *Surg. Clin. North Am.*, **53**, 1149, 1973.
60. Riddell, D. H., and Kirtley, J. A., Jr.: Stenosis of the sphincter of Oddi. Transduodenal sphincterotomy and some other surgical aspects. *Ann. Surg.*, **149**, 773, 1959.

Post-cholecystectomy Syndrome and Biliary Dyskinesia

61. Westphal, K.: Muskelfunktion nervensystem und pathologie der gallenwege. I. Untersuchungen uber den schmerzanfall der gallenwege und seine ausstrahlen reflexe. *Z. Klin. Med.* (Berlin), **96,** 22, 1923.

62. Bodvall, B.: The postcholecystectomy syndromes. *Clin. Gastroenterol.,* **2,** 103, 1973.

63. Christiansen, J., and Schmidt, A.: The postcholecystectomy syndrome. *Acta Chir. Scand.* **137,** 789, 1971.

64. Jacobsson, B.: Determination of pressure in the common bile duct at and after operation. *Acta Chir. Scand.,* **113,** 483, 1957.

65. Bodvall, B., and Ekdahl, P. H.: The conjugation of C^{14}-labeled cholic acid in liver homogenates from patients with and without postoperative biliary distress. *Acta Chir. Scand.,* **127,** 101, 1964.

66. Glenn, F., and Johnson, G. Jr.: Cystic duct remnant, a sequela of incomplete cholecystectomy. *Surg. Gynecol. Obstet.,* **101,** 331, 1955.

67. Womack, N. A., and Crider, R. L.: The persistence of symptoms following cholecystectomy. *Ann. Surg.,* **126,** 31, 1947.

68. Bodvall, B., and Overgaard B.: Computer analysis of postcholecystectomy biliary tract symptoms. *Surg. Gynecol. Obstet.,* **124,** 723, 1967.

69. Laursen, T., and Schmidt, A.: Increase in serum-GPT and serum-LDH after administration of morphine to patients suffering from bile-duct dyskinesia. *Scand. J. Clin. Lab.,* **18** [Suppl 92], 175, 1966.

70. Sorensen, B.: Morfintransaminase prven ved dyskinesia bilaris. *Ugeskr. Laeger,* **126,** 1393, 1964.

71. Grage, T. B., Lober, P. H., Imamoglu, K., et al.: Stenosis of the sphincter of Oddi; a clinicopathologic review of 50 cases. *Surgery,* **48,** 304, 1960.

72. Lehmann, K.: Results of surgical treatment of the postcholecystectomy syndrome. *Acta Chir. Scand.,* **112,** 40, 1956.

73. Comfort, M. W., and Walters, W.: Intermittent jaundice due to neuroma of cystic and common bile ducts. *Ann. Surg.,* **93,** 1142, 1931.

74. Zeff, R. H., Pfeffer, R. B., Adams, P. X., et al.: Reoperation for amputation neuroma of the cystic duct. *Am. J. Surg.,* **131,** 369, 1976.

75. Florcken, H.: Gallenblasenregeneration mit steinrezidiv nach cholecystektomie. *Dtsche. Chir.* (Leipzig), **113,** 604, 1912.

76. Manier, J. W., Cohen, W. N., and Printen, K. J.: Dysfunction of the sphincter of Oddi in a postcholecystectomy patient. *Am. J. Gastroenterol.,* **62,** 148, 1974.

77. Schein, C. J., and Beneventano, T. C.: Choledochal dynamics in man. *Surg. Gynecol. Obstet.,* **126,** 591, 1968.

78. Best, R. R., Hicken, N. F., and Finlayson, A. I.: The effect of dehydrocholic acid upon biliary pressure and its clinical application. *Ann. Surg.,* **110,** 67, 1939.

Biliary Stricture

79. Cattell, R. B., and Braasch, J. W.: Primary repair of benign strictures of the bile duct. *Surg. Gynecol. Obstet.,* **109,** 531, 1959.

80. Cosman, B., and Porter, M. R.: Benign stricture of the bile ducts. *Ann. Surg.,* **152,** 730, 1960.

81. Hermann, R. E.: Diagnosis and management of bile duct strictures. *Am. J. Surg.,* **130,** 519, 1975.

82. Walters, W. Nixon, J. W., Jr., and Hodgins, T. E.: Strictures of the common bile duct. Five to 25-year followup of 217 operations. *Ann. Surg.,* **149,** 781, 1959.

83. Glenn, F.: The importance of technique in cholecystectomy. *Surg. Gynecol. Obstet.,* **101,** 201, 1955.

84. Hermann, R. E.: A plea for a safer technique of cholecystectomy. *Surgery,* **79,** 609, 1976.

85. Aust, J. B., Root, H. D., Urdaneta, L., et al: Biliary stricture. *Surgery, 62,* 601, 1967.

86. Warren, K. W., Poulantzas, J. K., and Kung, A.: A Y-tube splint in the repair of biliary strictures. *Surg. Gynecol. Obstet., 122,* 785, 1966.

87. Braasch, J. W., Warren, K. W., and Blevins, P. K.: Progress in biliary stricture repair. *Am. J. Surg., 129,* 34, 1975.

88. Barner, H. B.: Choledochoduodenostomy with reference to secondary cholangitis: 15-year review of 24 cases. *Ann. Surg., 163,* 74, 1966.

89. Degenshein, G. A.: Choledochoduodenostomy: an 18-year study of 175 consecutive cases. *Surgery, 76,* 319, 1974.

90. Farrar, T., Painter, M. W., and Betz, R.: Choledochoduodenostomy in the treatment of stenosis in the distal common duct. *Arch. Surg., 98,* 442, 1969.

91. Hurwitz, A., and Degenshein, G. A.: The role of choledochoduodenostomy in common duct surgery: reappraisal. *Surgery, 56,* 1147, 1964.

92. Wexler, M. J., and Smith, R.: Jejunal mucosal graft. A sutureless technic for repair of high bile duct strictures. *Am. J. Surg., 129,* 204, 1975.

93. Hertzer, N. R., Gray, H. W., Hoerr, S. O., et al.: The use of T-tube splints in bile duct repairs. *Surg. Gynecol. Obstet., 137,* 413, 1973.

94. Kolff, J., Hoeltge, G., and Hermann, R. E.: Silastic T-tube splints for biliary repair. *Am. J. Surg., 129,* 236, 1975.

95. Stone, R. M., Cohen, Z., Taylor, B. R., Langer, B., and Tovee, E. B.: Bile duct injury. Results of repair using a changeable stent. *Am. J. Surg., 125,* 253, 1973.

96. Goff, R. D., Eisenberg, M. M., and Woodward, E. R.: Interlobar intrahepatic approach to biliary tract reconstruction. *Ann. Surg. 165,* 624, 1967.

Neoplasms

4

Benign Tumors

Benign tumors of the gallbladder and bile ducts are rare lesions. Papillomas and polyps, adenomas, adenomyomas, lipomas, fibromas, and hemangiomas have been reported.[1-3] Of these, the polyp or papilloma occurs most frequently. In 1915 Irwin and MacCarthy[4] reported 85 cases of papillomas of the gallbladder found in 2,168 cholecystectomy specimens, an incidence of 3.9%. In more recent studies a 1% to 4.2% incidence of benign tumors in the gallbladder has been reported.[5,6]

Benign tumors of the bile ducts are even more rare. The two most comprehensive reviews of the world literature on this subject were by Chu[2] in 1950 and by Dowdy and associates[3] in 1962. These two reviews have identified only 98 cases of benign tumors of the bile ducts reported in the literature up to 1962, 73 of which appeared to be authentic and were confirmed histologically.

Pathology

Most benign tumors found in the gallbladder are papillomas or polyps.[5,6] Table 4-1 gives the incidence of these rare lesions in one reported series, that from Memorial-Sloan Kettering Hospital, New York, for 1937 through 1964.[5] They are usually solitary lesions, but may be multiple (Figure 4-1). They are rarely larger than 0.5 to 1.0 cm. The cause is unknown and probably not related to the formation of gallstones.

Because there has been a difference of opinion in the surgical literature over what constitutes a "true" papilloma, it has been defined as follows: "A vascular connective tissue stalk covered by a single layer of tall columnar epithelial cells. Repeated branching and rebranching of the stalk generally occurs, resulting in a multiple villus-like process, each of which is also covered by a single layer of columnar or cuboidal epithelium."[5] Carcinoma-in-situ may be found with some frequency. Papillomas are thus thought to be potentially premalignant lesions.[7,8]

An adenomyoma of the gallbladder, the next most common benign tumor, is usually a larger lesion. It has been defined as "a system of acinar tubular structures lined by cuboidal or columnar cells in a scanty connective tissue stroma interlacing with smooth muscle bundles"[5,9] (Figure 4-2).

TABLE 4-1 Benign tumors of the gallbladder (Memorial Hospital, New York,
1937–1964)

Tumor	No.
Papilloma	12
Adenomyoma	5
Lipoma	1
Hemangioma	1
Total	19

SOURCE Data from Arbab and Brasfield.[5]

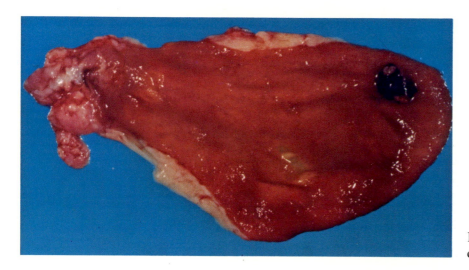

FIGURE 4-1. Operative specimen
of a papilloma of the gallbladder.

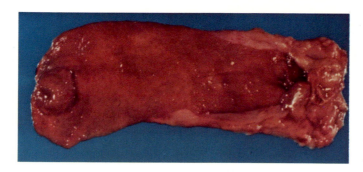

FIGURE 4-2. Operative specimen
of an adenomyoma of the gallbladder.

These lesions may be congenital or may be a type of hamartoma; they
seem to be associated more frequently with gallstones and cholecystitis.
Malignant changes rarely occur.

The benign tumors reported in the bile ducts have been found in all
locations from the intrahepatic ducts all the way to the ampulla of Vater.[2,3]
They seem to be more common in the distal bile duct, especially in the ampullary region, than in the proximal bile ducts. Table 4-2 gives the locations
in one reported series, that from the Hermann Hospital, Houston, Texas,
for 1950 through 1960.[3] Occasionally multiple lesions have been found.[10,11]
The types of tumor reported in the Hermann Hospital series included papillomas, polyps, adenomas, fibroadenomas, granular cell myoblastomas,
and a variety of less common lesions (Table 4-3). In addition to the more
common lesions, such as papillomas and polyps, we have seen several pa-

TABLE 4-2 Location of benign tumors of the bile ducts (Hermann Hospital, Houston, 1950–1960)

Location	No.
Intrahepatic and common hepatic ducts	8
Junction cystic–hepatic duct	4
Cystic duct	3
Common bile duct	11
Ampulla of Vater	13
Multiple	4
Total	43

SOURCE Data from Dowdy et al.[3]

TABLE 4-3 Benign tumors of the bile ducts (Hermann Hospital, Houston, 1950–1960)

Tumor	No.
Papilloma	16
Polyp	4
Adenoma	11
Fibroadenoma	4
Adenomyoma	1
Leiomyoma	1
Granular cell myoblastoma	4
Neuroma	1
Hamartoma	1
Total	43

SOURCE Data from Dowdy et al.[3]

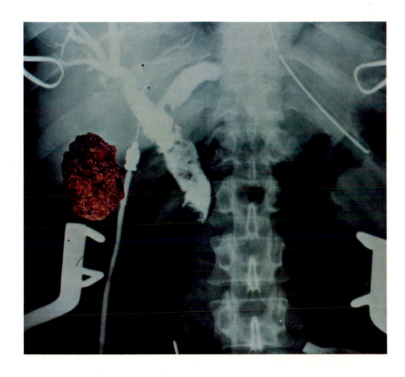

FIGURE 4-3. Operative specimen of a benign papillary adenoma (villous tumor) of the papilla of Vater superimposed on the operative cholangiogram.

tients with papillary adenomas (villous tumors) of the papilla of Vater (Figure 4-3). Carcinoma-in-situ has been found with some frequency in papillomas and papillary adenomas. Cattell and Pyrtek reported several cases in which benign tumors became malignant.[7] This potential for malignant development should be assessed by careful frozen-section study of all lesions thought to be benign found in the gallbladder or bile ducts. Malignant tumors of the bile ducts, of course, are much more common than are benign lesions.

Diagnosis
Clinical Features. Benign tumors of the gallbladder are almost always asymptomatic. They are usually found by oral cholecystography (Figures 4-4 and 4-5) and may be confused with a solitary gallstone, or they are found incidentally at surgery. These tumors may be present in patients with cholecystitis but are rarely the cause of the inflammation.

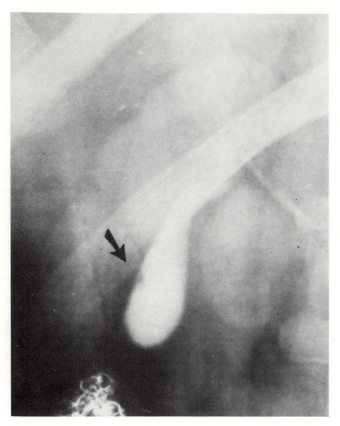

FIGURE 4-4.   Oral cholecystogram showing a polyp of the gallbladder.

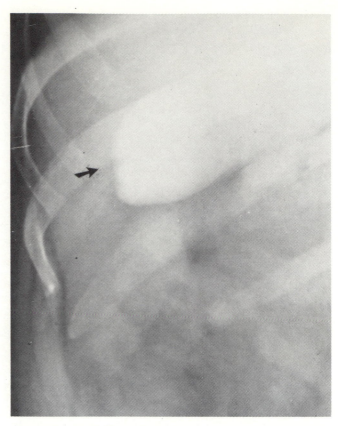

FIGURE 4-5.   Oral cholecystogram showing an adenomyoma of the gallbladder.

Jaundice is the most frequent symptom in patients with benign tumors of the bile ducts. The jaundice may be constant or intermittent and is usually accompanied by pain in the right upper abdomen or typical biliary colic. Fever, chills, and symptoms of cholangitis are present in about 25% of patients; hemobilia has been described in some.[3] Some patients may lose weight because they are unable to eat or to digest fats adequately. Wright[11] has reported intermittent pancreatitis in a patient with a benign polyp of the distal common bile duct.

Diagnostic Studies.   Diagnostic studies should include routine laboratory tests of liver function. Oral cholecystography or intravenous cholangiography is of value if the patient is not jaundiced. When jaundice is present, as it is in most patients who have a benign tumor of the bile ducts, ERC or percutaneous transhepatic cholangiography should be performed to locate the site of biliary obstruction. At endoscopy (duodenoscopy), tumors protruding through the orifice of the papilla of Vater may be seen, and a biopsy may be performed pre-operatively (Figure 4-6). Because malignant tumors are frequently a cause of obstruction of the bile ducts and benign tumors of the bile ducts are rare, it is unlikely that the diagnosis of a benign tumor of the extrahepatic bile ducts will be made very often pre-operatively.

Treatment
Benign Tumors of the Gallbladder.   For benign tumors of the gallbladder, cholecystectomy is the treatment of choice and is curative.[12–14] Operative cholangiography should always be performed to assess the bile ducts for patency and for the presence of other lesions.

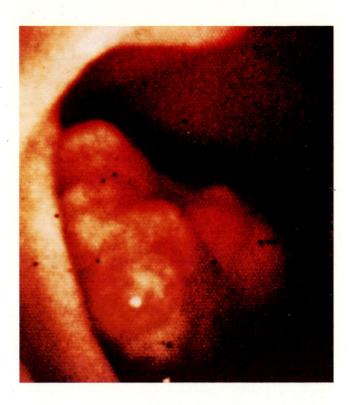

FIGURE 4-6. Photograph taken through an endoscope showing a polypoid tumor projecting through the orifice of the papilla of Vater.

Benign Tumors of the Bile Ducts. Benign tumors of the bile ducts may be difficult to palpate and locate at operation because they are often soft or spongy. Probes may be passed through the lesion when the duct is opened above or below the tumor. The pre-operative cholangiogram is of great help in locating the tumor mass.

When a soft tissue mass occludes the bile ducts and does not infiltrate the wall of the duct, ulcerate, nor appear to be as vascular or firm as the usual carcinoma, one should suspect the rare presence of a benign tumor. The duct should be opened and the lesion excised locally and widely for biopsy and frozen section. This will usually entail local resection of the bile duct itself with duct-to-duct reconstruction.

For tumors at the ampulla of Vater, wide local excision of papillomas and papillary adenomas should result in cure if no evidence of malignancy is seen. Often, because of the infrequency of benign tumors and the relative frequency of carcinomas of the distal bile duct or ampulla of Vater, a pancreatoduodenectomy (Whipple operation) is performed with wide resection of the lesion, distal bile duct, and head of the pancreas. If a benign tumor is found to be the cause of the biliary obstruction, cure should result. If a benign tumor cannot be resected, a biliary–intestinal bypass procedure can be performed.

Results. Chu[2] has reported the successful excision of benign bile duct tumors in 2% of 55 patients; Dowdy and associates[3] reported successful excision of 75% of the benign tumors in their series of patients. The overall operative mortality was approximately 10%; the highest mortality (40%) occurred in those patients who had radical resections of a benign tumor. The tumor or another tumor in the bile ducts recurred in 12% of the patients.

The ideal treatment for benign tumors of the gallbladder and bile ducts is local excision of the lesion. If the benign nature of the tumor can be confirmed, radical operative resections should be avoided.

Carcinoma of the Gallbladder
Caldwell B. Esselstyn, Jr.

Cancer of the gallbladder accounts for approximately 6500 deaths annually in the United States.[15] It is the fifth most common malignancy of the gastrointestinal tract, accounting for 4% of all cancer deaths[16,17] The prognosis is almost uniformly grave.

Pathology

In most reported series, the tumor is either grossly evident at surgery or incidentally diagnosed at the time of cholecystectomy after histological study of the gallbladder (Figure 4-7). The diagnosis is rarely made pre-operatively because of the lack of specific symptoms. The histological type is usually adenocarcinoma (Figure 4-8), ranging from well differentiated to anaplastic, with an occasional rare epidermoid cancer.

Fahim and associates[18] have described the mode of spread of carcinoma of the gallbladder. It may be lymphatic, vascular, neurological, or ductal, or it may extend directly into the liver and adjacent viscera.

The association of this neoplasm with gallstones is well recognized; in most reported series it is between 60% and 85%.[19-22] No causal relationship between carcinoma of the gallbladder and gallstones has as yet been established. It is not known whether the presence of stones and the chronic irritation or inflammation they cause predispose to cancer or whether the development of cancer causes the precipitation of stones.

Diagnosis

Clinical Features. The major difficulty in achieving an early or pre-operative diagnosis of carcinoma of the gallbladder is the absence of any specific symptoms. Patients most frequently complain of upper abdominal pain which is imprecise and not unlike that of cholecystitis. The second most common finding is jaundice; the third is an abdominal mass.

Pre-operative Studies. Pre-operative roentgenographic studies are of minimal value. Cholecystograms infrequently visualize and, if they do, usually reveal only cholelithiasis. Upper gastrointestinal roentgenographic series using barium may show gastric or duodenal compression, or duodenal obstruction if the disease is advanced. Laboratory studies will confirm hyperbilirubinemia and an elevated alkaline phosphatase level in patients with obstructive jaundice. Unfortunately, laboratory values cannot differentiate between inflammatory disease, stones, or neoplastic lesions.

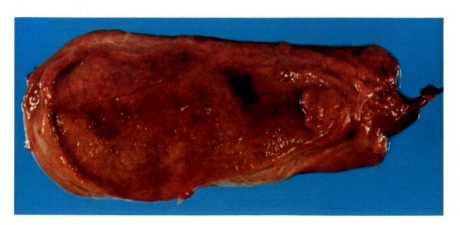

FIGURE 4-7. Operative specimen of a gallbladder with a carcinoma infiltrating and obstructing the lumen at the ampulla. The tumor was not recognized preoperatively or intraoperatively until the gallbladder had been removed.

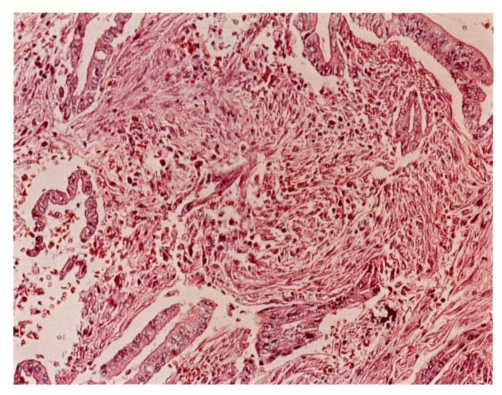

FIGURE 4-8.   Photomicrograph of the gallbladder wall showing adenocarcinoma.

Isotopic liver scans, ultrasound, CT, and selective angiography may detect filling defects in the liver or suggest a mass, but these tests are expensive and imprecise and delay the definitive diagnosis obtained at abdominal exploration.

Operative Diagnosis.   In many patients the cancer is simply an incidental finding at histological examination of the gallbladder specimen after cholecystectomy. In other patients, a large tumor mass of the gallbladder is evident at operative exploration.

Treatment
Unsuspected Carcinomas.   Most patients with carcinoma of the gallbladder will have cholecystectomy as their definitive treatment, simply because the diagnosis is not recognized until the gallbladder specimen is reviewed histologically. Their cancers are inapparent by gross examination at surgery. If the tumor has not infiltrated or extended beyond the wall of the gallbladder, most surgeons would not advise re-exploration for further nodal or hepatic wedge resection. In occasional reports, however, this recommendation has been made.

Most reviews contain one or two 5-year survivors in this group of inapparent gallbladder cancers, but long-term survival or cure is still rare.

Overt Carcinoma   The prognosis is even less favorable for patients who have overt or obvious cancer of the gallbladder identified at surgery; most of these patients die within the year.[23]

Radical Operations.   Surgeons are divided about the role of radical operations for cancer of the gallbladder. The poor survival of patients with early lesions confined to the gallbladder and the high incidence of local recur-

83

rence has suggested to Moossa and associates[20] that immediate gross and microscopic evaluation of all suspicious gallbladder specimens be obtained at cholecystectomy, and a further resection performed if cancer is identified. Adson[24] also believes that many patients have been under-treated in the past. He advocates more frequent use of extended right hepatic lobectomy in selected patients. Although one might argue that prophylactic cholecystectomy in all patients with stones would achieve earlier diagnosis and decrease the death rate from carcinoma of the gallbladder, the mortality from prophylactic surgery would probably offset any potential cures.[25-28]

Until more definitive data are available to justify the morbidity and mortality of the extended procedures, cholecystectomy will remain the procedure of choice for inapparent carcinomas of the gallbladder. As a surgical principle, opening of the gallbladder during routine cholecystectomy should be avoided to prevent possible tumor spillage and seeding. Palliative decompressive procedures should be imployed when appropriate for carcinomas that have extended into the liver or adjacent structures.

Adjuvant Therapy. Recent studies have emphasized the possible value of adjuvant chemotherapy, intraoperative radiation therapy, or both for carcinoma of the gallbladder.[15,23,29] These studies are still in the investigative stage.

Carcinoma of the Bile Ducts
Avram M. Cooperman

Malignant tumors of the bile ducts are uncommon. The incidence is approximately 1/125,000 persons.[30] Autopsy studies in series of cancer patients disclosed this lesion in 2.9% of necropsies.[31]

The bile ducts begin as small ductules in the liver which join to form a major right and left duct; these then unite to form the common hepatic duct, which is joined by the cystic duct to form the common bile duct. In this discussion, the bile duct above the bifurcation of the hepatic ducts is designated the proximal or upper duct, the duct from the bifurcation to below the cystic duct is the middle third, and the duct below this is the lower third.

Pathology

The most common malignant bile duct tumor is an adenocarcinoma; it accounts for 97% of all malignancies. The most common type is an infiltrating and scirrhous lesion (Figure 4-9). Polypoid tumors are more frequent in the lower third of the duct, but are uncommon when compared to infiltrating lesions. Of 14 cases reported by Ingis and Farmer,[32] 5 were scirrhous adenocarcinoma, 2 were adenocarcinoma with fibrous reaction, 6 were poorly to well-differentiated adenocarcinomas, and only 1 was a papillary adenocarcinoma. Rarer tumors include embryonal rhabdomyosarcoma[33] and carcinoid tumors.[34]

Pathogenesis. As with most cancers, bile duct tumors most frequently arise de novo, without pre-existing or underlying disease.[35] There are, however, a few diseases that precede, co-exist with, or may cause the development of bile duct cancers. These include chronic ulcerative colitis, *Clonorchis sinensis,* hepaticolithiasis, benign papillomas, choledochal cysts, and perhaps sclerosing cholangitis.

Chronic ulcerative colitis has an increased association with bile duct cancer from 10 to 50 times that of the normal population. Recently Akwari et al.[36] reported 13 cases from the Mayo Clinic and reviewed 41 other reported cases. The mean age of the patients at the onset of colitis was 19 to 26 years, the entire colon was usually involved, 25% of the patients also

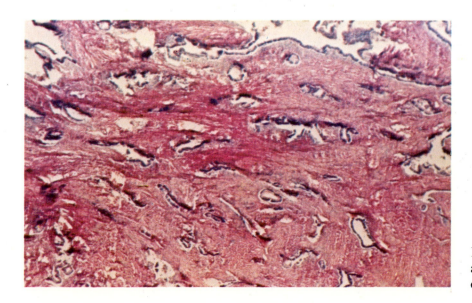

FIGURE 4-9. Histological appearance of an adenocarcinoma of the bile ducts.

had liver disease (type and extent not specified), and bile duct cancers developed about 14 years after the onset of the colitis. Colectomy did not appear to prevent the development of bile duct tumors; 60% to 70% of these tumors were in the proximal bile ducts.

A higher incidence of bile duct cancer and cholangiocarcinomas has been reported with *Clonorchis sinensis,* a Chinese liver fluke.[37]

Occasional reports have suggested that choledocholithiasis, chronic inflammation, chronic biliary obstruction, and adenomatous hyperplasia (a late inflammatory change) may lead to carcinoma of the bile ducts, but this association has not been consistent.[38] Whether the carcinogenic agent may be the stones, inflammation, dilatation, or coincidence is not clear, but usually two or more of these conditions coexist.

As early as 1911, 6 cases of bile duct cancer in which cholangitis and papillomatosis coexisted with the bile duct tumors were described.[39] At least 14 subsequent reports have suggested an association between papillomas and bile duct cancers. Most recently, diffuse ductal papillomatosis and focally invasive carcinoma were found in 1 patient.[40]

Irwin and Morison,[41] in 1944, showed an association between congenital choledochal cysts and bile duct carcinoma. Since then 36 cases have been reported.[42] In some patients, stones were also present in the cyst.

Diagnosis

Signs and Symptoms. Regardless of location in the bile duct, the presenting symptoms of these cancers—jaundice, pruritis, and weight loss—are similar. Less frequently, anorexia, pain, nausea, and vomiting are present. Cholangitis and fever occur infrequently. This is particularly true for proximal lesions in which reflux behind the obstruction is uncommon. In some instances the early non-specific signs mimic chronic liver disease.[43]

Physical Examination Specific, positive physical findings are infrequent. Hepatomegaly and jaundice may be present but do not help differentiate bile duct, intrahepatic, or periampullary malignancies. A palpable gallbladder (Courvoisier's sign) implies the obstruction is at or below the cystic duct. Splenomegaly and ascites are late findings and reflect a decompensated liver or carcinomatosis.

Laboratory Studies. The earliest laboratory abnormality is an elevated serum alkaline phosphatase level. Since this is derived from many sources, fractionation may be necessary to confirm the source. One stimulus to the production of this canalicular enzyme is partial or complete obstruction. The alkaline phosphatase level in bile duct cancers is at least three to five times normal. Most of the circulating enzyme represents newly synthesized alkaline phosphatase and not refluxed secretions.

The serum bilirubin level is elevated in at least 80% of patients. In long-standing obstruction or tumors obstructing both ducts, the level frequently exceeds 10 mg/dl. The SGOT is mildly elevated (two to three times normal). Less frequently, anemia, increased serum cholesterol levels, and occult blood are found in the stools.[32]

Roentgenographic Studies. The diagnosis, initially suspected by the history and laboratory findings, is supported further by roentgenographic studies that delineate the bile ducts. The level of bilirubin usually precludes adequate visualization of the ducts by oral cholecystography. An intravenous cholangiogram may be attempted but, for similar reasons, visualization is usually inadequate.

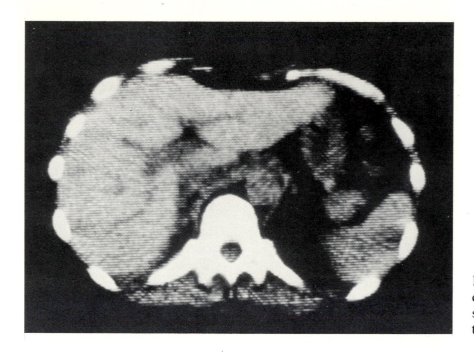

FIGURE 4-10. CT of dilated bile ducts in the liver in a patient with obstructive jaundice from carcinoma of the distal bile duct.

Two other noninvasive diagnostic tests are ultrasonography and CT. We have had limited experience using ultrasonography in diagnosing bile duct tumors. For distal duct tumors, a proximal dilated duct or gallbladder may be detected, but the accuracy and value of this test are still unknown.

CT has several potential advantages. It allows visualization of the liver, porta hepatis, and head of the pancreas, and it is noninvasive (Figure 4-10). We have localized and diagnosed several bile duct tumors by CT. The absolute value and accuracy of this test, however, are still to be determined.[44]

In most hospitals the diagnosis will be suggested by transhepatic cholangiography or ERC. The relative value of each has been compared in one prospective study.[45] Although both are valuable (more than 80% accurate), transhepatic cholangiography has been more effective for diagnosing extrahepatic lesions and ERC for intrahepatic obstructions. Both tests helped localize the obstruction in 95% of cases. Whether one or both of these tests will be used depends on the availability and expertise at each hospital. I prefer CT or ultrasound study initially. If dilated bile ducts are seen, then a skinny-needle percutaneous cholangiogram is performed (Figure 4-11). If the ducts are not dilated, then ERC is performed (Figure 4-12).

Treatment

Operative Strategy In most patients, the diagnosis will be strongly suspected by the preceding roentgenographic studies. The definitive diagnosis may be more difficult to establish. An operation will be necessary in most patients to establish the diagnosis, to resect the tumor, or to relieve biliary and hepatic obstruction if resection is not possible. The procedure to be employed will depend on the intraoperative findings, the location of the tumor, the general condition of the patient and, to a lesser extent, on the philosophy of the surgeon. Philosophical issues aside, it is unusual for middle or upper duct tumors to be resected because the hepatic artery and portal vein course very close to the bile duct, and tumors that infiltrate and extend beyond the duct in this region frequently involve these structures. Braasch[46] has stated that at surgery distant metastases are present in one third of bile duct cancers, perineural invasion in 30% to 50%.

87

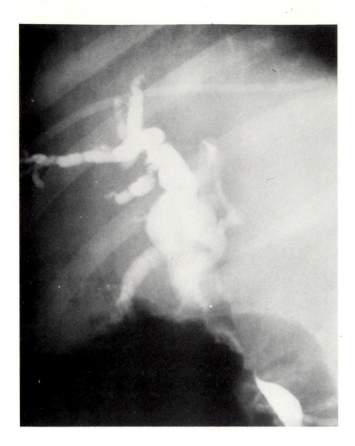

FIGURE 4-11. Percutaneous transhepatic cholangiogram in a patient with a carcinoma of the distal common bile duct.

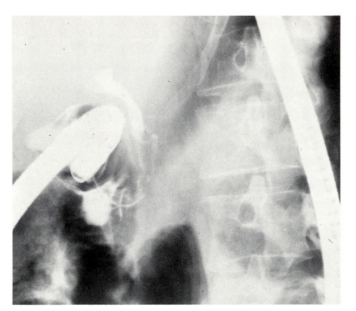
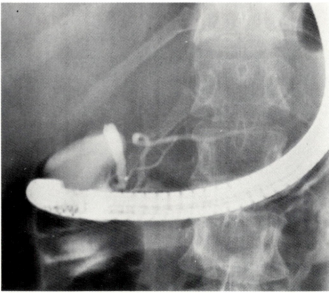

FIGURE 4-12. ERC showing obstructing lesions in the middle and lower bile ducts, later identified at operation to be carcinomas.

Any incision that affords access to the porta hepatis is satisfactory. Most surgeons use an upper midline, right upper abdominal oblique, or right paramedian incision. Confirming the diagnosis of bile duct cancer histologically may be extremely difficult. When the cancer is obvious, regional or hepatic metastases will provide tissue diagnosis. Not infrequently, a thickened common bile duct and hepatic duct are palpated.

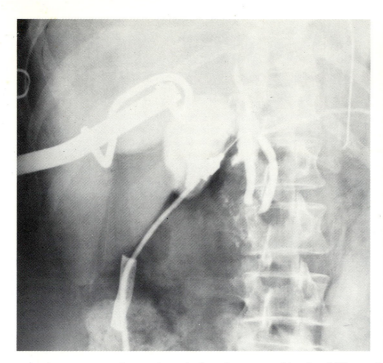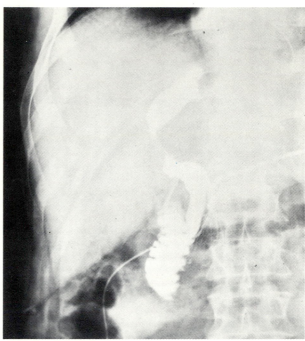

FIGURE 4-13.   Operative cholangiograms showing biliary obstruction from carcinomas of the bile ducts.

At this stage, I prefer to do an operative cholangiogram, using a but-
terfly needle inserted into the common duct, directed toward the hilus. An
alternative is a cholecystocholangiogram through the gallbladder. A clue to
the diagnosis may be absence of reflux into the proximal duct. If this is
found, a noncrushing clamp may be placed across the distal duct and dye
forced to reflux proximally. Operative cholangiography provides a detailed
study of the duct and its abnormalities (Figure 4-13).

I next incise the duct longitudinally and excise a segment of duct wall
for frozen-section study. Commonly, scirrhous reaction or fibrosis without
malignant cells is seen, and it may be difficult to distinguish neoplasm from
sclerosing cholangitis. When this is encountered, the medical and drug his-
tories must be reconsidered. Even then the diagnosis may be difficult and
the correct diagnosis may only be established by the subsequent clinical
course.

If the location of the lesion precludes direct biopsy, duct washings or
scrapings guided by choledochoscopy may establish the diagnosis. Finally,
if all these maneuvers are negative (they frequently are), the treatment
must be based on surgical judgment. A recent advance has been intraoperative choledochoscopy.[47] Many tumors that appear unicentric and localized will in fact be multicentric and incurable. We use a Stortz-Hopkins
rigid scope in all cases. Rarely, carcinoma of the gallbladder or carcinoma
arising in the cystic duct may spread through the common duct and into the
hepatic ducts. Both the gallbladder and cystic duct should be palpated to
exclude a primary source of these lesions.

Upper Duct Cancers.   The relationship of the hepatic artery, portal vein,
and bile duct is especially close in the upper duct. Scirrhous tumors are
common in this area. Locating the bile duct may be difficult since it may be
surrounded by thick inflammatory tissue that obscures normal structures.
The gallbladder frequently is collapsed or contracted due to the proximal

89

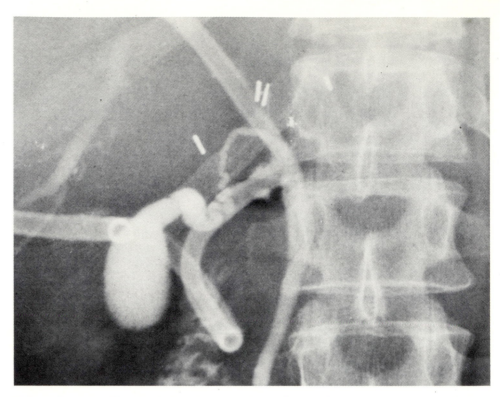

FIGURE 4-14.   T-tube cholangiogram of a patient with an unresectable carcinoma of the bile duct which has been dilated and held open by placement of a T-tube through the lesion while postoperative radiation or cobalt therapy is given.

obstruction. The bile duct should be entered, if possible, in the middle or lower third and probes and dilators should be passed upward toward the hilus. It is helpful to have had the ductal anatomy delineated pre-operatively by ERC.

If there is proximal dilatation of the ducts and the cancer is not resectable, intubation (tube decompression) may be attempted from below by dilating the cancer and passing a T- or Y-tube up into the dilated ducts (Figure 4-14). Radiation therapy can then be given post-operatively for palliation. Resection of the lateral segment of the left lobe of the liver and hepatojejunostomy (Longmire's procedure) may also be performed to decompress the obstructed system, but we rarely utilize this procedure. If there is no proximal dilatation or if the ducts appear beaded and small, then multicentricity of the tumor or direct spread into the liver is likely and little can be done.

Recently, we have utilized percutaneous transhepatic decompression as another palliative method for the treatment of advanced tumors.[48] Under angiography or CT a catheter is placed through the liver into the duct above the obstruction (Figure 4-15). This technique is particularly valuable when bulky hilar metastases preclude intubation from below or when the dissection is difficult. Percutaneous decompression may be performed post-operatively as easily and satisfactorily as intraoperatively.

Very rarely (in less than 4% of all cases), resection of upper duct cancers is possible.[49] This may involve resection of a lobe of the liver, hepatic artery, or portal vein. There are few reported cases (probably less than 24), but it is likely that more of these procedures have been done than have been reported. Morbidity and mortality are high and life expectancy remains limited, particularly when resection is done for palliation.[50] At the

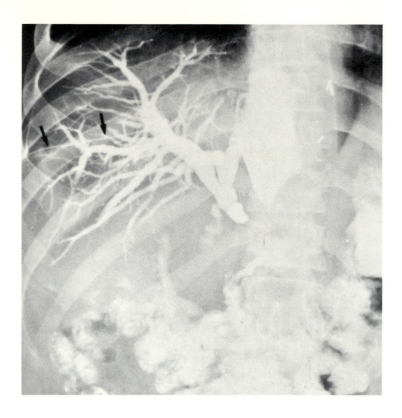

FIGURE 4-15. Percutaneous transhepatic cholangiogram has been performed and a transhepatic catheter (arrows) has been placed into the obstructed biliary system for drainage in a patient with recurrent carcinoma of the bile ducts and carcinomatosis. Another operative procedure was deemed inadvisable.

Cleveland Clinic, no resectable upper duct cancers have as yet been encountered.

Two additional techniques have been suggested. An exchangeable U-tube may be passed through the liver, through the area of tumor, and into the common bile duct to allow bile to re-enter the digestive tract as well as to stent the tumor.[51,52] Recently, Iwasaki et al.[53] reported on small-field, single-dose (3,000- to 5,000-rad) intraoperative radiotherapy for unresectable lesions. Only three patients were treated and obstruction did improve.

Middle Duct Cancer. The limiting factors that apply to resective surgery for upper duct lesions also hold true for middle third cancers. Technically, resection or decompression is easier because dilated extrahepatic ducts may be easily located above middle duct tumors.

When resection is possible, choledochoscopic examination of the upper duct is first done to ensure a unicentric origin of tumor. The gross and microscopic examinations should identify tumor-free margins. For reconstruction, end-to-end ductal anastomosis is usually not possible (and theoretically may be undesirable). I prefer a Roux-Y hepatojejunostomy using a long (50- to 60-cm) defunctionalized limb.

If resection is not possible, then a Roux limb frequently can be brought above the obstruction and used to decompress the duct above the cancer. Alternatively, the cancer can be dilated from below: a catheter or T-tube is passed up through the area of tumor to decompress the obstructed system through this stent. Radiation therapy can be given postoperatively to the area of the tumor if it is marked by silver clips (Figure 4-16).

Distal Duct Tumors. Although distal bile duct tumors are surrounded by pancreas and duodenum, resection for cure is infrequent. In large series of patients with bile duct tumors few had lower duct lesions.[54] When resec-

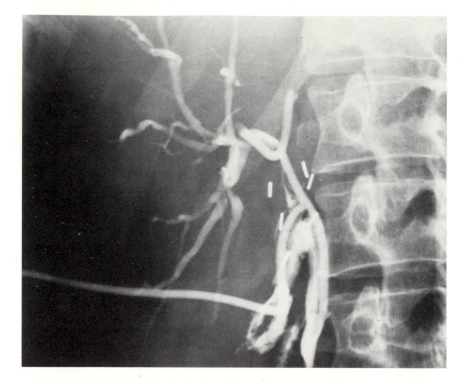

FIGURE 4-16. Y-tube cholangiogram showing the biliary system in a patient with carcinoma of the bile duct. The area of tumor is marked by silver clips. Subsequent radiation therapy successfully controlled this lesion so that the Y-tube could be removed. No recurrence of the lesion has been noted in a 4-year follow-up period.

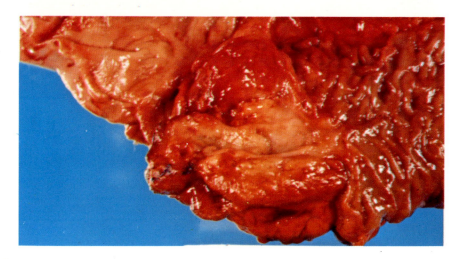

FIGURE 4-17. Operative specimen from a patient with carcinoma of the distal bile duct resected by a pancreatoduodenal resection (Whipple's operation). The close-up photograph shows the area of the lesion. Note the infiltration and thickening in the wall of the distal bile duct.

tion is possible, a pancreatoduodenal resection should be performed (Figure 4-17). The technic of this operation is discussed in Chapter 6. When curative resection is not possible, a biliary–enteric bypass using either gallbladder or common bile duct joined to jejunum or duodenum should be fashioned.

Chemotherapy and Radiotherapy. As with other gastrointestinal adenocarcinomas, chemotherapy of carcinoma of the bile ducts has had limited success. Intravenous, oral, and intra-arterial administration each has its own enthusiasts.[46] Despite occasional responders, optimism for the use of these agents cannot yet be endorsed.

Radiotherapy, both wide and narrow field, has been utilized for many patients and is still being investigated.[53,55] We have had occasional or temporary success with control of the local tumor for periods of several years in some patients.

Results. Despite the location, the long-term outlook for bile duct cancers is poor. In a review of 173 patients with bile duct cancers only 25 survived more than 1 year, 42% died within 1 month of surgery, and 103 died within 6 months.[46] The outlook and survival are worse for proximal lesions and better for distal tumors.[56-59] In the series of Ingis and Farmer,[32] the mean survival was twice as long for distal tumors (20 months). Surprisingly good results have been reported by Terblanche et al.[52] using prolonged intubation with the U-tube. Five patients have survived 2.5 to 5 years after this procedure.

References

Neoplasms

1. Cattell, R. B., Braasch, J. W., and Kahn, F.: Polypoid epithelial tumors of the bile ducts. *N. Engl. J. Med.,* **266,** 57, 1962.
2. Chu, P. T.: Benign neoplasms of the extrahepatic biliary ducts, review of the literature and report of a case of fibroma. *Arch. Pathol.,* **50,** 84, 1950.
3. Dowdy, G. S., Olin, W. G., Jr., Shelton, E. L., Jr., et al.: Benign tumors of the extrahepatic bile ducts. *Arch. Surg.,* **85,** 503, 1962.
4. Irwin, H. C., and MacCarthy, W. C.: Papilloma of the gallbladder: report of 85 cases. *Ann. Surg.* **61,** 725, 1915.
5. Arbab, A. A., and Brasfield, R.: Benign tumors of the gallbladder. *Surgery,* **61,** 535, 1967.
6. Kane, C. F., Brown, C. H., and Hoerr, S. O.: Papilloma of the gallbladder: report of eight cases. *Am. J. Surg.,* **83,** 161, 1952.
7. Cattell, R. B., and Pyrtek, L. J.: Premalignant lesion of the ampulla of Vater. *Surg. Gynecol. Obstet.* **90,** 21, 1950.
8. Oh, C., and Jemerin, E. E.: Benign adenomatous polyps of the papilla of Vater. *Surgery,* **57,** 495, 1965.
9. Shepard, V. D., Walters, W., and Dockerty, M. B.: Benign neoplasms of the gallbladder. *Arch. Surg.,* **45,** 1, 1942.
10. Eiss, S., DiMaio, D. and Caedo, J. P.: Multiple papillomas of the entire biliary tract: case report. *Ann. Surg.,* **152,** 320, 1960.
11. Wright, R. B.: Relapsing pancreatitis: report of a case with unusual features. *Br. J. Surg.,* **45,** 394, 1958.
12. Greco, J. G., and Harkins, H. N.: Polyposis of the gallbladder. *Am. J. Surg.,* **63,** 398, 1944.
13. Kerr, A. B., and Lendrum, A. C.: A chloride-secreting papilloma in gallbladder; tumour of heterotopic intestinal epithelium containing Paneth cells and enterochromaffine cells and associated with massive chloride loss: with critical review of papilloma of the gallbladder. *Br. J. Surg.,* **23,** 615, 1936.
14. Mayo, C. H.: Papillomas of the gallbladder. *Ann. Surg.,* **62,** 193, 1915.

Carcinoma of the Gallbladder

15. Bossart, P. A., Patterson, A. H., and Zirtel, H. A.: Carcinoma of the gallbladder: a report of seventy-six cases. *Am. J. Surg.,* **103,** 366, 1962.
16. Hardy, M. A., and Volk, H.: Primary carcinoma of the gallbladder: a ten year review. *Am. J. Surg.,* **120,** 800, 1970.
17. Holmes, S. L., and Mark, J. B. D.: Carcinoma of the gallbladder. *Surg. Gynecol, Obstet.,* **133,** 561, 1971.
18. Fahim, R. B., McDonald, J. R., Richards, J. C., et al.: Carcinoma of the gallbladder: a study of its modes of spread. *Ann. Surg.,* **156,** 114, 1962.
19. Beltz, W. R., and Condon, R. E.: Primary carcinoma of the gallbladder. *Ann. Surg.,* **180,** 180, 1974.
20. Moossa, A. R., Anagnost, M., Hall, A. W., et al.: The continuing challenge of gallbladder cancer. Survey of thirty years' experience at the University of Chicago. *Am. J. Surg.,* **130,** 57, 1975.

21. Piehler, J. M., and Crichlow, R. W.: Primary carcinoma of the gallbladder. *Arch. Surg.,* **112,** 26, 1977.
22. Weiskopf, J., and Esselstyn, C. B., Jr.: Carcinoma of the gallbladder: a twenty-five year review. *Am. J. Gastroenterol.,* **65,** 522, 1976.
23. Iwasaki, Y., Ohto, M., Todoroki, T., et al.: Treatment of carcinoma of the biliary system. *Surg. Gynecol. Obstet.,* **144,** 219, 1977.
24. Adson, M. A.: Carcinoma of the gallbladder. *Surg. Clin. North Am.,* **53,** 103, 1973.
25. Milner, L. R.: Cancer of the gallbladder, its relationship to gallstones. *Am. J. Gastroenterol.,* **39,** 480, 1963.
26. Arminski, T. C.: Primary carcinoma of the gallbladder: a collective review with the addition of twenty-five cases from Grace Hospital, Detroit, Michigan. *Cancer,* **2,** 379, 1949.
27. Klein, J. B., and Finck, F. M.: Primary carcinoma of the gallbladder: review of 28 cases. *Arch. Surg.,* **104,** 769, 1972.
28. Pemberton, L. B., Diffenbaugh, W. F., and Strohl, E. L.: The surgical significance of carcinoma of the gallbladder. *Am. J. Surg.,* **122,** 381, 1971.
29. Treadwell, T. A., and Hardin, W. J.: Primary carcinoma of the gallbladder. The role of adjunctive therapy in its treatment. *Am. J. Surg.,* **132,** 703, 1976.

Carcinoma of the Bile Ducts
30. Silverberg, E., and Grant, R. N.: Cancer statistics 1970. *Cancer* **20,** 11, 1970.
31. Sako, K., Seitzinger, G. L., and Garside, E.: Carcinoma of the extrahepatic bile ducts: review of the literature and report of six cases. *Surgery,* **41,** 416, 1957.
32. Ingis, D. A., and Farmer, R. G.: Adenocarcinoma of the bile ducts. Relationship of anatomic location to clinical features. *Am. J. Dig. Dis.,* **20,** 253, 1975.
33. Majmudar, B., and Kumar, V. S.: Embryonal rhabdomyosarcoma (sarcoma botryoides) of the common bile duct: a case report. *Hum. Pathol.,* **7,** 705, 1976.
34. Bergdahl, L.: Carcinoid tumours of the biliary tract. *Aust. N.Z. J. Surg.,* **46,** 136, 1976.
35. Neibling, H. A., Dockerty, M. B., and Waugh, J. M.: Carcinoma of the extrahepatic bile ducts. *Surg. Gynecol. Obstet.,* **89,** 429, 1949.
36. Akwari, O. E., VanHeerden, J. A., Adson, M. A., et al.: Bile duct carcinoma associated with ulcerative colitis. *Rev. Surg.,* **33,** 289, 1976.
37. Hou, P. C.: The relationship between primary carcinoma of the liver and infestation with *Clonorchis sinensis. J. Pathol. Bacteriol.,* **72,** 239, 1956.
38. Falchuk, K. R., Lesser, B. P., Galdabini, J. J., et al.: Cholangiocarcinoma as related to chronic intrahepatic cholangitis and hepatolithiasis: case report and review of the literature. *Am. J. Gastroenterol.,* **66,** 57, 1976.
39. Yamagiwa, K.: Zur kenntnis des primären parenchymatösen Leberkarzinoms (Hepatoma). *Virchow's Arch. [Pathol. Anat.]* **206,** 437, 1911.
40. Neumann, R. D., LiVolsi, V. A., Rosenthal, N. S., et al.: Adenocarcinoma in biliary papillomatosis. *Gastroenterology,* **70,** 779, 1976.
41. Irwin, S. T., and Morison, J. E.: Congenital cyst of the common bile duct containing stones and undergoing cancerous change. *Br. J. Surg.,* **32,** 319, 1944.
42. Fujiwara, Y., Ohizumi, T., Kakizaki, G., et al.: A case of congenital choledochal cyst associated with carcinoma. *J. Pediatr. Surg.,* **11,** 587, 1976.
43. Pelleya-Kouri, R., Dusol, M., Jr., Orta, D., et al.: Bile duct carcinoma mimicking chronic liver disease. *Arch. Intern. Med.,* **136,** 1051, 1976.
44. Cooperman, A. M., Haaga, J. R., Reich, N., et al.: Computed tomography: an aid to the abdominal surgeon. *Surg. Annu.* **10,** 73, 1978.
45. Elias, E., Hamlyn, A. N., Jain, S., et al.: A randomized trial of percutaneous transhepatic cholangiography with the Chiba needle versus endoscopic retrograde cholangiography for bile duct visualization in jaundice. *Gastroenterology,* **71,** 439, 1976.

46. Braasch, J. W.: Carcinoma of the bile duct. *Surg. Clin. North Am.,* **53,** 1217, 1973.

47. Tompkins, R. K., Johnson, J., Storm, F. K., et al.: Operative endoscopy in the management of biliary tract neoplasms. *Am. J. Surg.,* **132,** 174, 1976.

48. Johnson, R. W., and Wray, C. H.: Carcinoma of the bile duct. *J. Med. Assoc. Ga.,* **64,** 431, 1975.

49. Longmire, W. P., Jr., McArthur, M. S., Bastounis, E. A., et al.: Carcinoma of the extrahepatic biliary tract. *Ann. Surg.,* **178,** 333, 1973.

50. Fortner, J. G., Kallum, B. O., and Kim, D. K.: Surgical management of carcinoma of the junction of the main hepatic ducts. *Ann. Surg.,* **184,** 68, 1976.

51. Terblanche, J.: Is carcinoma of the main hepatic duct junction an indication for liver transplantation or palliative surgery? A plea for the U tube palliative procedure. *Surgery,* **79,** 127, 1976.

52. Terblanche, J., Saunders, S. J., and Louw, J. H.: Prolonged palliation in carcinoma of the main hepatic duct junction. *Surgery,* **71,** 720, 1972.

53. Iwasaki, Y., Ohto, M., Todoroki, T., et al.: Treatment of carcinoma of the biliary system. *Surg. Gynecol. Obstet.,* **144,** 219, 1977.

54. Warren, K. W., Mountain, J. C., Lloyd-Jones, W.: Malignant tumours of the bile ducts. *Br. J. Surg.,* **59,** 501, 1972.

55. Hudgins, P. T., and Meoz, R. T.: Radiation therapy for obstructive jaundice secondary to tumor malignancy. *Int. J. Radiat. Biol.,* **1,** 1195, 1976.

56. Klatskin, G.: Adenocarcinoma of the hepatic duct at its bifurcation within the porta hepatis. An unusual tumor with distinctive clinical and pathological features. *Am. J. Med.,* **38,** 241, 1965.

57. Praderi, R. C.: Twelve years' experience with transhepatic intubation. *Ann. Surg.,* **179,** 937, 1974.

58. Ross, A. P., Braasch, J. W., and Warren, K. W.: Carcinoma of the proximal bile ducts. *Surg. Gynecol. Obstet.,* **136,** 923, 1973.

59. Yarbrough, D. R., III: Carcinoma of the extrahepatic biliary tract. *J. Sc. Med. Assoc.,* **72,** 80, 1976.

Injuries of the Gallbladder and Bile Ducts

5

Ezra Steiger

Introduction

Most injuries of the biliary system are iatrogenic and occur in the operating room. The etiology, diagnosis, and methods of treating these complications of biliary surgery are discussed in other chapters. In addition, however, the biliary tract can be injured from non-operative abdominal trauma in association with other intra-abdominal injuries or, rarely, as an isolated injury. Penetrating injuries from gunshot and knife wounds are more common than blunt injuries and, according to some reports, account for approximately 90% of all injuries of the extrahepatic biliary system.[1] In children, blunt injuries are the more common cause of injury.[2] The increasing incidence of all types of abdominal trauma, especially blunt injuries from high-speed automobile accidents, makes it imperative that surgeons be able to diagnose and treat trauma of the biliary system.[3]

Pathology

The gallbladder, right and left hepatic ducts, common hepatic duct, and common bile duct can all be injured. Injuries of the gallbladder are the most common injuries reported, accounting for more than 80% of all injuries.[2-4] Bile duct injuries occur in less than 20% of cases reported. Injuries of the vascular structures in the portal triad and of the liver, kidney, inferior vena cava, and duodenum are frequently associated with injuries of the biliary system. Isolated biliary injuries are rare; additional organ damage in the right upper quadrant should be searched for if biliary tract trauma is present. The involvement of other organs increases the seriousness of the injury.

Diagnosis

Clinical Features—Immediate Diagnosis. If bile is found in fluid from a peritoneal tap in a patient with a penetrating injury of the abdomen or in a patient who has had blunt trauma, a liver, biliary tract, or intestinal perforation is usually present.[5] At the time of exploratory laparotomy for trauma, if retroperitoneal bile staining, free bile, or bile mixed with blood and blood clots are found in the peritoneal cavity or the lesser peritoneal cavity, a full exploration of the biliary system should be performed. If a

97

major vascular injury of the porta hepatis is also present, vascular control of the hepatoduodenal ligament, the hepatic artery and portal vein, or the underlying vena cava with vascular clamps should be performed while exploring the extrahepatic biliary system. Occlusion of the hepatic artery or portal vein for 15 to 20 min, either with vascular clamps or by manual compression, can safely be accomplished in normothermic patients without liver cell damage.

Hepatic artery injuries can be managed safely by ligating the injured common hepatic artery or its branches when necessary. In the post-operative period after hepatic artery ligation, antibiotics, nasal oxygen, and supplemental glucose administration are important considerations. If the hepatic artery is ligated, it should be recalled that the cystic artery is an end artery and a cholecystectomy should be performed.

After initial control and repair of associated vascular injuries, attention can then be directed to the biliary injuries. A Kocher maneuver is essential to fully explore the distal common duct, where a significant percentage of common duct injuries from blunt abdominal trauma occur.[6,7] Visual inspection alone should not be relied on; an operative cholangiogram is helpful in localizing the site and extent of any injury. For this reason, at laparotomy facilities should be available to obtain an operative cholecysto-cholangiogram or a common duct cholangiogram with a 23-gauge needle if the gallbladder is not present or cannot be utilized (Figure 5-1).

Delayed Diagnosis. In many patients with isolated injuries of the bile system, diagnosis is delayed because of the initial lack of presenting symptoms. Usually there is a history of blunt trauma, often from a steering wheel in an automobile crash, with a relatively short period of right upper abdominal pain and hypotension that readily responds to conservative measures. After a period of days to weeks, the clinical picture of biliary ascites may develop. This is characterized by abdominal distension with fluid, jaundice, fever, anorexia, weight loss, and acholic stools. A collection confined to the lesser peritoneal cavity may present as an upper ab-

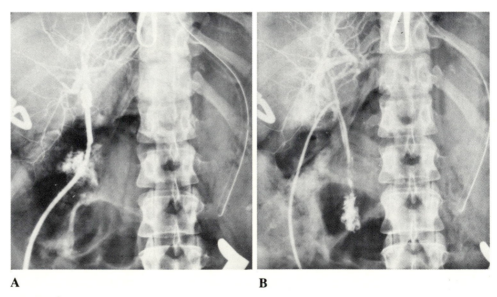

A   B

FIGURE 5-1.   (**A**) Operative cholangiogram in a patient with a transection injury of the upper bile ducts from blunt injury of the upper abdomen. (**B**) Duct-to-duct repair was performed over a T-tube stent.

dominal mass or the initial presentation may be that of a subhepatic abscess.

Paracentesis of bile-stained abdominal fluid will confirm the diagnosis.[5] The pre-operative assessment of bile duct continuity by ERC may be helpful; its use for the diagnosis of biliary tract injuries has not as yet been reported. It might not visualize the gallbladder, a common site of the bile leakage.

Once the presumptive diagnosis of bile ascites has been made, anemia, hypoalbuminemia, and fluid and electrolyte abnormalities should be corrected and the patient should be taken to the operating room as soon as possible. In most instances of bile accumulation in the peritoneal cavity, bile peritonitis exists and intestinal organisms can be cultured from the peritoneal fluid.[5] Pre-operative broad-spectrum antibiotics should be given until specific cultures are available.

Hemobilia Occasionally, the syndrome of right upper abdominal colicky pain, jaundice, and gastrointestinal bleeding will occur weeks or months after injury to the liver or intrahepatic biliary system. Hemobilia as a cause of the triad of pain, jaundice, and gastrointestinal bleeding should be kept in mind for any patient who has incurred a blunt injury to the liver.

The diagnosis can best be made by selective celiac and superior mesenteric angiography.[8] Visualization of the area of liver injury, the intrahepatic arterial fistula with the bile ducts, and dilated bile ducts filled with blood can often be seen on angiograms or on cholangiograms, confirming the diagnosis (Figures 5-2 and 5-3).

Treatment
Injuries to the Gallbladder. Trauma to the cystic duct, cystic artery, and gallbladder is usually best treated by cholecystectomy. Simple suture repair of a gallbladder laceration or cholecystostomy may be appropriate in certain instances.[4] The degree of the injury and the condition of the patient at the time of operative exploration dictates the best operative approach for gallbladder injuries. With gallstones or more extensive injuries, a cholecystectomy should be performed. A cholecystostomy may be performed if the patient is a poor operative risk.

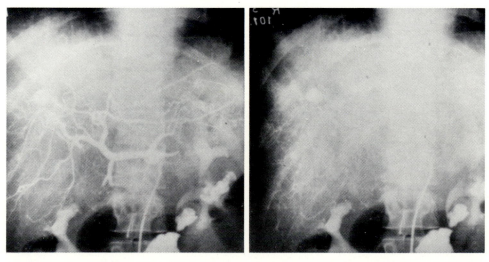

FIGURE 5-2. Selective celiac arteriogram showing a cavity or false aneurysm in the right lobe of the liver that communicated with the intrahepatic bile ducts in a patient with post-traumatic hemobilia.

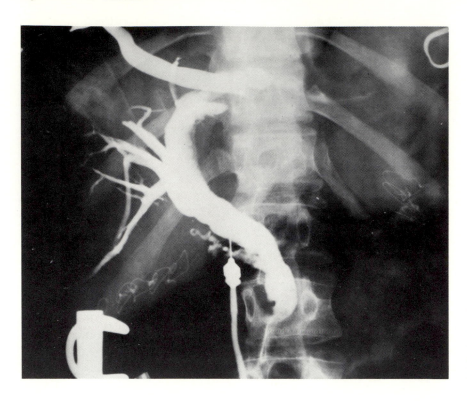

FIGURE 5-3. Operative cholangiogram of the same patient shown in Figure 5-2 demonstrates a dilated common hepatic and intrahepatic bile duct from repeated episodes of bleeding into the biliary system.

Injuries to the Bile Ducts. The immediate, conservative operative treatment for bile duct injury, if it is imperative that the operation be terminated rapidly, is placement of a tube into the bile duct for external diversion of the bile, and stenting of the injury. Even if the duct injury cannot be readily reconstructed, such as in distal duct avulsive injuries, drainage of the proximal duct with a straight tube can be used as a temporizing maneuver until definitive surgery can be accomplished at a later time. The distal portion of the injured bile duct need not be oversewn or ligated if complete biliary diversion has been achieved.[7,9]

If the patient is stable enough for definitive surgery, direct ductal repair can usually be accomplished when there is a simple laceration without severe surrounding inflammation or devitalized tissue. If the duct has been completely severed, an end-to-end repair of the duct using a T-tube stent brought out through a separate opening in the duct above or below the area of injury can be accomplished (Figure 5-4). Linear lacerations can be closed primarily over a T-tube stent. A generous Kocher maneuver is essential to achieve as much length as possible for repair under minimal tension.

If the injury is extensive or involves the retroduodenal common duct —a frequent occurrence—alternative methods of repair include choledochoduodenostomy or, preferably, Roux-Y choledochojejunostomy.[1,7] With a normal size bile duct, a stent brought out through the common duct or the limb of jejunum protects the anastomosis and assures adequate biliary decompression. These stents can be removed 3 to 6 weeks post-operatively, after a cholangiogram shows an intact biliary–enteric anastomosis and after a period of trial clamping of the tube. Although common duct defects and strictures have been repaired using jejunal mucosal grafts and pedicled gallbladder grafts,[9] their use in cases of biliary tract trauma has not been reported.[10,11] Cholecystoenterostomy might be tried if direct, definitive repair or internal drainage of a lower common duct injury is impossible. Postoperative drainage of the subhepatic space is always advisable.

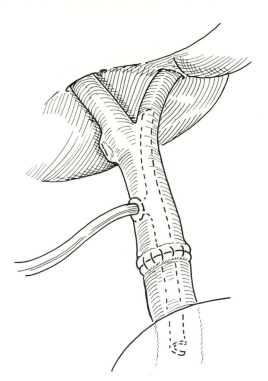

FIGURE 5-4. T-tube placed in the common hepatic duct above an injury to the duct has been repaired by choledochocholedochostomy. The external limb of the T-tube should be brought out above or below the duct repair, never through it.

Injuries of the Intrahepatic Ducts: Hemobilia. If intrahepatic injury of the bile duct occurs with significant subsequent hemobilia, two courses of operative treatment are available. The hepatic artery to the area of bleeding can be isolated and clamped to see if bleeding stops; if this is effective, it is ligated. If hepatic artery ligation is not sufficient to stop the bleeding, a partial or complete hepatic lobectomy may be necessary to control the bleeding. A T-tube stent in the bile duct is not essential postoperatively.

References

1. Diethrich, E. B., Beall, A. C., Jr., Jordan, G. L., Jr., et al.: Traumatic injuries to the extrahepatic biliary tract. *Am. J. Surg.,* **112,** 756, 1966.
2. Harman, S. W., and Greaney, E. M., Jr.: Traumatic injuries to the biliary system in children. *Am. J. Surg.,* **108,** 150, 1964.
3. Barnes, J. P., and Diamonon, J. S.: Traumatic rupture of the gallbladder due to nonpenetrating injury. *Tex. State J. Med.,* **59,** 785, 1963.
4. Smith, S. W., and Hastings, T. N.: Traumatic rupture of the gallbladder. *Ann. Surg.,* **139,** 517, 1954.
5. Means, R. L.: Bile peritonitis. *Am. Surg.,* **30,** 583, 1964.
6. Hinshaw, D. B., Turner, G. R., and Carter, R.: Transection of the common bile duct caused by nonpenetrating trauma. *Am. J. Surg.,* **104,** 104, 1962.
7. Rydell, W. B., Jr.: Complete transection of the common bile duct due to blunt abdominal trauma. *Arch. Surg.,* **100,** 724, 1970.
8. Hermann, R. E., and Hoerr, S. O.: Aids in the diagnosis of hemobilia. *Surg., Gynecol., Obstet.,* **125,** 55, 1967.
9. Sturmer, F. C., Jr., and Wilt, K. E.: Complete division of the common duct from external blunt trauma. *Am. J. Surg.,* **105,** 781, 1963.
10. Sandblom, P., Tabrizian, M., Rigo, M., et al.: Repair of common bile duct defects using the gallbladder or cystic duct as a pedicled graft. *Surg., Gynecol., Obstet.,* **140,** 425, 1975.
11. Wexler, M. J., and Smith, R.: Jejunal mucosal graft. A sutureless technic for repair of high bile duct strictures. *Am. J. Surg.,* **129,** 204, 1975.

Operative
Technics

6

Biliary Exploration

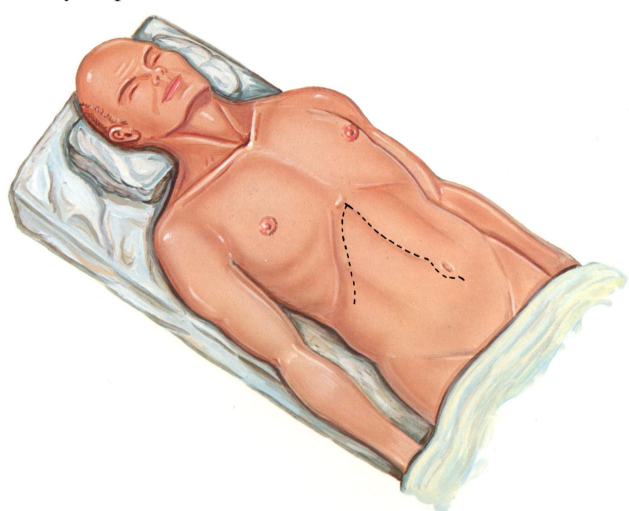

FIGURE 6-1.   The incisions I prefer for operations on the gallbladder and bile ducts. A subcostal incision is preferred for obese patients or those with a wide costal angle. A midline or right paramedian incision is used for slender patients with a narrow costal angle.

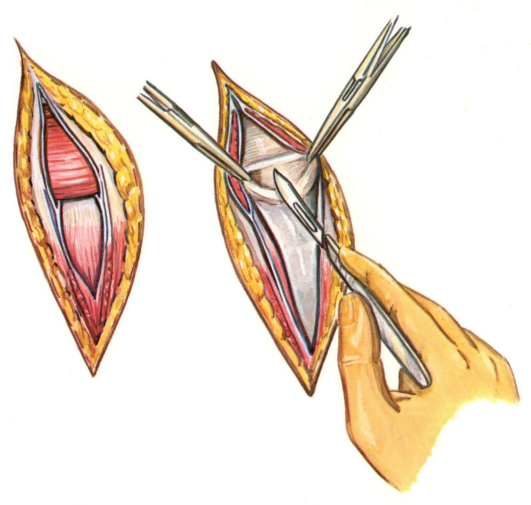

FIGURE 6-2.   A subcostal incision is carried down through rectus muscle, which is divided; Kocher clamps are placed on the deep fascial layer and peritoneum, and the peritoneal cavity is entered.

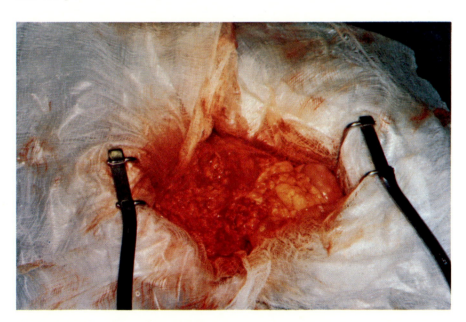

FIGURE 6-3.   The subcostal incision has been opened throughout its length and a self-retaining retractor has been placed laterally or inferiorly, so that it will be out of the field for a subsequent operative cholangiogram. Liner gauze sponges, made of gauze and a plastic material, are placed inside the wound to protect it from contamination.

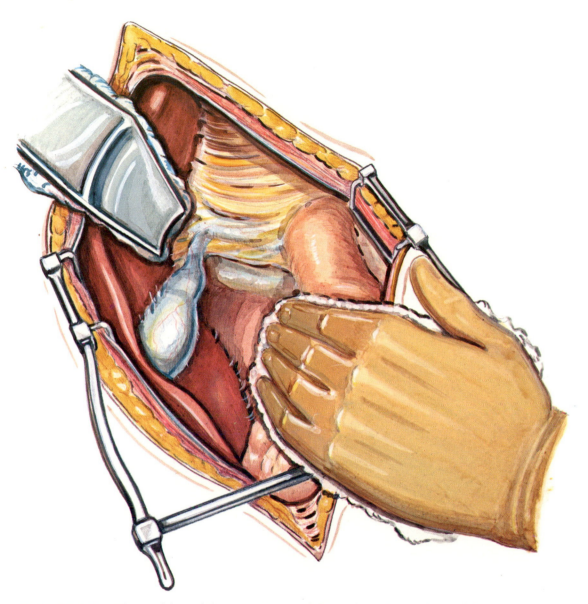

FIGURE 6-4. The position of the retractors and the assistant's hand for a biliary exploration. I use a Doyen retractor, a right-angle retractor with a flat blade, medial to the gallbladder to retract the liver. The assistant's left hand, on a gauze pad, retracts the duodenum medially and inferiorly to expose the subhepatic space.

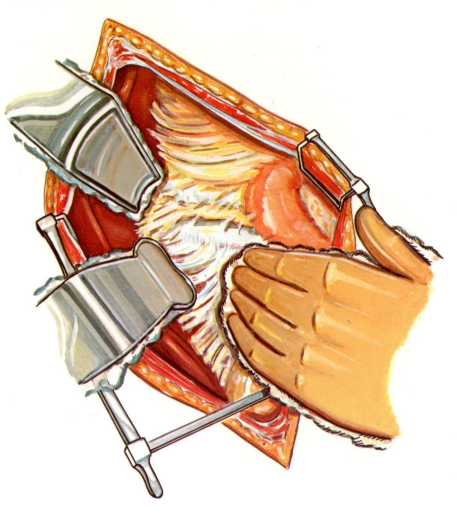

FIGURE 6-5. If the gallbladder has been previously removed, a Harrington retractor is placed over the gallbladder bed as a second major retractor to expose the subhepatic space.

Operative Cholangiography

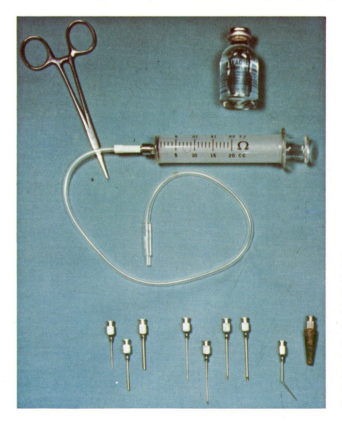

FIGURE 6-6. Operative cholangiography is an essential part of all operative procedures on the gallbladder and bile ducts; the instruments needed for operative cholangiography include an assortment of sharp and blunt needles, a length of intravenous tubing, a 20-ml syringe, and a water-soluble dye solution (we now use Renografin-60).

106

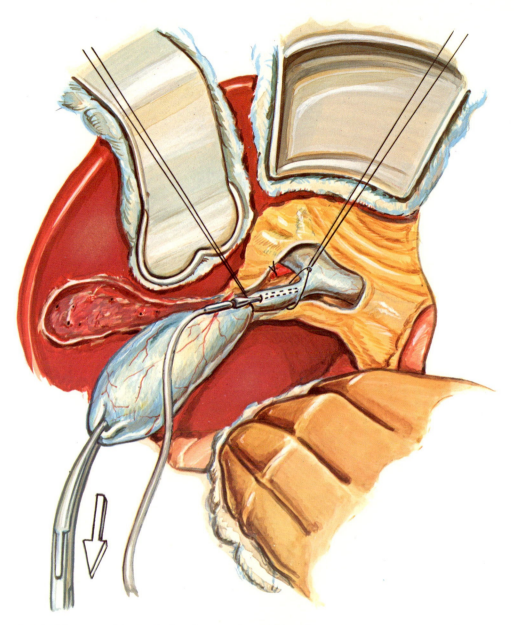

FIGURE 6-7.   The technic of operative cholangiography through the cystic duct when the gallbladder will be removed. After the gallbladder is dissected from its liver bed, the cystic duct is identified; any stones in the duct are milked back into the gallbladder, and an occlusive silk ligature is placed on the proximal cystic duct where it joins the gallbladder. Another silk ligature is passed around the distal cystic duct and left untied. The cystic duct is partially divided and an 18-gauge blunt needle, attached to a segment of tubing and a syringe, is inserted into the duct. The distal silk ligature is then tied around the duct and needle to hold it firmly in place.

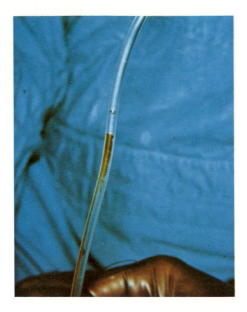

FIGURE 6-8.   Fifteen ml of Renografin-60 is used for the operative cholangiogram. Approximately 3 ml is used for an initial injection and an x-ray is taken. An additional 10 to 12 ml of dye is used for the second injection and a second x-ray is taken. Every effort must be made to remove air bubbles from the tubing prior to injection of the contrast medium.

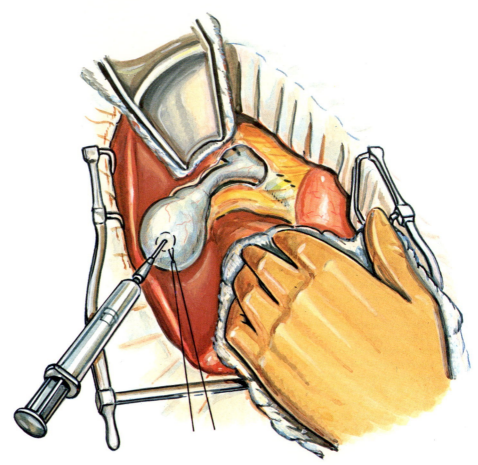

FIGURE 6-9.   A cholecystocholangiogram should be obtained whenever the gallbladder might be preserved for subsequent biliary–intestinal bypass. This technic is also applicable to the child undergoing exploration for biliary atresia. A 3-0 silk purse-string suture is placed in the fundus of the gallbladder. A 15- or 18-gauge needle is used to enter the gallbladder and empty it of bile. Approximately 15 ml of Renografin-60 is then instilled in the gallbladder, the needle and syringe are withdrawn, and the purse-string suture is tied. A hemostat is attached to the end of the silk suture as a handle for traction, and the cholecystocholangiogram is taken while the surgeon squeezes the dye out of the gallbladder into the bile ducts with his right hand.

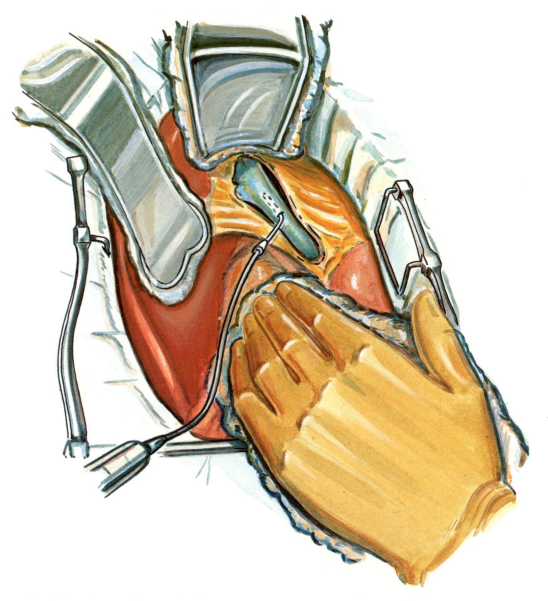

FIGURE 6-10.   If the gallbladder has been removed previously, a common duct cholangiogram can be obtained. A 21- or 23-gauge needle, attached to a length of tubing and a syringe with dye, is inserted into the common bile duct. A ''right angle needle'' is shown, which I occasionally find useful in positioning the needle into the bile duct. Again, it is important that there is no air in the system. Bile is aspirated into the tubing to be certain that the needle is in the common bile duct. Then 10 to 15 ml of dye is gently introduced into the bile duct and two roentgenograms are taken at intervals.

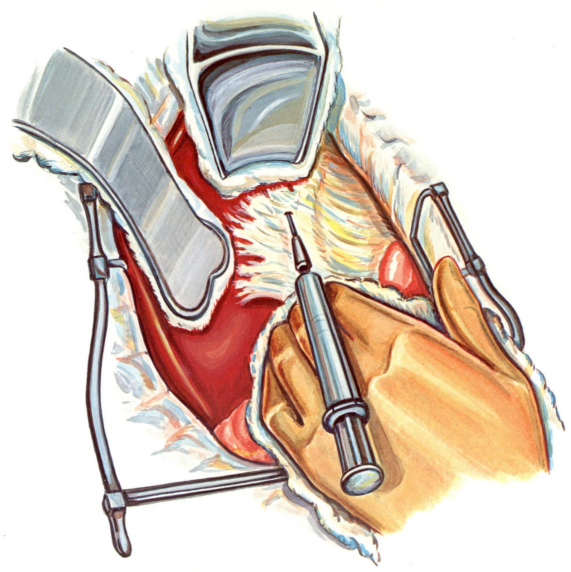

FIGURE 6-11.   The technic of operative cholangiography performed transhepatically. This technic is especially useful in patients who have had previous operations on the biliary system, when the anatomy or location of the bile ducts is obscure. It is especially useful for patients with a biliary stricture. In this drawing, the anatomy of the biliary system is unclear as the gallbladder has previously been removed. Direct needling into the porta hepatis in the region of the junction of the right and left hepatic ducts is performed with a 21-gauge needle and syringe. When bile is identified, dye will be placed into the intrahepatic biliary system and the cholangiogram will be obtained.

Portoenterostomy for Biliary Atresia

A preliminary exploration of the porta hepatis is performed through a subcostal incision. When neither the gallbladder nor the extrahepatic biliary system can be identified, the incision should be widely extended to fully expose the subhepatic space. The liver is elevated for maximal exposure of the porta hepatis.

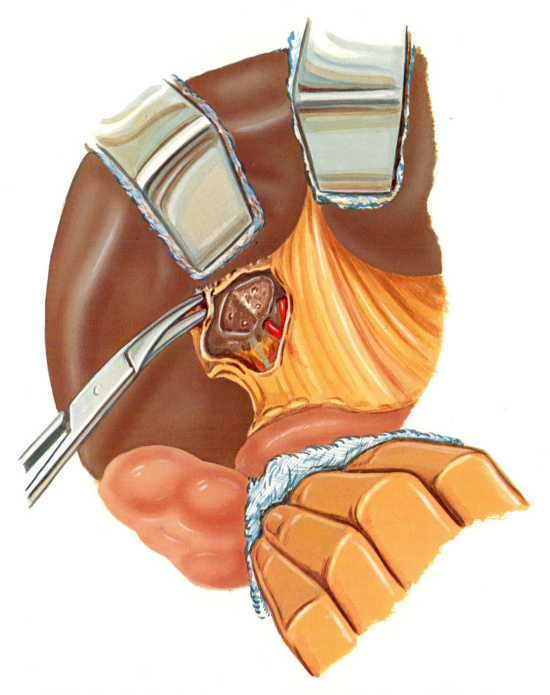

FIGURE 6-12.   The liver has been elevated and the dissection carried into the porta hepatis. No bile ducts can be seen. A segment of liver tissue 2 to 3 cm in width and 1 cm in depth is excised from the region of the confluence of the main hepatic ducts. Small duct-like structures are seen. Extensive needling into the liver may be performed as a preliminary maneuver to help identify any dilated intrahepatic bile ducts.

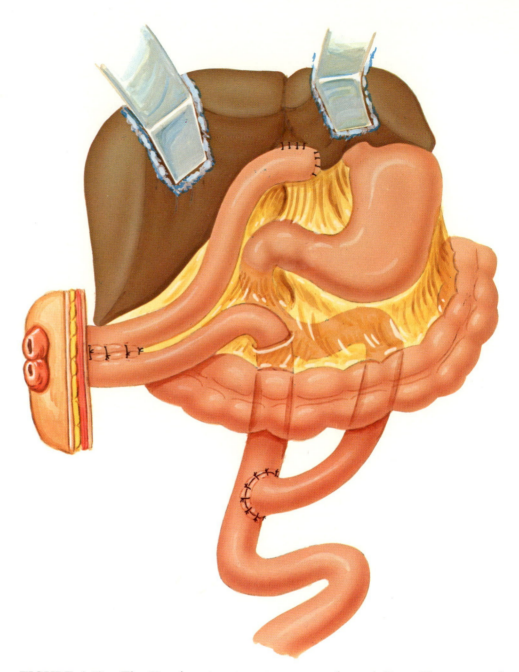

FIGURE 6-13.   The Kasai portoenterostomy procedure. A Roux-Y segment of jejunum is brought up under the transverse colon. The end of the jejunum is closed and an opening is created in the lateral wall, which is sewn to the area of denuded liver and hepatic ducts in the porta hepatis. The jejunum is anchored in place with interrupted 3-0 silk sutures placed so that the mucosa is opened widely to cover the entire denuded area of liver. The modification of the Kasai procedure by Suruga and by Lilly is shown. The Roux-Y jejunal segment is interrupted and brought externally to the skin as a divided loop jejunostomy to prevent reflux into the ascending limb of jejunum and cholangitis. Bile flow out the proximal jejunal segment can be monitored at the stoma. If bile flow appears and jaundice subsides, at approximately 6 months the loop jejunostomy can be closed, thereby reconstructing the jejunal segment in the abdomen.

Operations for Choledochal Cyst

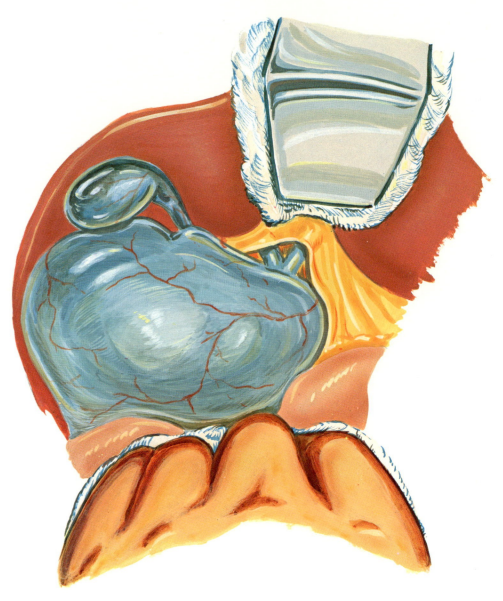

FIGURE 6-14.   A large type A choledochal cyst in the subhepatic space. Gall-bladder and hepatic ducts are normal.

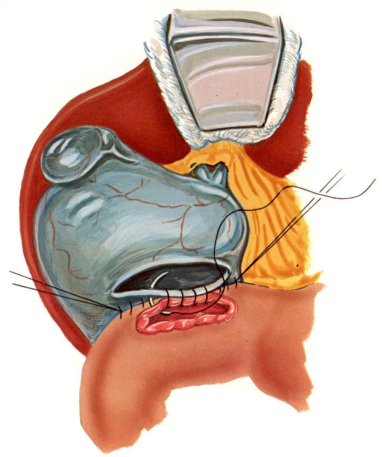

FIGURE 6-15.   After operative cholangiography has been performed and the duodenum mobilized, a choledochoduodenostomy is performed. A posterior row of interrupted 3-0 silk sutures has been placed. An inner row of interrupted or continuous 3-0 chromic catgut sutures is used for the inner layer of the anastomosis.

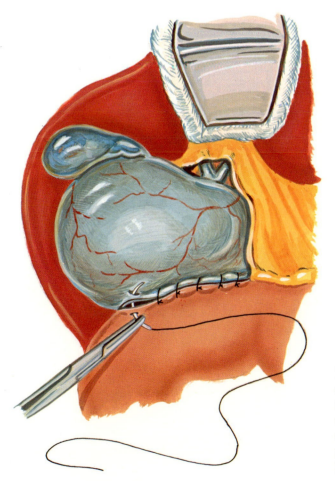

FIGURE 6-16.   The choledochoduodenostomy is completed by continuing the inner row of sutures anteriorly, then placing a final outer row of silk sutures. The anastomosis should be approximately two fingerbreadths (3 to 4 cm).

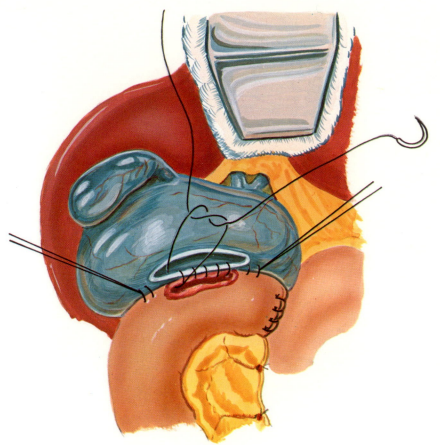

FIGURE 6-17. Alternatively, a choledochojejunostomy is made utilizing a defunctionalized Roux-Y segment of jejunum. The jejunal segment has been brought up to the undersurface of the choledochal cyst and the anastomosis is in progress. A row of interrupted 3-0 silk sutures has been placed as an outer row; an inner row of interrupted or continuous 3-0 chromic catgut sutures is being placed.

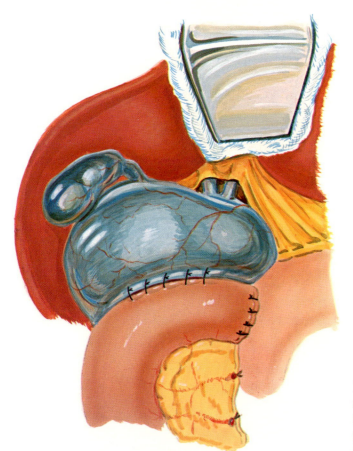

FIGURE 6-18. The choledochal cystojejunostomy anastomosis has been completed by continuing the inner row of chromic catgut sutures anteriorly and placing an additional, outer row of interrupted silk sutures.

115

Cholecystectomy

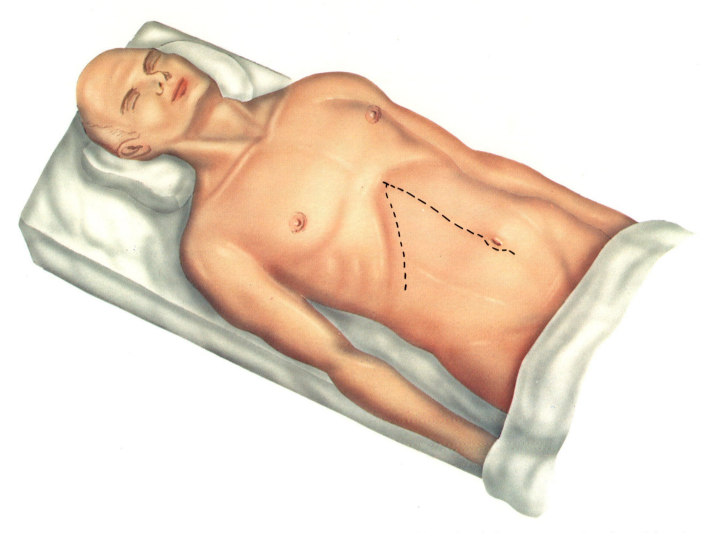

FIGURE 6-19.   The preferred incisions for cholecystectomy. I prefer a right sub-costal incision in most patients, especially the obese. I use a midline upper abdominal incison or upper right paramedian incision only in thin patients. It is essential to carry the incision up to the xiphoid process to expose the upper bile ducts.

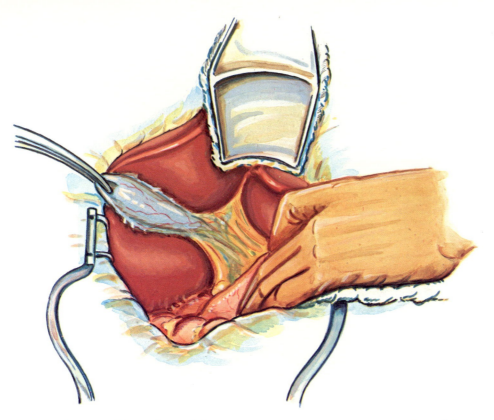

FIGURE 6-20.   The subcostal incision has been opened and a self-retaining retractor placed with the bar of the retractor inferiorly or laterally. The assistant's left hand on a laparotomy pad reflects the duodenum downward and medially. A Doyen retractor is medial to the gallbladder to expose the subhepatic space. A Kelly clamp is placed on the gallbladder for gentle traction. A large laparotomy tape in the right gutter, lateral to the duodenum, is used to depress the hepatic flexure of the colon and occlude the right lateral gutter if there should be spillage of bile during the operative dissection.

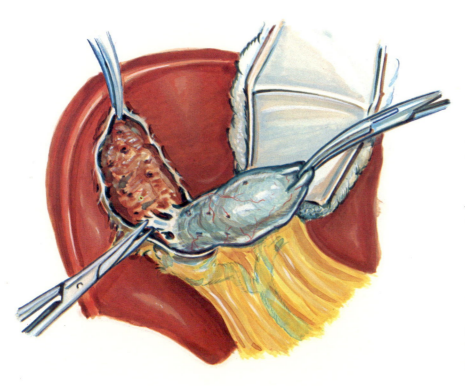

FIGURE 6-21.   With gentle traction on the fundus of the gallbladder, the peritoneal reflection is scored with a knife on both sides of the gallbladder; the gallbladder is then dissected by scissors dissection from its liver bed, from the fundus toward the duct. This is the safest technic of cholecystectomy and the one I use for all patients, whether the operation is done for acute or for chronic cholecystitis. As the gallbladder is removed, small bleeding vessels are encountered in the liver bed; they can be coagulated with the Bovie electrocautery unit. The dissection plane should stay close to the gallbladder. As the dissection proceeds, a moist laparotomy pad may be placed against the gallbladder bed in the liver and a Harrington retractor placed against the pad for tamponade of minor bleeding.

117

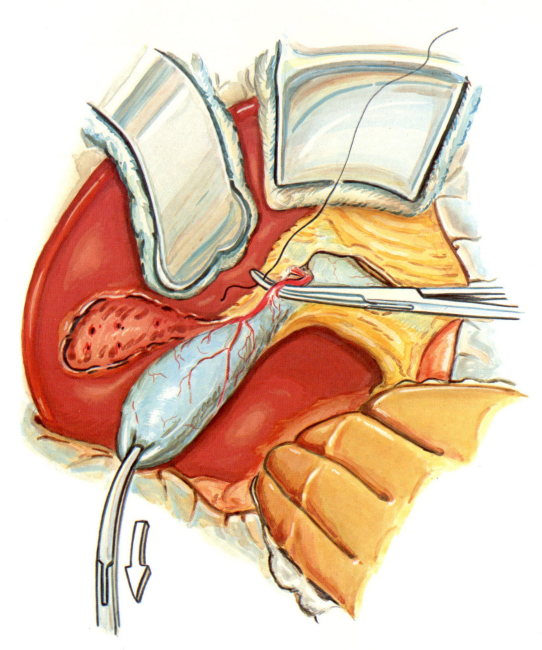

FIGURE 6-22.   As the dissection continues toward the ampulla of the gallbladder, if gentle traction is placed on the fundus of the gallbladder (arrow), the cystic artery will be made taut and will be felt by the palpating finger as a cord. At this point, a right angle clamp is passed under the cystic artery and a ligature is placed around the artery. The artery can be divided and the dissection of the ampulla of the gallbladder can be carried down to the cystic duct.

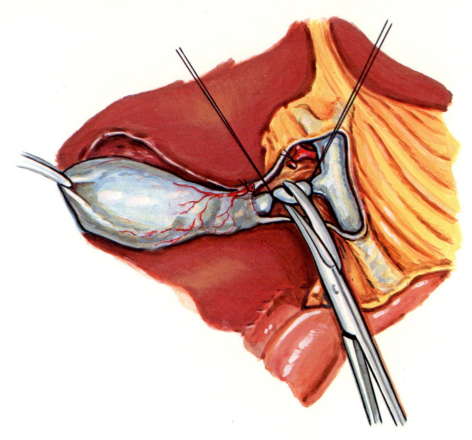

FIGURE 6-23.   The cystic duct is exposed. The ligated cystic artery can be seen. Any stones in the cystic duct are milked back into the gallbladder by the surgeon's fingers and a right angle clamp. A silk ligature is tied on the gallbladder side of the cystic duct and another silk ligature is placed around the distal cystic duct. Using a scissors, the surgeon partially transects the cystic duct for an operative cholangiogram.

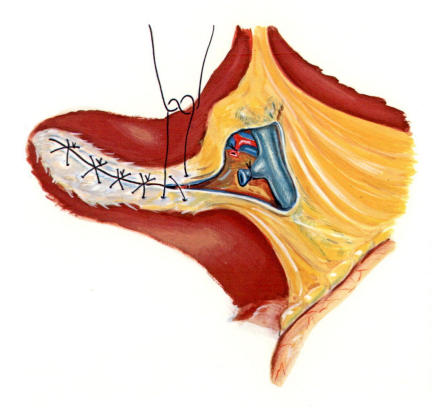

FIGURE 6-24.   After operative cholangiography has been completed, the cystic duct can be clamped, ligated, and divided. A 2-0 silk ligature is used to ligate the cystic duct 0.5 to 1.0 cm from its junction with the common hepatic duct. The peritoneal reflection overlying the bed of the gallbladder in the liver is then closed with interrupted figure-of-eight 3-0 silk sutures, after it is certain that hemostasis of the liver bed has been achieved.

119

Retrograde Method of Cholecystectomy

Although it is always safest to remove the gallbladder from the fundus toward the duct, some surgeons prefer to remove the gallbladder from the duct toward the fundus. These drawings depict this method.

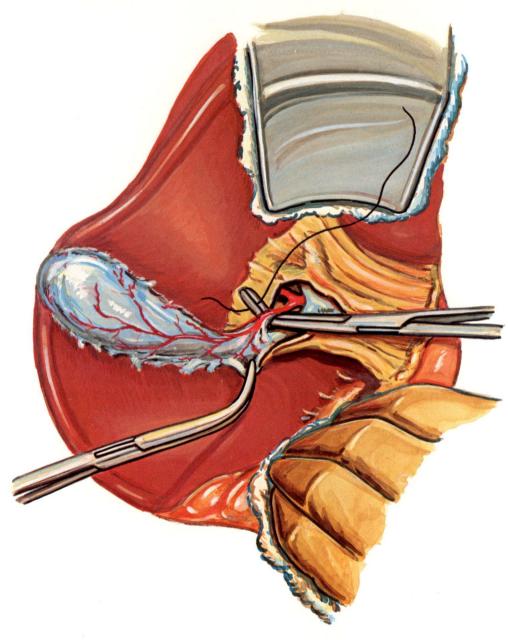

FIGURE 6-25. The subhepatic space is exposed as previously shown. A right angle clamp is placed on the ampulla of the gallbladder to make the cystic artery and cystic duct taut. The cystic artery is palpated with the surgeon's finger, a right angle clamp is placed under the artery, and a ligature is placed about the artery. The cystic artery is then ligated and divided.

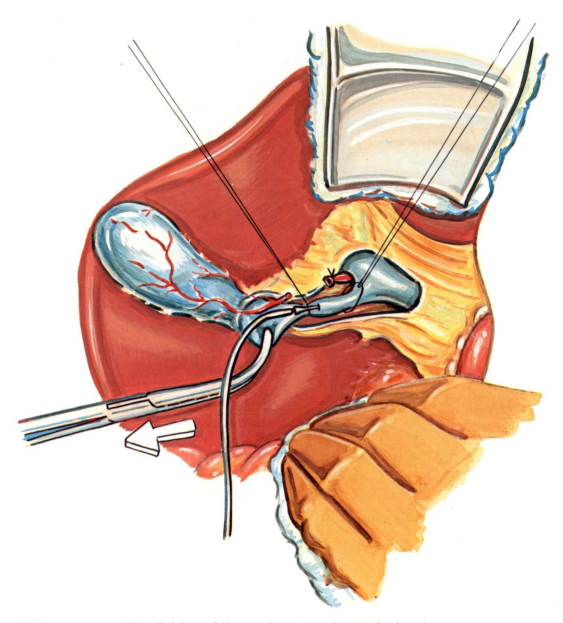

FIGURE 6-26. With division of the cystic artery, the cystic duct becomes apparent and can be traced from its junction with the common hepatic duct to the gallbladder. Silk ligatures may be placed about the cystic duct after any stones in the duct have been milked back up into the gallbladder. An operative cholangiogram is then performed through a small opening in the cystic duct. It is important that no ducts be divided or ligated until this operative cholangiogram has been seen.

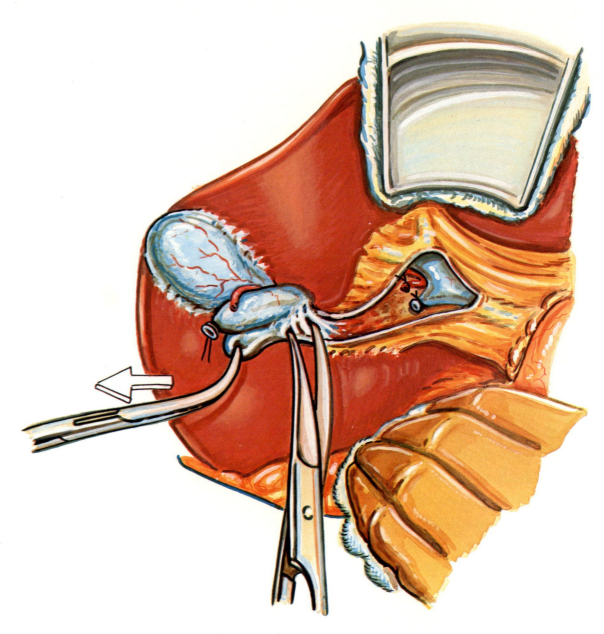

FIGURE 6-27.   After a satisfactory operative cholangiogram, the cystic duct can be ligated with a silk ligature and divided. The gallbladder is then dissected from its liver bed, retrograde from the duct toward the fundus. The liver bed is closed as before.

Drains

In the past, almost all surgeons drained the subhepatic space routinely after cholecystectomy or after operations on the bile ducts. Recently, many surgeons have abandoned routine drainage of the subhepatic space, especially after uncomplicated cholecystectomy. I no longer use drainage routinely after cholecystectomy; however, I continue to drain patients who have had acute cholecystitis or in whom there was gross spillage of bile during the operative procedure. In addition, if there has been troublesome bleeding or any evidence of bile leakage following completion of the operative procedure, a Penrose or suction tube drain should be placed and brought out through a separate stab incision below the subcostal incision.

Cholecystostomy

Cholecystostomy is reserved for patients with hydrops of the gallbladder and extreme inflammation which obscures the normal anatomy and makes cholecystectomy hazardous. Additionally, cholecystostomy under local anesthesia may be used for the extremely ill patient who might not tolerate cholecystectomy or general anesthesia.

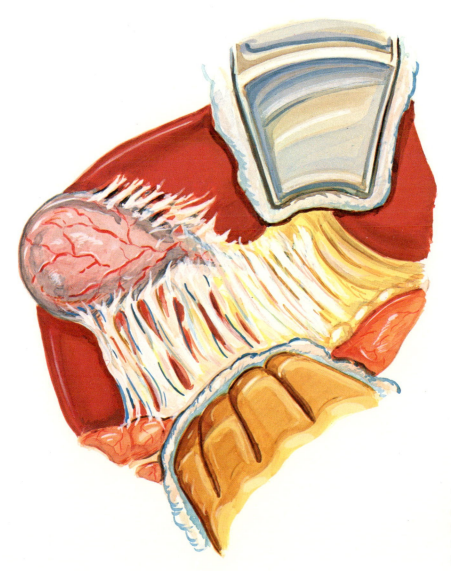

FIGURE 6-28. An acutely inflamed, distended gallbladder with multiple inflammatory adhesions obscures the normal subhepatic and hepatoduodenal anatomy.

123

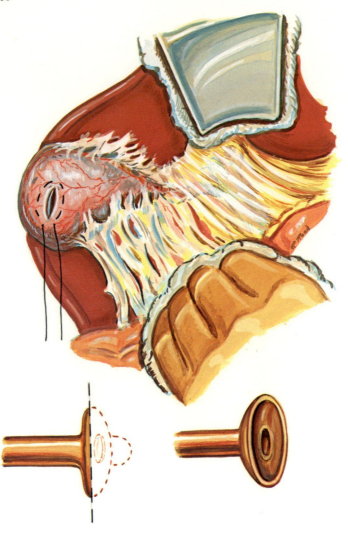

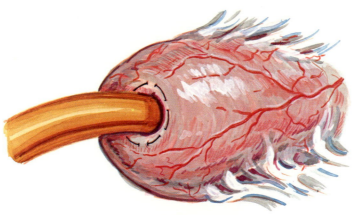

FIGURE 6-29. A purse-string suture of 2-0 chromic catgut is placed in the fundus of the gallbladder and a stab incision is made through the encircling suture; a large (No. 30 or No. 32) mushroom catheter is utilized. I prefer to cut off the end of the mushroom catheter.

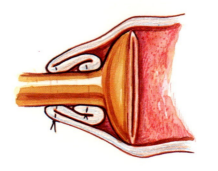

FIGURE 6-30. After the bile has been aspirated and any stones removed, the catheter is placed in the fundus of the gallbladder. The purse-string suture is tied down and, frequently, a second purse-string suture is placed to further invert or seal the cholecystostomy tube. The tube is then brought out through the subhepatic incision or adjacent to it, either above or below, depending on the placement of the incision and the anatomy of the patient. A drain may be used to drain the subhepatic space, depending on the degree of infection, amount of bile leakage, or likelihood of subhepatic infection.

Common Bile Duct Exploration

The incisions for common bile duct exploration are the same as those for cholecystectomy or biliary exploration. A subcostal incision is preferred, although a midline or right paramedian incision can be utilized in thin patients.

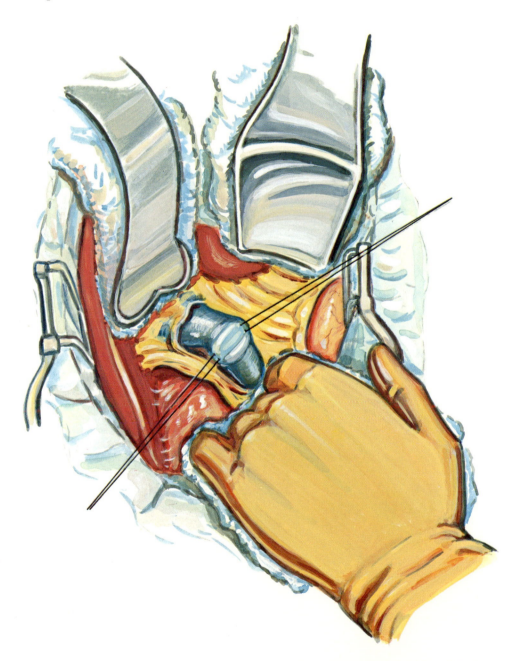

FIGURE 6-31. After the subhepatic space is dissected and the common bile duct identified, two traction sutures of 3-0 silk are placed in the common bile duct opposite each other prior to opening of the duct; the assistant's left hand retracts the duodenum downward and medially to provide critical exposure of the subhepatic space. It is important that the retraction on the liver is not too vigorous, lest the entire operative field disappear up under the rib cage, making visualization difficult.

125

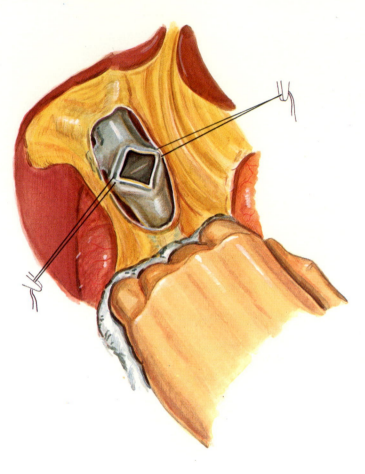

FIGURE 6-32.   The common bile duct is opened longitudinally between the two traction sutures. This incision should be made in the mid-common duct at approximately the level of the junction of the cystic duct with the common hepatic duct. The incision can be extended up or down as dictated by the operative situation.

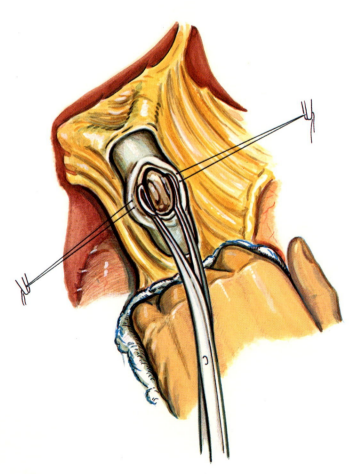

FIGURE 6-33.   A stone is removed from the common bile duct by a common duct forceps.

126

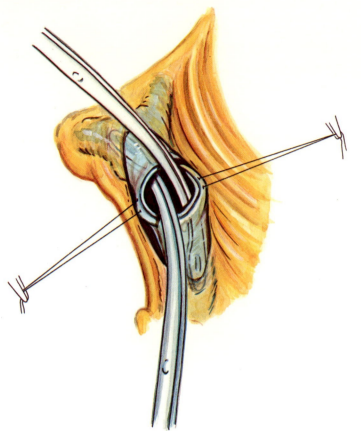

FIGURE 6-34. Curved and angled bile duct forceps are passed up into the intrahepatic ducts and down into the distal bile duct and ampulla of Vater to remove additional stones. A Kocher maneuver with mobilization of the duodenum from its retroperitoneal position is essential so that the surgeon's left hand can palpate the distal bile duct as the stone forceps and Bake's sounds are passed into the distal duct and through the papilla of Vater into the duodenum.

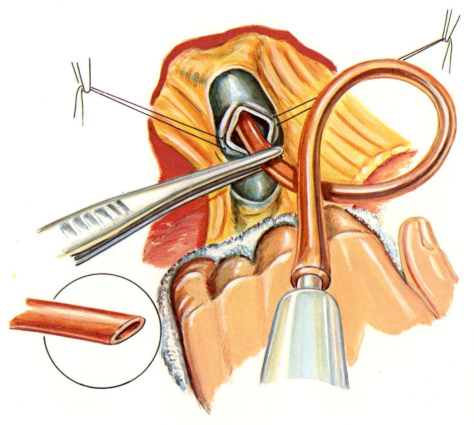

FIGURE 6-35. After all stones are removed, the common bile duct is irrigated with saline solution both up into the intrahepatic ducts and down into the distal common bile duct. A No. 18 straight rubber catheter with the end cut off is used for irrigation.

127

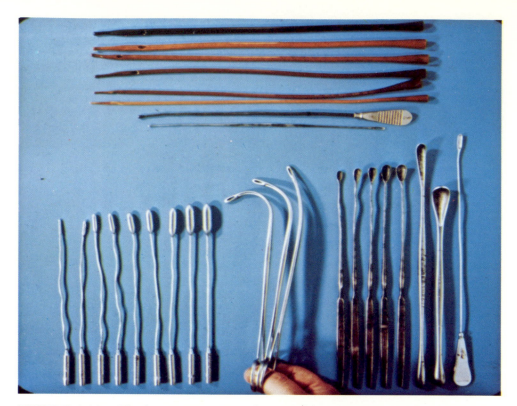

FIGURE 6-36.   The instruments I use for operative exploration of the bile ducts include stone forceps with various angles in the center of the photograph, Bake's sounds and dilators on the left, and stone scoops and spoons on the right. Woven catheters and probes are shown in the upper center.

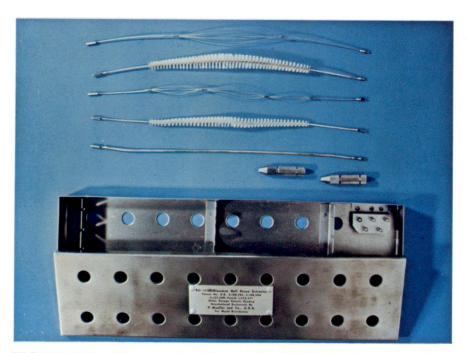

FIGURE 6-37.   These woven (Glassman) nylon brushes are useful if stones impacted in the distal bile duct cannot be totally removed. The brushes may be passed through the distal bile duct into the duodenum and out through a stab incision in the lateral wall of the duodenum. As they are passed through the distal bile duct they brush out any residual stone fragments that may be embedded in the wall of the distal duct. Surprisingly, these brushes do little or no damage to the wall of the common bile duct.

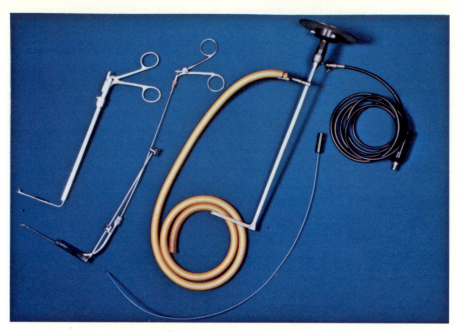

FIGURE 6-38. The Stortz-Hopkins choledochoscope with its attachments. The choledochoscope is extremely useful in difficult explorations or re-explorations of the bile ducts for stones, especially if the bile ducts are dilated.

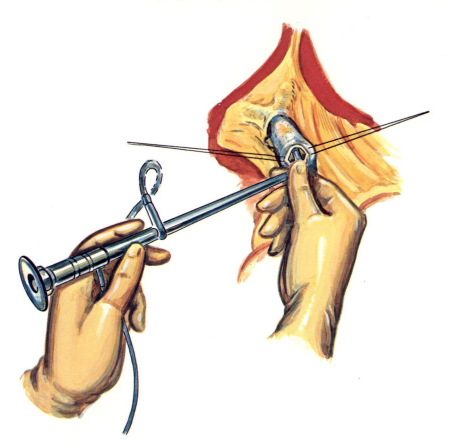

FIGURE 6-39. The choledochoscope is introduced through the choledochotomy incision and is held in the surgeon's hands. With a continuous stream of water irrigating the ducts, the light source gives excellent visualization of the intrahepatic biliary system. With a 6-cm scope, one can see up into the intrahepatic bile ducts or down into and through the ampulla of Vater. The rigid choledochoscope is more useful than the flexible scope because the tip can be directed. Attachments to the scope permit extraction of stones, biopsy of lesions, and cauterization of bleeding points.

129

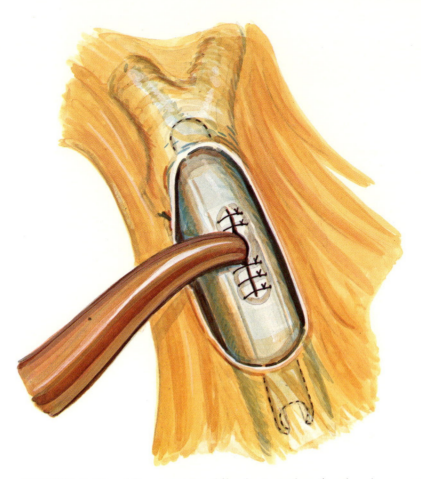

FIGURE 6-40.   After common bile duct exploration has been completed, a T-tube is placed in the duct for post-operative drainage. Interrupted 3-0 chromic catgut sutures hold the T-tube in place.

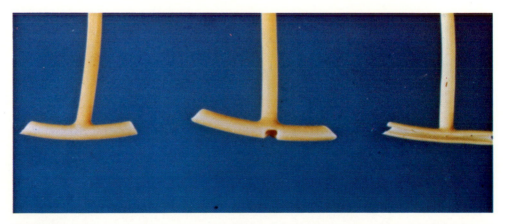

FIGURE 6-41.   I prefer to use a "split back" T-tube rather than a solid tube or one in which a wedge has been cut out of the back wall. Removing the back wall of the T-tube permits the tube to collapse upon itself when it is removed from the duct 8 or 10 days after surgery. Immediately following placement of a T-tube in the bile duct, a T-tube cholangiogram should be obtained to be certain that all stones have been removed from the bile ducts and no additional pathological changes have been overlooked.

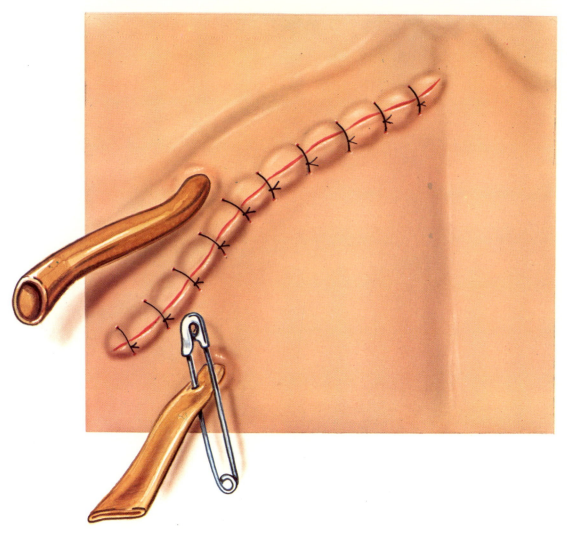

FIGURE 6-42. The placement of a T-tube and Penrose drain through separate stab incisions.

Sphincteroplasty

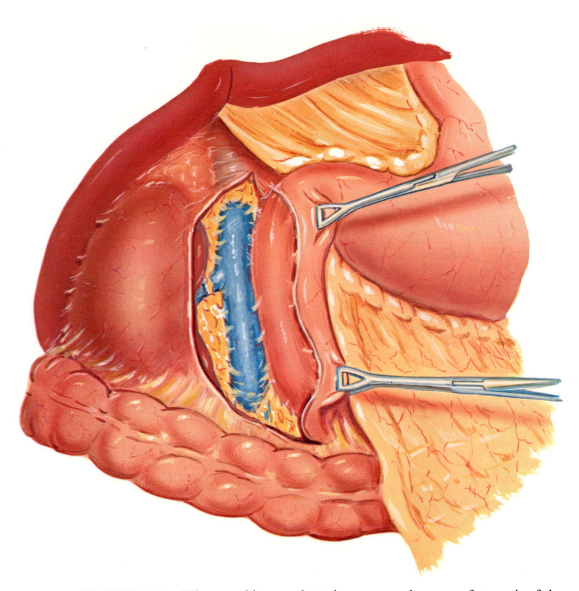

FIGURE 6-43.   When a sphincteroplasty is necessary because of stenosis of the sphincter of Oddi or a stone impacted in the distal bile duct, the initial maneuver should be wide mobilization of the descending duodenum from its retroperitoneal position, a Kocher maneuver. Gentle retraction of the duodenum may be achieved by Babcock clamps placed on the descending duodenum while the surgeon elevates the duodenum by blunt or sharp dissection, anterior to the vena cava. A Kocher maneuver should be part of all explorations of the distal bile duct so that the surgeon can palpate the distal duct and pass probes or instruments with his left hand.

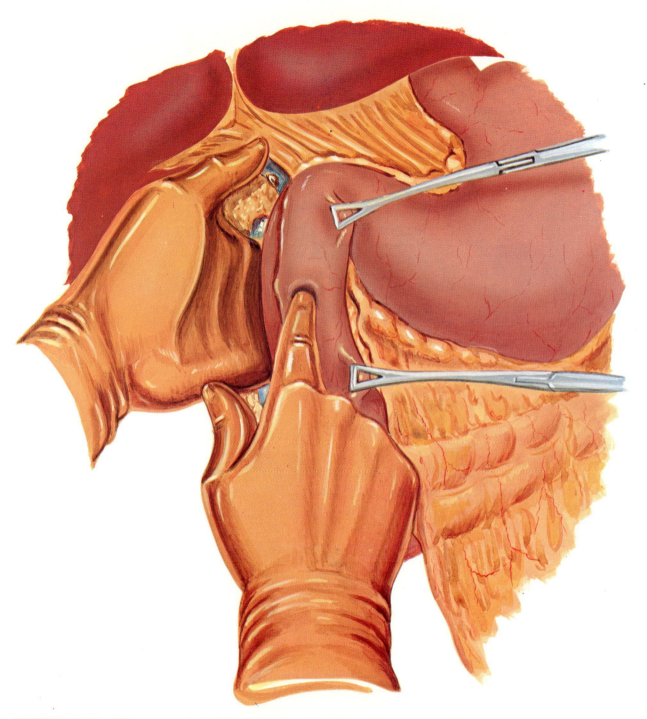

FIGURE 6-44.   The surgeon's left hand is placed behind the descending duodenum and distal bile duct; with the right forefinger, he palpates for the papilla of
Vater. A previous operative cholangiogram will portray just where the bile duct
enters the duodenum.

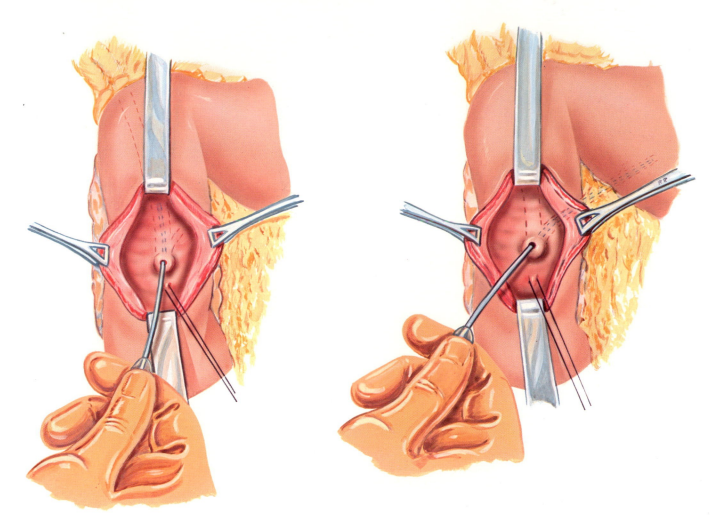

FIGURE 6-45. A longitudinal duodenotomy is performed. Babcock clamps placed on the lateral walls of the duodenum and small right angle retractors in the duodenum expose the lumen. Laparotomy tapes passed up and down the duodenum are used to occlude the flow of duodenal juice. The papilla of Vater can be palpated as a "pimple" on the medial wall of the duodenum and, if observation continues for several seconds or longer, the flow of bile or pancreatic juice from this orifice can be seen. A traction suture of 3-0 silk is placed below the papilla of Vater to bring the medial wall of the duodenum anteriorly. A small probe is passed both up the distal bile duct and, if possible, into the distal pancreatic duct.

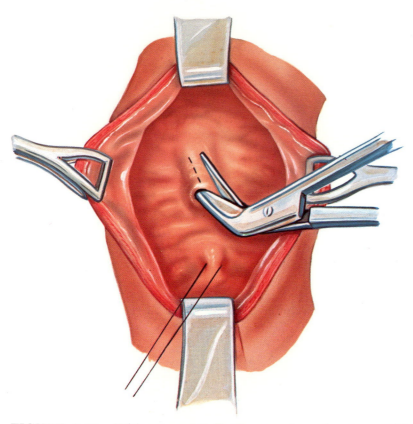

FIGURE 6-46. With an angled Pott's vascular scissors, a sphincterotomy is begun by cutting the choledochal sphincter in its superior–lateral region at approximately 11 o'clock. This incision is kept lateral to avoid injury to the medial opening of the pancreatic duct.

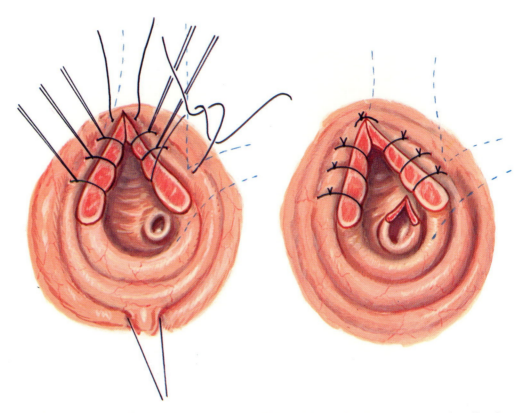

FIGURE 6-47. The incision is continued for at least 2.0 to 2.5 cm up the distal bile duct. As the incision proceeds, interrupted fine chromic catgut sutures are used to unite the duodenal and common bile duct mucosa. If small hemostats are left on these sutures as traction sutures, exposure is aided. As this incision is lenthened and the opening between distal bile duct and duodenum is made larger, this procedure becomes a sphincteroplasty rather than a sphincterotomy. If the opening is long enough (2.5 cm or longer), it is a true choledochoduodenostomy of the distal bile duct and duodenum. It is essential to place a suture at the apex of the incision, the point where leakage between the back wall of the duodenum and common bile duct might potentially occur. If the septum between the pancreatic duct orifice and common bile duct is thickened, a sphincterotomy of the pancreatic sphincter can also be performed.

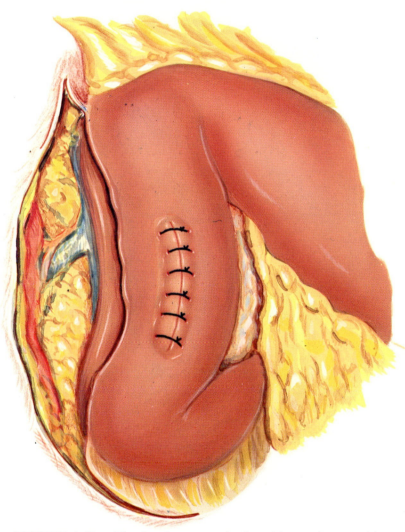

FIGURE 6-48.   The duodenotomy is closed in two layers with a running 3-0 chromic catgut suture to the inner layer of mucosa and interrupted sutures of 3-0 silk to the seromuscular layer. Drainage of the subhepatic space is optional.

Choledochocholedochostomy

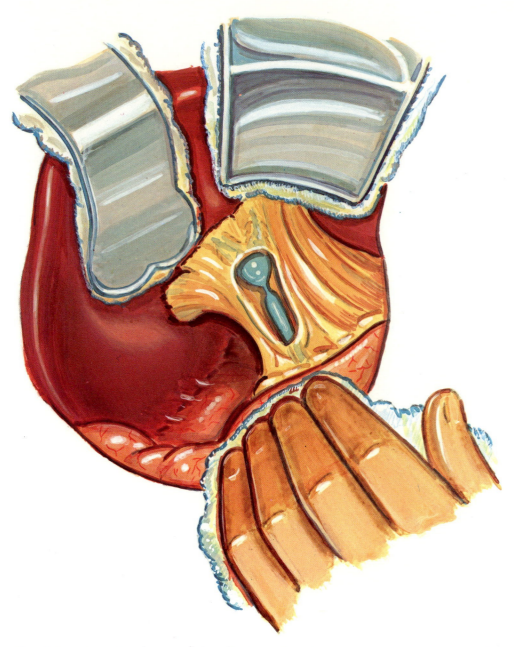

FIGURE 6-49.   A stricture of the bile duct. Careful dissection of the bile duct is essential to expose the duct above and below the strictured area. The bile duct above and below the stricture appears to be usable for a duct-to-duct repair.

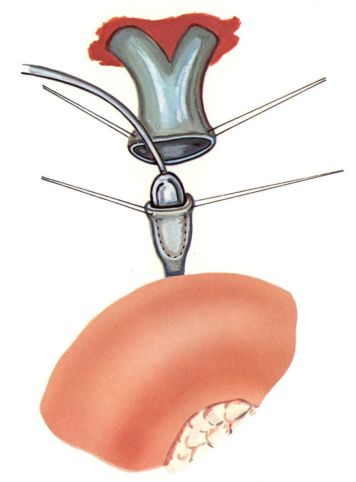

FIGURE 6-50. The area of the stricture has been excised. It is essential to remove all scarred duct tissue. Traction sutures are placed on both the upper and lower ducts. The lower duct is gently and gradually dilated with Bake's dilators to achieve maximal size.

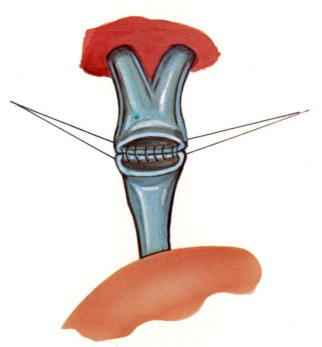

FIGURE 6-51. A choledochocholedochostomy is then performed with interrupted 3-0 chromic catgut sutures.

139

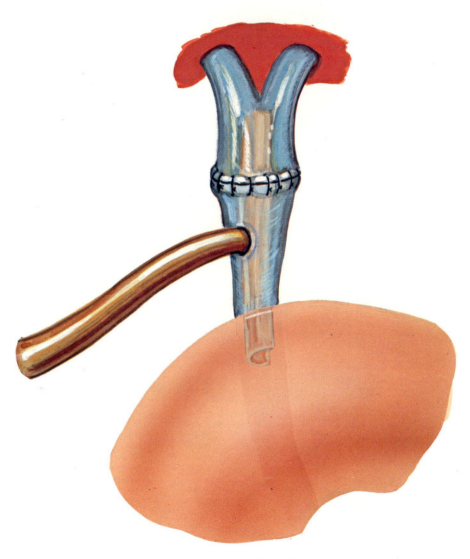

FIGURE 6-52.   The anastomosis is splinted with a T-tube brought out through a stab incision in the duct above or below the suture line, *never* through the suture line. In performing choledochocholedochostomy, it is not usually possible to make a two-layered anastomosis. It is advisable to use a T-tube splint for the anastomosis for continued dilatation of the lower bile duct. The T-tube is left in place 6 weeks.

Choledochoduodenostomy

I prefer choledochoduodenostomy to choledochojejunostomy for stricture of the bile duct if the duodenum is mobile and this operative procedure is technically possible. A choledochoduodenostomy is a simpler operative procedure involving only one anastomosis and is more physiological in that bile is returned to the duodenal segment for participation in acid inhibition and normal digestive function.

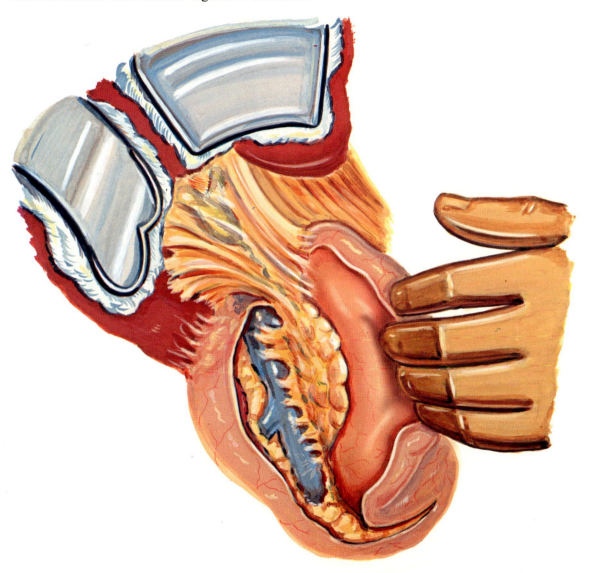

FIGURE 6-53. Extensive adhesions in the porta hepatis and hepatoduodenal ligament from previous surgical procedures and inflammation. A generous Kocher maneuver is performed to mobilize the duodenum and the hepatoduodenal area.

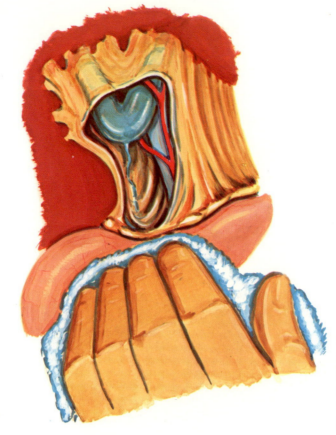

FIGURE 6-54. The hepatoduodenal adhesions have been divided with the pulsations of the hepatic artery as a guide, and a scarred, strictured bile duct is identified. The proximal hepatic ducts are dilated.

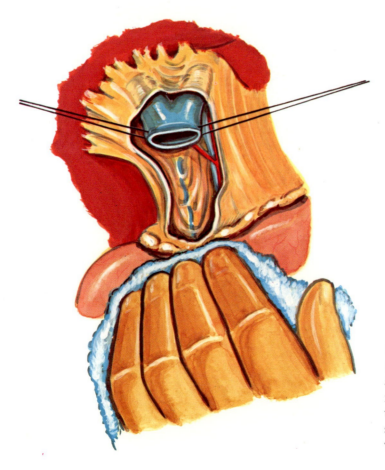

FIGURE 6-55. The stricture and surrounding scar tissue are excised and the dissection is carried up to normal, dilated proximal bile ducts. Since the distal bile duct is extremely scarred, a choledochoduodenostomy will be performed.

142

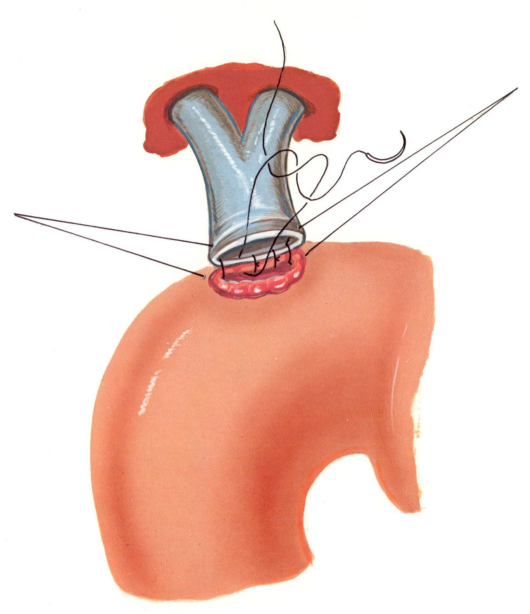

FIGURE 6-56.   Construction of an end-to-side choledochoduodenostomy. The opening should be made as wide as possible, at least 2.0 to 2.5 cm in diameter. A series of interrupted 3-0 silk sutures are placed as a posterior row. An inner row of interrupted 4-0 chromic catgut sutures are placed for mucosal approximation.

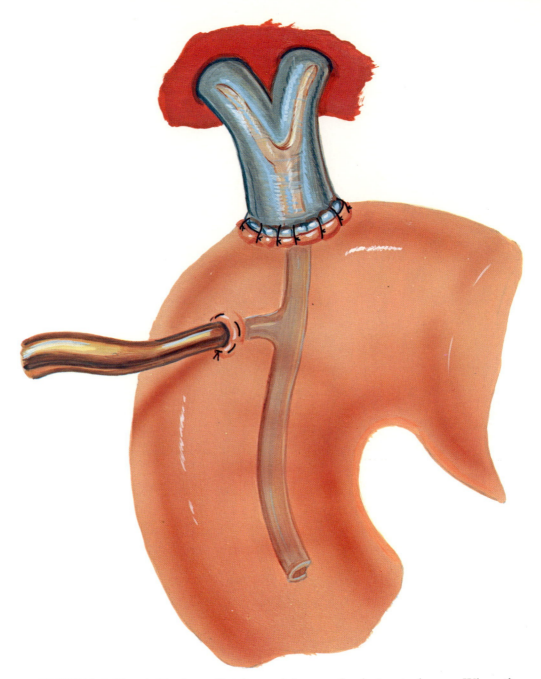

FIGURE 6-57. A T-tube splint is used frequently, but not always. When the common bile duct is greatly dilated, I do not splint it. However, if it is only moderately dilated, splinting the anastomosis protects it from bile leakage.

A Y-tube has been placed through a choledochoduodenostomy for a high biliary stricture. A separate stab incision is made in the wall of the duodenum, and a right-angle clamp is placed through this stab incision and out the area of anastomosis to grasp the long limb of the T-tube. The T- or Y-tube is then brought out through the stab incision and is placed through the anastomosis. The anastomosis is completed with interrupted 4-0 chromic catgut sutures to the mucosal layer and 3-0 silk sutures to the outer layer. A purse-string suture of 2-0 chromic catgut is used to encircle the T-tube as it exists from the duodenum to prevent leakage at this point. It is important to emphasize again that the external limb of the T-tube should not be brought out through the area of the anastomosis. T-tube or Y-tube splints are left in place 5 to 6 weeks post-operatively.

Side-to-Side Choledochoduodenostomy

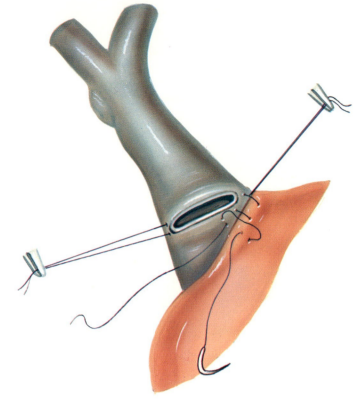

FIGURE 6-58. For patients with multiple, recurrent common bile duct stones, a choledochal cyst, or malignant (unresectable) obstruction of the distal bile duct, a side-to-side choledochoduodenostomy may be made by the identical technic described for end-to-side choledochoduodenostomy. A side-to-side choledochoduodenostomy has the *potential* disadvantage of leaving a bypassed segment of distal bile duct, which may collect debris or stones or harbor a low-grade infection. In my experience, cholangitis is rarely a problem after choledochoduodenostomy, whether performed end-to-side or side-to-side, unless the anastomosis becomes strictured. The anastomosis should be large—at least 2.5 cm in diameter.

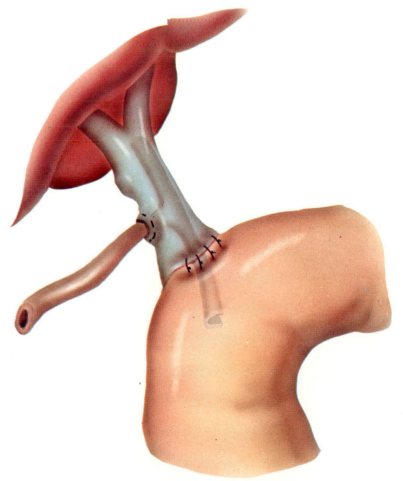

FIGURE 6-59. A T-tube splint is used if the bile duct is not greatly dilated or thickened. The external arm of the T-tube is brought out above or below, never through the anastomosis.

145

Choledochojejunostomy

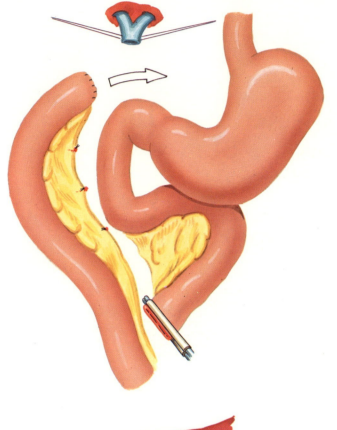

FIGURE 6-60. Choledochojejunostomy with a Roux-Y, defunctionalized jejunal segment in progress.

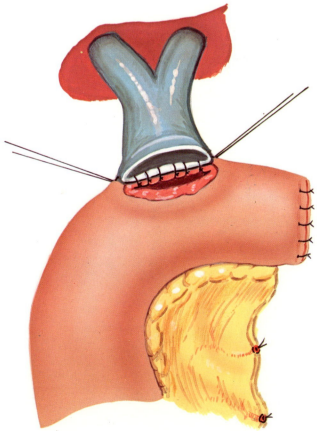

FIGURE 6-61. The end of the jejunal segment is closed with a stapling device and a second row of interrupted 3-0 silk sutures. The side of the jejunal segment is opened and sewn to the end of the proximal bile duct. A two-layer anastomosis is created with interrupted 3-0 silk sutures for the outer row and interrupted 4-0 chromic catgut sutures for the inner, mucosal row.

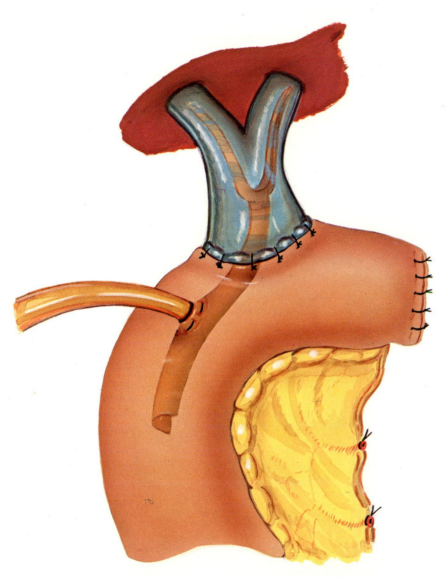

FIGURE 6-62.   A Y-tube splint in place after completion of the choledochojejunostomy. This splint is passed out the lateral wall of the jejunum through a separate stab incision, protected by a purse-string suture of 2-0 chromic catgut. The
choledochojejunostomy anastomosis has been completed with 4-0 chromic catgut
sutures to the inner, mucosal layer and interrupted 3-0 silk sutures to the seromuscular layer.

Hepatojejunostomy: "Mucosal Graft" Technic

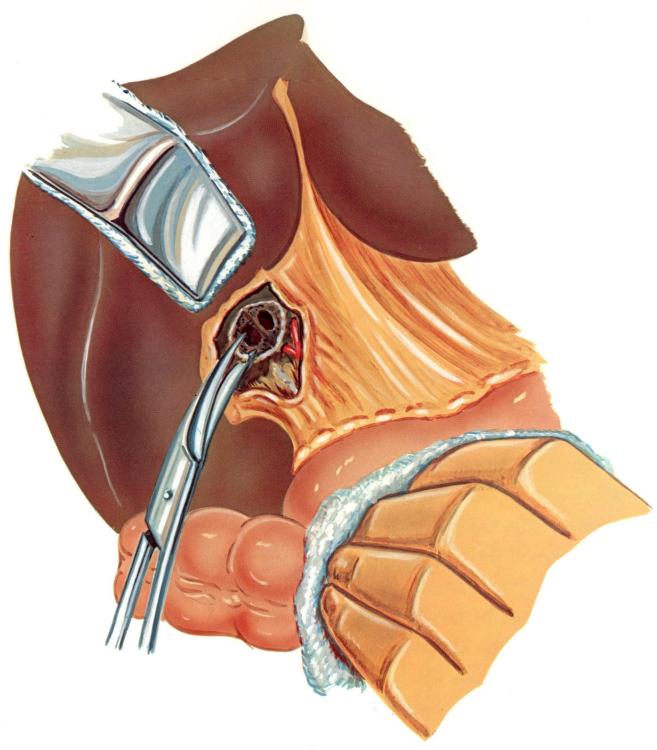

FIGURE 6-63.   In patients with high, intrahepatic, and difficult strictures of the biliary system, after operative cholangiography has identified the stricture, a 2 × 3 cm core of liver tissue is dissected away to identify the dilated right and left main bile ducts in the liver.

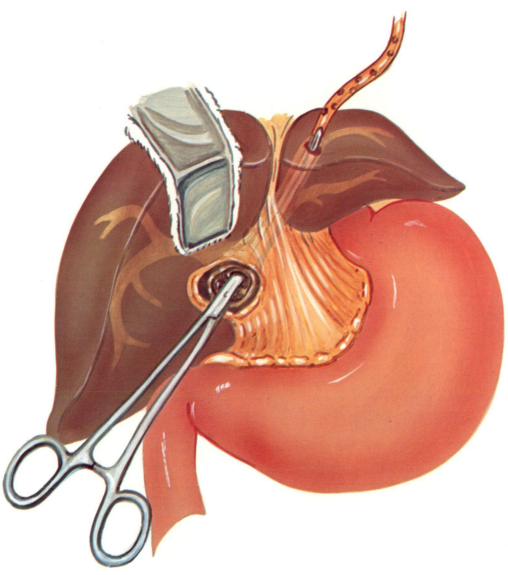

FIGURE 6-64.   A long, curved gallbladder forceps is passed up into the left intra-hepatic bile duct and thrust out the anterior surface of the left lobe of the liver; a stab wound is made in the abdominal wall and a No. 18 or No. 20 multiperforated rubber (or silastic) French catheter is grasped and brought down through the abdominal wall, the left lobe of the liver, and left main bile duct.

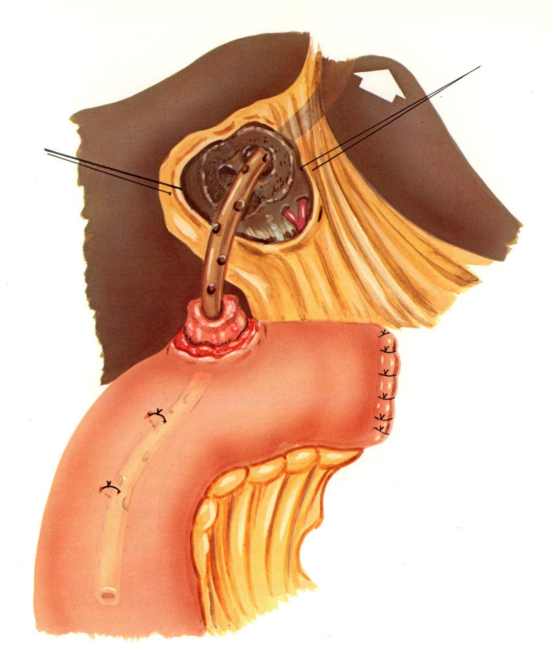

FIGURE 6-65. A Roux-Y jejunal segment is constructed and the end is closed. A button of seromuscular wall of the jejunum is cut away so that mucosa ''pouts'' up. The mucosa is then incised and the jejunum opened. The multiperforated catheter is then passed through the jejunal opening and is sewn to the wall of the jejunum with 2-0 chromic catgut sutures.

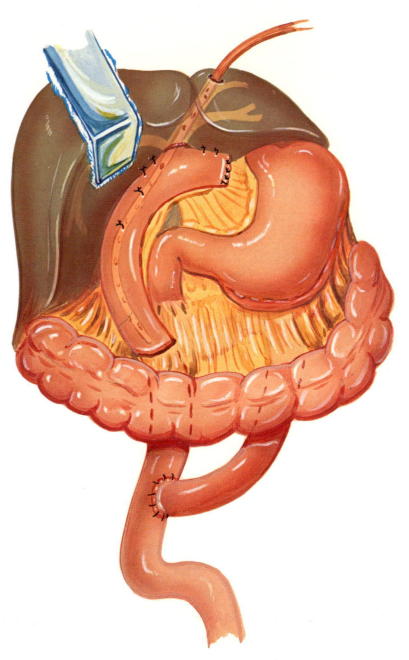

FIGURE 6-66.   With traction on the tube, the jejunum is pulled up flush against the undersurface of the liver to "graft" the mucosa of the jejunum to the opened bile ducts. The jejunum is held in place by gentle fixation of the catheter to the skin. A series of interrupted 3-0 silk sutures is then placed around the "mucosal graft" to suture the jejunum to the undersurface of the liver. This technic, reported and used extensively for biliary stricture repair by Sir Rodney Smith of London, provides mucosa-to-mucosa approximation in the repair of difficult intrahepatic strictures without the need for accurate suturing of the mucosa in this difficult intrahepatic position. The straight catheter splints the anastomosis and should be left in place for approximately 6 months or longer. The catheter can then be removed or replaced by another catheter, immediately passed into the same position. The replacement of these catheters at roughly 6-month intervals ensures continued patency of the hepatojejunostomy and prevents the accumulation of bile sludge on the catheter, which would occlude the anastomosis. The subhepatic space should be drained post-operatively.

151

Exocrine Pancreas

II

General Introduction

7

Surgical Anatomy

The pancreas is a glandular organ of the digestive system with both exocrine and endocrine functions. The surgical anatomy and endocrine physiology of the islet cells of the pancreas and the surgical management of insulinomas and other endocrine tumors of the pancreas have been described by Edis et al.[1] The following chapters cover the surgical anatomy, physiology, and management of problems of the exocrine pancreas.

Anatomists and surgeons have divided the pancreas into several parts: the head, uncinate process, neck, body, and tail (Figure 7-1). It measures 4.5 to 6 cm in width in its widest portion (the head and uncinate process) and 3.5 to 4.5 cm in its midportion, gradually tapering to a narrow tip. It is 3.5 to 4.5 cm thick in the region of the head, gradually becoming thinner toward the tail, and is 20 to 25 cm in length.[2,3]

Location and Relationships

The pancreas lies in a fixed position in the retroperitoneum, extending transversely across the upper abdomen at the level of the second lumbar vertebra and obliquely upward from the duodenal C-loop to the hilar region of the spleen. Posteriorly, the head of the pancreas overlies the inferior vena cava at the level of the right renal vessels; the neck of the pancreas lies over the aorta and the superior mesenteric vessels. The uncinate process extends to and behind the superior mesenteric vein as it passes over the third part of the duodenum. The body of the pancreas passes just above the ligament of Treitz and the duodenojejunal junction, above the left renal vessels, and over the left adrenal gland. The body and tail of the pancreas partially enclose the splenic artery and vein in a groove on its posterior surface. The tail of the pancreas lies in the hilus of the spleen[2-5] (Figure 7-2). The common bile duct passes through the head of the pancreas in its most distal third before entering the medial wall of the duodenum. Anteriorly, the pancreas is covered by the stomach, the greater omentum, and sometimes the transverse colon.

Pancreatic Ducts

The major pancreatic duct, the duct of Wirsung, runs longitudinally through the upper central pancreas, originating from multiple smaller ducts in the tail, body, neck, and head of the gland; it passes obliquely downward

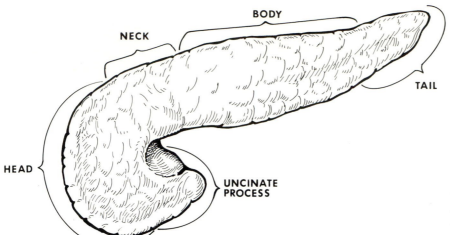

FIGURE 7-1. Parts of the pancreas: the head, uncinate process, neck, body, and tail.

parallel to the distal common bile duct in the head of the pancreas and joins the common bile duct at the ampulla of Vater to pass through the medial wall of the duodenum.[2,3,5,6] The lesser pancreatic duct, the duct of Santorini, joins with the duct of Wirsung in the neck of the pancreas and empties separately into the duodenum about 2.5 to 3 cm proximal to the papilla of Vater. Variations in the anatomy of these two ducts are common[6] (Figure 7-3). In about 10% of the patients, the duct of Santorini is the major pancreatic duct. Anatomical variations in the junction of the common bile

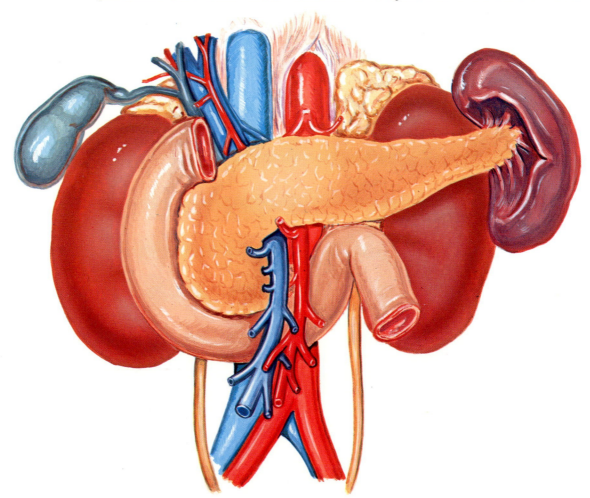

FIGURE 7-2. Relationship of the pancreas to other structures in the upper abdomen.

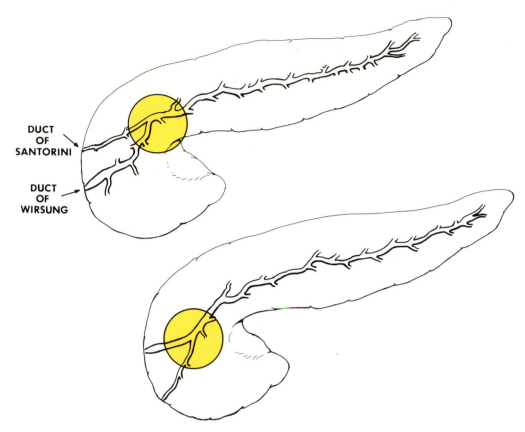

DUCT
OF
SANTORINI

DUCT
OF
WIRSUNG

FIGURE 7-3. Duct of Wirsung is the main pancreatic duct in 90% of patients; duct of Santorini is the main pancreatic duct in 10% of patients. The area where these two ducts unite in the neck of the pancreas (yellow circle) is a site of frequent congenital stenosis or of narrowing and tortuosity of the pancreatic duct system.

duct and duct of Wirsung, the size of the ampulla of Vater, and their entry into the duodenum are also common;[7] they have been described in Chapter 1 (Figure 7-4). The terminus of the pancreatic duct is surrounded by a small but well-defined sphincter integrally related to the choledochal sphincter[2] (Figure 7-5).

Arteries and Veins

The major arteries that supply the pancreas are (1) the superior and inferior pancreatoduodenal arteries (often paired) from the gastroduodenal and superior mesenteric arteries, (2) the superior pancreatic (dorsal pancreatic) artery, or arteries arising from the splenic or celiac artery, (3) an inferior pancreatic artery from the superior mesenteric, which frequently joins with the superior pancreatic artery to form the pancreatic magna artery, and (4) branch arteries from the splenic artery[8] (Figure 7-6). The veins that drain the pancreas flow into the splenic vein or the superior mesenteric vein, or they join the portal vein directly.

Pancreatic Lymphatics

The lymphatics of the pancreas follow predominantly the vascular channels of the gland and the common bile duct.[2-5,9,10] Lymph node groups draining the pancreas include the subpyloric nodes, common bile duct nodes, celiac nodes, mesocolic and superior mesenteric nodes, suprapancreatic nodes, and splenic nodes (Figure 7-7).

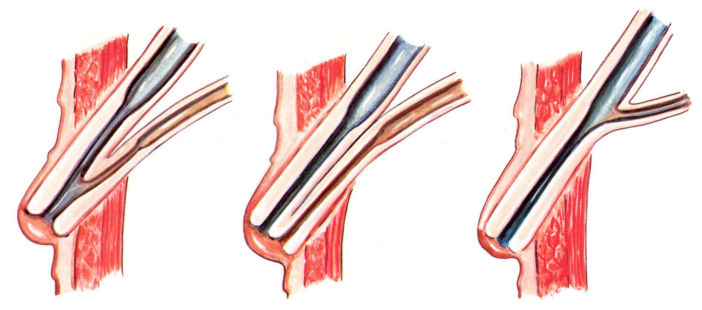

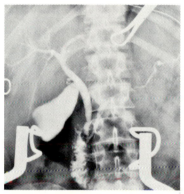

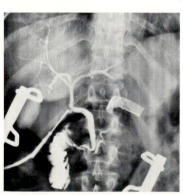

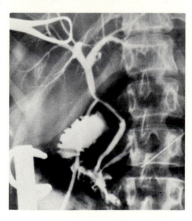

FIGURE 7-4. Distal common bile duct and duct of Wirsung join one another in a variable pattern to enter the duodenum through the papilla of Vater; the three most common patterns are shown in these operative cholangiograms. Although the two ducts usually join to form an ampulla of Vater, this union is a distal one in about 60% to 70% of patients. From anatomical studies it has been determined that a true "common channel" exists in only about 15% of patients; in about 10% to 15% of patients the two ducts open separately into the duodenum.

Nerve Supply of the Pancreas

It is important to mention and briefly discuss the innervation of the pancreas. The major and most disabling symptom of both chronic pancreatitis and carcinoma of the pancreas, especially of the body and tail, is severe pain. A main goal in the treatment of chronic pancreatitis and carcinoma of the pancreas is the relief of pain.

The pancreas is innervated by the sympathetic nervous system via the splanchnic nerves and by the parasympathetic nervous system via the vagus nerve.[3,5,10] Both the splanchnic nerves and the vagus nerve are preganglionic fibers terminating in the celiac ganglion plexus of nerves (Figure 7-8).

Pancreatic secretion is predominantly under parasympathetic (vagal) control. Pancreatic pain sensation is transmitted over sympathetic fibers to the celiac ganglion and from there to the greater, lesser, and least splanchnic nerves. Relief of pain can therefore be achieved by celiac ganglionectomy or by interruption of the splanchnic nerves.

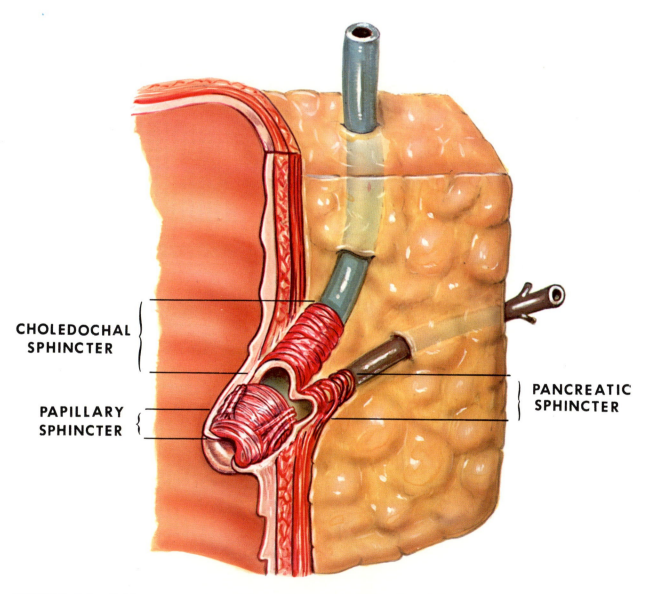

FIGURE 7-5. Sphincter complex of the sphincter of Oddi. The choledochal sphincter, pancreatic sphincter, and papillary sphincter can all be identified as separate entities by careful anatomical dissection.

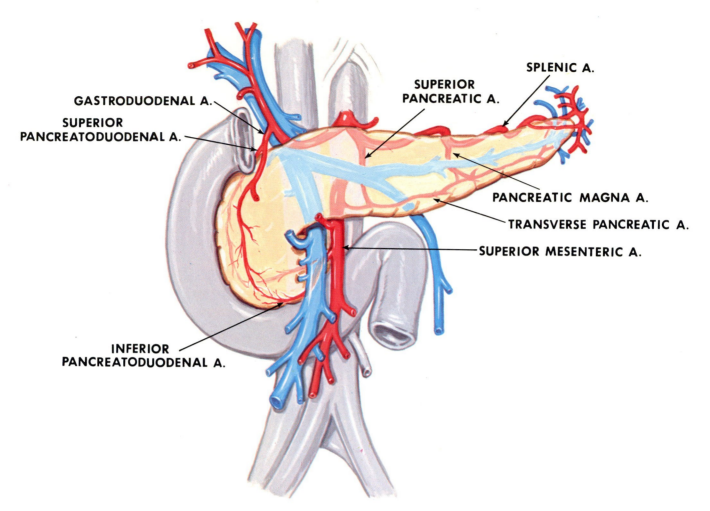

FIGURE 7-6. Major arteries and veins of the pancreas.

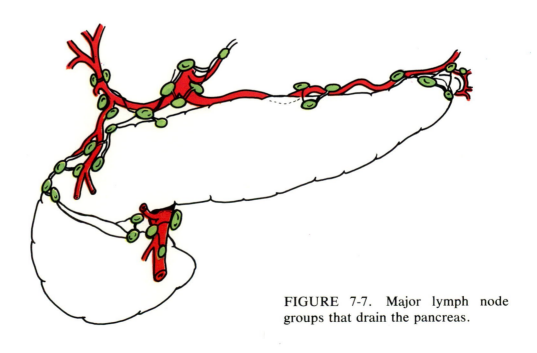

FIGURE 7-7. Major lymph node groups that drain the pancreas.

160

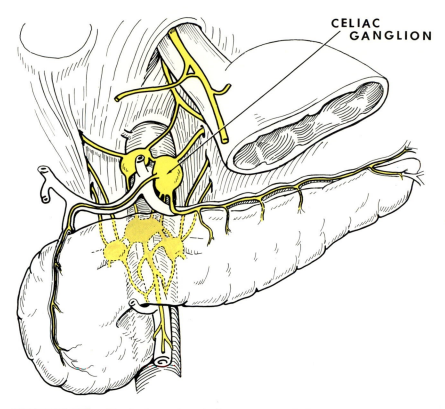

CELIAC
GANGLION

FIGURE 7-8.   Both the splanchnic nerves and the posterior (right) vagus nerve terminate in the celiac ganglion; they are thus pre-ganglionic nerves. Post-ganglionic nerve fibers originate in the celiac ganglion and innervate the pancreas.

Physiology of Pancreatic Exocrine Function

Acinar Cell

The pancreatic acinar cell is the basic cell unit of the exocrine pancreas.[11] Both hormonal and neurological stimuli act upon the cell to produce a wide variety of enzymes. These enzymes appear to originate in the zymogen granules of the acinar cell (Figure 7-9). The acinar cells are arranged around terminal ducts, so that each cell faces on a ductule (Figure 7-10). Pancreatic secretion is a continuous process, although appropriate stimulation can dramatically increase the release of enzymes and the secretion of pancreatic juice.[12-15] The zymogen granules are released from the acinar cells into the ducts, whence they flow into larger ducts and into the duodenum. Pancreatic flow pressures in the pancreatic duct system vary from 30 to 50 cm H_2O; the average is 30 cm H_2O, a pressure consistently higher than flow pressures in the bile ducts.[15-17]

Secretion of Pancreatic Juice

Hormonal and neurogenic stimuli control the secretion of pancreatic juice. The hormone pancreozymin is produced in the duodenal mucosa in response to the presence of hydrochloric acid, proteins, and fats, and promotes the excretion by the acinar cells of an enzyme (zymogen) rich, viscid pancreatic juice.[13-15,17,18] Similarly, vagal stimulation also causes the release of stored pancreatic enzymes from the acinar cell in a protein-rich, thick pancreatic juice.

The hormone secretin, which is also produced in the duodenal mucosa in response to hydrochloric acid, principally stimulates the release of

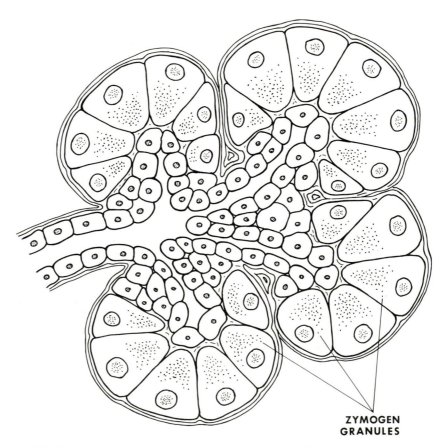

ZYMOGEN
GRANULES

FIGURE 7-9.   Typical arrangement of acinar cells around terminal ducts so that each acinar cell faces on a duct for discharge of its enzymes (zymogen granules).

162

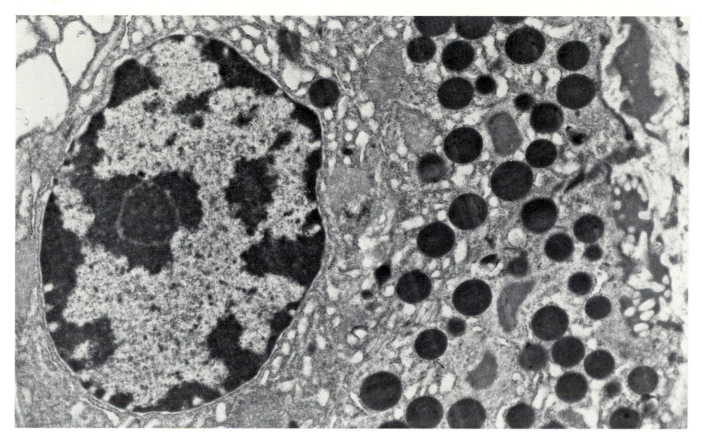

FIGURE 7-10.   Electron micrograph of a pancreatic acinar cell. A large nucleus and multiple zymogen granules are seen. ×18,900.

a thin, watery pancreatic juice low in pancreatic enzymes (zymogen granules) but high in bicarbonate content. This thin, watery secretion may come from the central pancreatic ductal cells as well as from the acinar cells.

Composition of Pancreatic Juice

The amount of pancreatic juice produced daily varies from 700 to 2000 ml, depending on the state of hydration, health of the patient, and stimuli to secrete pancreatic juice. Pancreatic juice is a clear, watery secretion that is alkaline in pH (8.0 to 8.7) and contains minerals, enzymatic proteins, and a small quantity of mucous. The consistency varies from a thin, watery fluid (during rapid rates of secretion or when stimulated by secretin) to a thicker, more viscid fluid (during periods of low flow or when stimulated by pancreozymin). The specific gravity of pancreatic juice varies from 1.007 to 1.042. The pancreas synthesizes a great deal of protein and may secrete 6 to 8 g of protein each day.[11] Table 7-1 lists the concentration of various substances in pancreatic juice obtained from human fistulas.[12,13,15,17,19]

The following enzymes are secreted by the pancreas:

1. *Amylase* is secreted in active form. Its function is to hydrolyze starch, amylodexins, and glycogen to maltose, glucose, and monosaccharides.
2. *Trypsin* is secreted in its inactive form, trypsinogen. It is activated in the duodenum on contact with the enzyme enterokinase or in the presence of active trypsin. It is a powerful proteolytic enzyme or protease.
3. *Chymotrypsin* is secreted in its inactive form, chymotrypsinogen. It is

163

TABLE 7-1   Range of concentration of various substances in human pancreatic juice

Substance	Concentration
Amylase	2000–80,000 Somogyi units/dl
Ash	520–860 mg/dl
Bicarbonate	60–75 meq/liter
Calcium	2.5–4.0 meq/liter
Chloride	60–80 meq/liter
Glucose	8.5–18.0 mg/dl
Lipase	300–3000 units/dl
Magnesium	0.3 meq/liter
Phosphatase, alkaline	0.8–12.7 Bodansky units/dl
Phosphorus	0.026–1.22 meq/liter
Potassium	4.1–5.6 meq/liter
Proteins	600–800 mg/dl
Sodium	130–145 meq/liter
Solids, organic	1240–1540 mg/dl
Sulfate	8.4 meq/liter
Trypsinogen	7.1–40 IU/dl
Trypsin inhibitor	10–60 IU/dl

SOURCE   Data from Busch[12,] Sunderman and Sunderman,[15] and Haverback et al.[19]

activated by trypsin, not by enterokinase. It is a powerful, proteolytic enzyme.

4. *Carboxypeptidases A and B* are secreted in their inactive forms, procarboxypeptidases. They are activated by trypsin and constitute the third group of proteolytic enzymes secreted by the pancreas.

5. *Leucine aminopeptidase* is a proteolytic enzyme with particularly high concentration in the pancreas. Concentrations in pancreatic juice are low.

6. *Trypsin inhibitor* is produced in normal patients in quantities sufficient to inhibit the spontaneous activation of trypsin in pancreatic juice or in serum.[19-21]

7. *Lipase* is secreted in its active form. It hydrolyzes fats into fatty acids and glycerol. Lipase activity is increased in the presence of bile salts, albumin, calcium, alcohol, and decarboxylated amino acids.

8. *Nucleases* are secreted in their active forms, ribonuclease and deoxyribonuclease. They hydrolyze nucleic acids.

9. *Elastase* splits and hydrolyzes elastic tissue, hemoglobin, fibrin, and albumin.

10. *Collagenase* attacks collagen.

11. *Lecithinase* is a phospholipase that digests lecithin, yielding lysolecithin and a fatty acid.

Activation of Proteolytic Enzymes

It is clear that pancreatic juice contains a variety of potentially damaging proteolytic enzymes in their inactive forms. When these enzymes become activated in the interstitial area of the pancreas, in the retroperitoneum, or in any area other than in the intestinal tract, cellular inflammation and necrosis occur. Much research has gone into those mechanisms whereby activation of the proteolytic enzymes occurs or can be prevented.

The activation of trypsinogen to trypsin appears to be the key to activation of all the proteases. This activation is retarded by trypsin inhibitor, normally present in pancreatic juice and in serum, by low levels of ionized calcium, and by an alkaline pH. It is promoted by decreases in trypsin inhibitor, high levels of ionized calcium, acidification, and incubation for periods of 48 to 72 hr with bile and blood, especially in the presence of infection.[19-24]

References

Surgical Anatomy

1. Edis, A. J., Ayala, L. A., and Egdahl, R. H.: *Manual of Endocrine Surgery.* New York, Springer-Verlag, 1975.
2. Anson, B. J., and McVay, C. B.: *Surgical Anatomy,* 2 vols., 2nd ed. Philadelphia, Saunders, 1971.
3. Hess, W.: *Surgery of the Biliary Passages and the Pancreas.* Princeton, N.J., Van Nostrand, 1965.
4. Carey, L. C.: *The Pancreas.* St. Louis, Mosby, 1973.
5. Howard, J. M., and Jordan, G. L.: *Surgical Diseases of the Pancreas.* Philadelphia, Lippincott, 1960.
6. Kelly, T. R., and Troyer, M. L.: Pancreatic ducts and postoperative pancreatitis. *Arch. Surg., 87,* 614, 1963.
7. Barraya, L., Pujol Soler, R., and Yvergneaux, J. P.: La region oddienne: anatomie millimetrique. *Presse Med., 55,* 2527, 1971.
8. Pierson, J. M.: The arterial blood supply of the pancreas. *Surg. Gynecol. Obstet., 77,* 426, 1943.
9. Dumont, A. E., Doubilet, H., and Mulholland, J. H.: Lymphatic pathway of pancreatic secretion in man. *Ann. Surg., 152,* 403, 1960.
10. Netter, F. H.: The Ciba Collection of Medical Illustrations, Liver, Biliary Tract and Pancreas with Supplement, vol. 3, part III. Summit, N. J., Ciba, 1962.

Physiology of the Pancreatic Exocrine Function

11. Webster, P. D.: Pancreatic acinar cells and their clinical significance. *Viewpoints Dig. Dis., 4,* 1972.
12. Busch, H.: *Chemistry of Pancreatic Diseases.* Springfield, Ill., Thomas, 1959.
13. Harper, A. A.: Progress report. The control of pancreatic secretion. *Gut, 13,* 308, 1972.
14. Haverback, B. J.: Exocrine function of the pancreas. Reappraisal of some physiological and biochemical principles. *J.A.M.A., 193,* 279, 1965.
15. Sunderman, F. W., and Sunderman, F. W., Jr.: *Measurements of Exocrine and Endocrine Functions of the Pancreas.* Philadelphia, Lippincott, 1961.
16. Howard, J. M., and Jordan, G. L.: *Surgical Disease of the Pancreas.* Philadelphia, Lippincott, 1960.
17. Zimmerman, L. M., Levine, R. (eds.): *Physiologic Principles of Surgery.* Philadelphia, Saunders, 1957.
18. Perrier, C. V., and Janowitz, H. D.: Progress in gastroenterology. The pancreas. *Gastroenterology, 42,* 481, 1962.
19. Haverback, B. J., Dyce, B., Bundy, H., et al.: Trypsin, trypsinogen, and trypsin inhibitor in human pancreatic juice. *Am. J. Med., 29,* 424, 1960.
20. Dyce, B., and Haverback, B. J.: Serum trypsin inhibitors in the normal and in patients with acute pancreatitis. *Am. J. Gastroenterol., 34,* 481, 1960.
21. Morgan, A., Robinson, L. A., and White, T. T.: Postoperative changes in the trypsin inhibitor activities of human pancreatic juice and the influence of infusion of trasyiol on the inhibitor activity. *Am. J. Surg., 115,* 131, 1968.
22. Hermann, R. E., Mitve, A., and Knowles, R. C.: The effect of bile on the activation of trypsin in pancreatic juice. Unpublished data.
23. Perrier, C. V., and Janowitz, H. D.: Progress in gastroenterology. The pancreas. II. *Gastroenterology, 44,* 493, 1963.
24. Webster, P. D. and Zieve, L: Alterations in serum content of pancreatic enzymes. *N. Engl. J. Med., 267,* 604, 1962.

Congenital Anomalies

8

Introduction

The pancreas develops from two diverticula of the primitive fetal foregut, the dorsal and ventral anlagen, which fuse to form the pancreas (Figure 8-1). The ventral anlage rotates behind the foregut to form a part of the head of the pancreas and uncinate process; the dorsal anlage forms the major part of the head of the pancreas and the body and tail. Identification of these anlagen is possible from the fourth or fifth week through the seventh week of fetal development.[1] Each anlage contains a duct; these ducts fuse in the neck of the pancreas. The duct from the ventral anlage persists as the larger duct, the duct of Wirsung, and the duct from the dorsal anlage becomes the smaller duct of Santorini. The place where these ducts fuse in the neck of the pancreas is an area of partial narrowing or tortuosity with the potential for congenital pancreatic duct stenosis or partial obstruction.

Annular Pancreas

Pathology

Annular pancreas is a relatively rare anomaly of pancreatic development whereby the developing dorsal and ventral anlagen of the pancreas encircle the duodenum with a narrow rim of pancreatic tissue (Figure 8-2). This tissue may contain all elements of the pancreas, including acinar cells, ducts, and islet cells.[2-4] The pancreatic tissue is intimately adherent or fused to the duodenal wall (Figure 8-3). The annulus may be complete or incomplete (partial) and its separation from the duodenum is hazardous or impossible. Histological studies of the annulus may show normal pancreatic tissue or, in many adults studied, may show some degree of pancreatitis and pancreatic fibrosis.[1,4,5] In addition, there may be a significant degree of duodenal stenosis and obstruction if the annulus is complete.[6,7] If the annulus is incomplete, duodenal narrowing may be minimal (Figure 8-4).

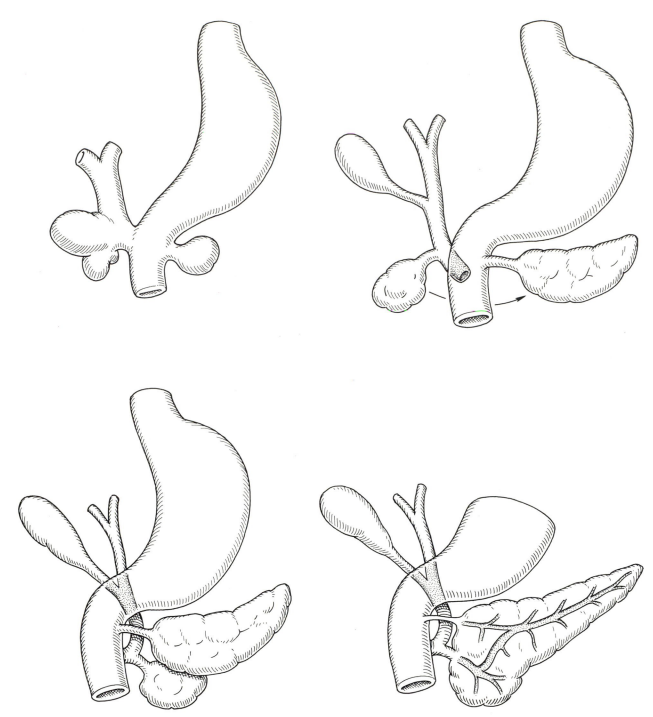

FIGURE 8-1.   Development of the fetal pancreas from two diverticuli of the fetal foregut.

Diagnosis

Annular pancreas may be diagnosed at any time from infancy through adulthood. Less than one-half of all cases are found in childhood, the majority in infancy (33% in the first year of life).[4] More than one-half of all patients do not have symptoms until their adult years. The diagnosis is uncommon during the teenage years, for unexplained reasons, but the incidence of the disease increases again during ages 20 through 50 years. In approximately 15% of patients annular pancreas is diagnosed after age 50.[5] In children the incidence in both sexes is the same; in adults the problem appears to be more common in males (66%).

168

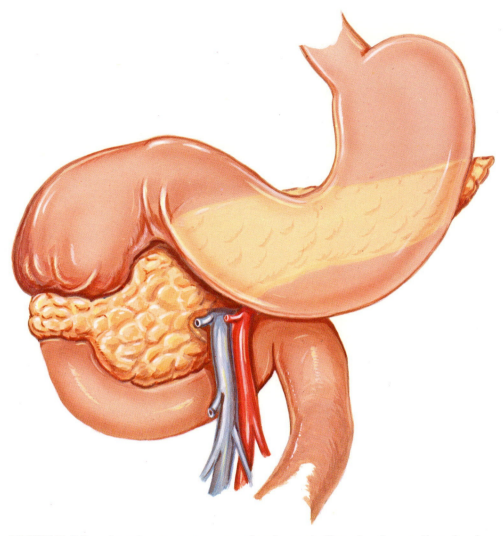

FIGURE 8-2. Annular pancreas completely encircling the descending duodenum with obstruction and narrowing of this segment. The proximal duodenum is partially obstructed and distended.

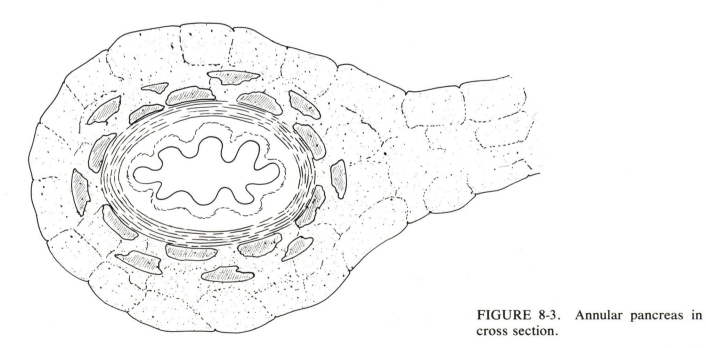

FIGURE 8-3. Annular pancreas in cross section.

169

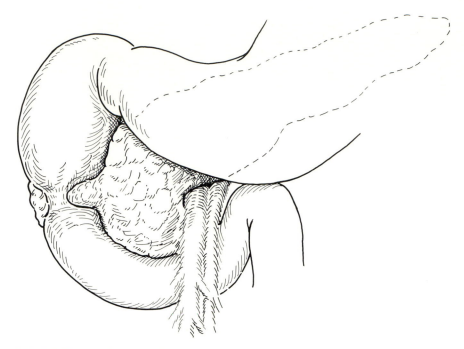

FIGURE 8-4.   Incomplete annular pancreas.

The difference in presentation of annular pancreas between infancy and adulthood depends on whether the annulus is complete or partial and on the degree of duodenal obstruction. In infants—in whom the annulus is usually complete and there is a severe degree of duodenal stenosis—acute obstructive symptoms with vomiting, inability to take feedings, and, occasionally, jaundice may occur.[6,7] A dilated duodenal bulb and stomach ("double-bubble sign") may be seen on a plain roentgenogram of the abdomen (Figure 8-5). A small amount of barium given to the infant confirms the presence of duodenal obstruction (Figure 8-6).

The differential diagnosis in an infant includes duodenal atresia, duodenal stenosis without annular pancreas, malrotation with Ladd's bands obstructing the duodenum, and duodenal webs or intraluminal diverticula.

In the adult, although the annulus may be complete, the degree of duodenal obstruction is less severe or chronic. Adults with annular pancreas usually have symptoms of duodenal ulcer from antral stasis and secondary hyperacidity, or symptoms of pancreatitis from inflammation of the annular ring or pancreatic duct obstruction.[5,8] When performing operations for duodenal ulcer with the duodenum open, one should always insert a finger down the duodenum to check for the presence of duodenal stenosis and annular pancreas. In the adult, narrowing of the duodenum is not always apparent on pre-operative upper gastrointestinal roentgenographic series with barium (Figure 8-7). The use of hypotonic duodenography or duodenoscopy may be helpful in making the diagnosis prior to surgery.

Treatment

Operative relief of the duodenal stenosis is the only effective treatment for annular pancreas. In the past, attempts made to divide the annulus have resulted in serious complications. Division of the annulus may result in pancreatic ductal injury, leakage of pancreatic juice, and a pancreatic fistula; duodenal obstruction will frequently not be relieved because of intrinsic duodenal stenosis.[3]

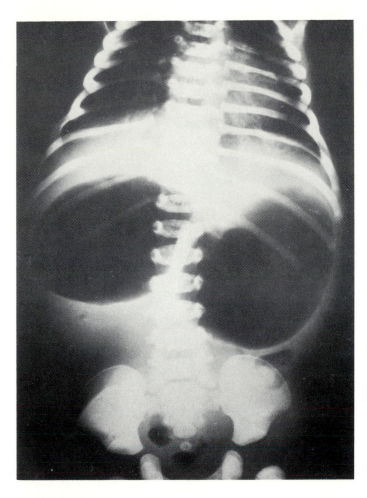

FIGURE 8-5. ''Double-bubble sign'' in an infant with an annular pancreas obstructing the duodenum.

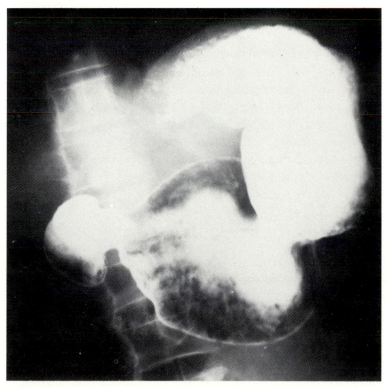

FIGURE 8-6. Complete duodenal obstruction in an infant with an annular pancreas.

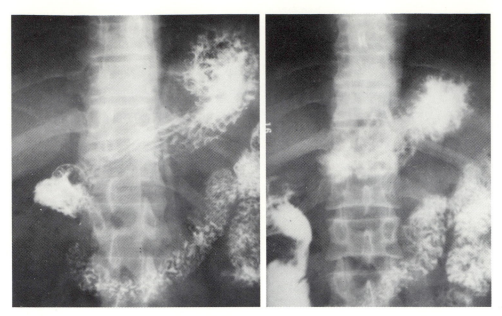

FIGURE 8-7.   Adult with an incomplete annular pancreas and minimal obstruction of the descending duodenum.

The treatment of choice is bypass of the obstructed duodenum accomplished by one of the following methods: duodenojejunostomy, joining the proximal duodenum side to side to the jejunum (Figure 8-8); duodenoduodenostomy around the annulus, if the duodenum can be mobilized adequately (Figure 8-9); or, occasionally, gastrojejunostomy (Figure 8-10).[2,3,6–8] If there has been evidence of a duodenal ulcer in an adult patient and gastrojejunostomy is performed, it is wise to protect the gastrojejunostomy by the addition of a vagotomy.

The mortality from operations to correct annular pancreas in past years has been high in 1- or 2-week-old infants (43%) because of the frequency of other severe, associated anomalies.[6,7] In recent years, with better recognition of other problems, improved methods of fluid and electrolyte replacement, and improved cardiorespiratory support, mortality has decreased. In adults the mortality from bypass procedures has always been reasonably low and should remain so. Long-term results with adequate bypass of the obstructed duodenum have been good.

Ectopic Pancreas

Accessory or ectopic pancreatic tissue can often be identified in several locations: the antrum of the stomach, the duodenum, the jejunum, and a Meckel's diverticulum. The true incidence of ectopic pancreatic tissue is unknown since there are no symptoms and the size of the ectopic pancreas is usually small.[1]

Pathology

Ectopic pancreatic tissue usually contains pancreatic acinar cells about a small duct or ducts. Islet cells are identified less frequently but have been found in ectopic locations as well. In the antrum of the stomach, ulceration of the ectopic pancreas is a frequent finding.

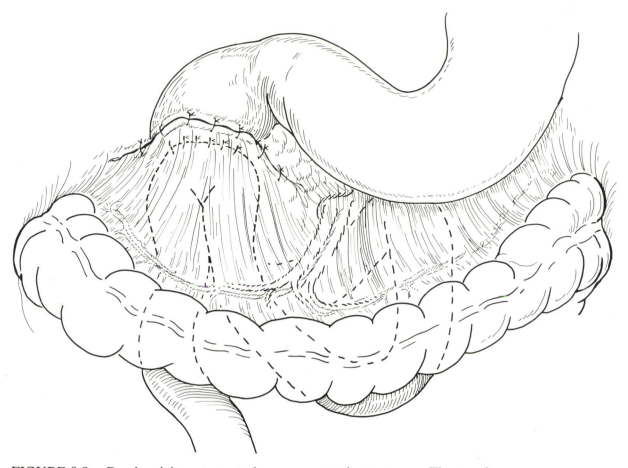

FIGURE 8-8. Duodenojejunostomy to bypass an annular pancreas. The proximal, obstructed duodenum is joined side to side to the jejunum under the transverse mesocolon.

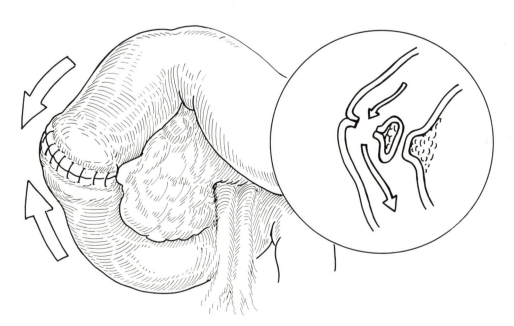

FIGURE 8-9. Duodenoduodenostomy constructed around an annular pancreas. The proximal, dilated duodenum is joined to the distal duodenum side to side to bypass the annular pancreas.

173

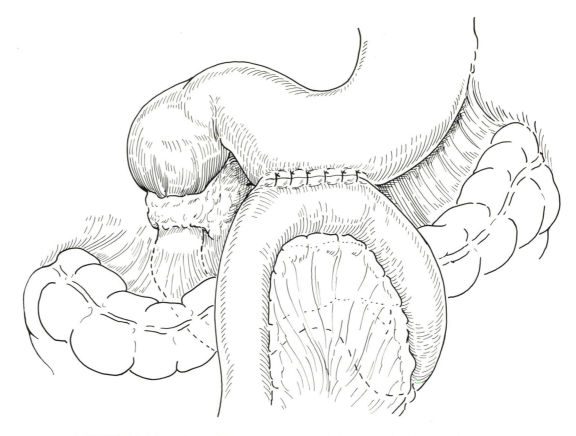

FIGURE 8-10. Gastrojejunostomy, a third method of bypassing duodenal obstruction from an annular pancreas.

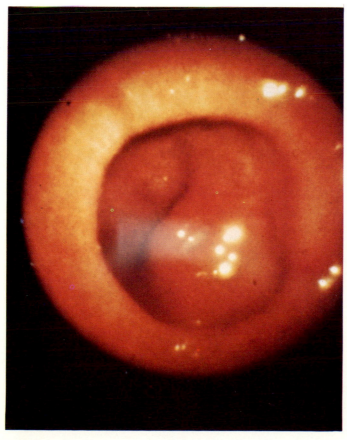

FIGURE 8-11. Ectopic pancreas found in the antrum of the stomach by gastroscopy.

Diagnosis

Since ectopic pancreatic tissue causes no symptoms in most patients, the diagnosis is usually made at operation when a biopsy is performed in an area of thickening in the antrum of the stomach or the duodenum. Symptoms of pain, peptic ulceration, and intussusception have been described with heterotopic pancreatic tissue. On upper gastrointestinal roentgenographic studies with barium, an area of ectopic pancreas in the stomach with ulceration may be confused with an ulcerating leiomyoma or leiomyosarcoma, a gastric ulcer, or localized carcinoma. The ulceration can frequently be seen at gastroscopy, and biopsies can confirm the diagnosis (Figure 8-11).

Treatment

The treatment of ectopic pancreas is surgical removal when necessary. Wedge excision of the lesion in the antrum of the stomach or in the duodenum is usually sufficient. In the jejunum, a segmental resection may be performed. In a Meckel's diverticulum, removal of the diverticulum is curative.

References

1. Gray, S. W., and Skandalakis, J. E.: *Embryology for Surgeons*. Philadelphia, Saunders, 1972.
2. Heymann, R. L., and Whelan, T. J., Jr.: Annular pancreas: demonstration of the annular duct on cholangiography. *Ann. Surg.*, **165**, 470, 1967.
3. Hyden, W. H.: The true nature of annular pancreas. *Ann. Surg.*, **157**, 71, 1963.
4. Reemtsma, K.: Embryology and congenital anomalies of the pancreas. In, J. M., Howard, and G. L. Jordan (eds.): *Surgical Diseases of the Pancreas*. Philadelphia, Lippincott, 1960.
5. Alexander, H. C.: Annular pancreas in the adult. *Am. J. Surg.*, **119**, 702, 1970.
6. Jackson, J. M.: Annular pancreas and duodenal obstruction in the neonate. *Arch. Surg.*, **87**, 379, 1963.
7. Shapiro, D. J., Dzurik, F. J., and Gerrish, E. W.: Obstruction of duodenum in the newborn infant due to annular pancreas. *Pediatrics*, **9**, 764, 1952.
8. Whelan, T. J., and Hamilton, G. B.: Annular pancreas. *Ann. Surg.*, **146**, 252, 1957.

Inflammatory Disease

9

Pancreatitis

Pancreatitis is a common cause of acute and chronic abdominal pain. It should be considered as a part of the differential diagnosis whenever a patient has upper abdominal or midabdominal pain that penetrates into the back. It is probably not diagnosed as often as it occurs because it is frequently associated with other abdominal or systemic illnesses.

Pancreatitis may be described or classified in a variety of ways: by the etiology of the disease (e.g., alcoholic pancreatitis, gallstone pancreatitis, post-traumatic pancreatitis); by the stage of the disease (from acute to chronic in a time sequence); by its severity (edematous, hemorrhagic, or necrotizing); or by its complications (pseudocyst, pancreatic ascites). All these descriptive terms are attempts to classify an inflammatory process that is still incompletely understood after many years of research and investigation.

At a symposium on pancreatitis in Marseilles, France, in 1963, four stages of the disease were defined:[1,2]

1. *Acute pancreatitis*—the first episode, frequently the most severe.
2. *Recurrent acute pancreatitis*—recurrent episodes of acute pancreatitis of moderate severity, without permanent damage to the pancreas. The gland is normal on testing or on operative exploration and biopsy between acute episodes.
3. *Recurrent chronic pancreatitis*—frequent, recurrent episodes of pancreatitis continued over a period of time. Fibrosis of the gland, acinar destruction, and ductal changes occur that are identifiable by altered pancreatic function studies, pancreatography, or operative exploration and biopsy.
4. *Chronic pancreatitis*—frequent to continuous episodes of pancreatitis lead to scarring of the pancreas, severe fibrosis, and intermittent ductal obstruction and dilatation. Pancreatic calcifications are usually seen on x-rays, pancreatic insufficiency is identified by steatorrhea and weight loss, and diabetes mellitus is frequently found.

Etiology

A variety of causes for pancreatitis have been identified. In approximately 80% to 85% of patients, a cause can be identified; in 15% to 20% no cause is apparent, and the disease is idiopathic[3-9] (Table 9-1).

TABLE 9-1   Causes of Pancreatitis

Biliary disease
Alcoholism
Trauma
Peptic ulcers
Operations on the pancreas, adjacent organs, or distant organs
Vascular ischemia
Metabolic problems: hyperparathyroidism, hyperlipemia, pregnancy, others
Systemic infections: viral and bacterial
Congenital or hereditary duct stenosis
Drug induced, toxins
Allergy
Emotions
Idiopathic

Biliary Disease.   This is the most common cause of pancreatitis in the United States. It accounts for about two-thirds of all cases admitted to private hospitals and about one-third of cases admitted to large charity hospitals and veterans' hospitals.[10-13] Gallstones probably cause pancreatitis in several ways: (1) by direct obstruction of the distal common bile duct–pancreatic duct complex at the ampulla of Vater, obstructing the flow of pancreatic juice; (2) by causing irritation and spasm of the sphincter of Oddi, thereby obstructing the flow of pancreatic juice; (3) by obstructing the ampulla of Vater, permitting a common channel of bile and pancreatic juice behind the point of obstruction; or (4) by introducing bacterial infection into the bile–pancreatic juice mixture, which changes the physiological characteristics and chemical properties of both bile and pancreatic juice and permits the flow of this incubated mixture into the higher pressure pancreatic duct system more readily under lower pressures[14-23] (Figure 9-1).

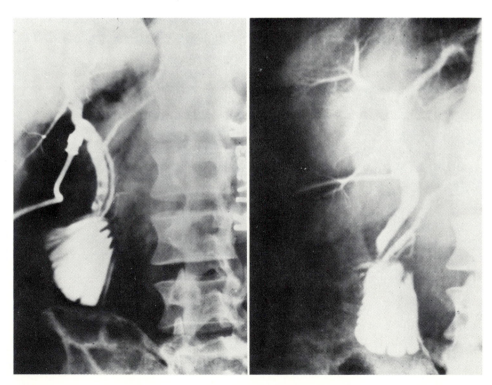

FIGURE 9-1.   Operative cholangiograms in a patient with pancreatitis showing stones in the common bile duct, spasm of the sphincter of Oddi, and reflux of cholangiographic dye into the pancreatic duct—all potential mechanisms for pancreatitis.

Acosta and Ledsesma[24] and Kelly,[25] working independently, have shown that in patients with gallstone pancreatitis the incidence of gallstones passed from the gallbladder into the common bile duct and through the sphincter of Oddi into the duodenum (recovered in the stool) is 80% to 85%.

Excessive Use of Alcohol. This is the second most common cause of pancreatitis and the *most* common cause of recurrent chronic and chronic pancreatitis in the United States.[2,5,6,11,26,27] It is the most common cause of pancreatitis in charity and veterans' hospitals. The exact relation of alcohol to the pancreas has been studied exhaustively.[28] There is some evidence that pancreatitis occurs more frequently in "binging" drinkers than in alcoholics who drink continuously, which may account for the inconstant relation between cirrhosis of the liver and pancreatitis in alcoholic patients. The intravenous infusion of alcohol in experimental animals has no evident toxic effect on the pancreas.[29] Alcohol administered directly into the duodenum causes increased pancreatic ductal pressure in dogs, but, conversely, apparently causes decreased pancreatic secretion. However, alcohol administered into the stomach causes both gastritis and pancreatic secretion through the acid–secretin mechanism.[30,31] Finally, results of recent studies have shown that excessive alcohol ingestion causes hyperlipemia and hypertriglyceridemia in many patients. Possibly pancreatitis develops in some patients after alcohol ingestion as a result of episodes of hyperlipemia. The exact mechanism of this cause of pancreatitis is being studied further.

Trauma. Trauma to the pancreas with direct injury to the gland, usually from a blunt injury, disruption of the pancreatic ducts, bleeding, and necrosis of acinar tissue is a cause of pancreatitis.[32]

Peptic Ulcer Disease. This disease may cause pancreatitis by direct penetration of the ulcer into the pancreas, causing secondary inflammatory changes, or may cause duodenitis and spasm of the sphincter of Oddi with stimulation of secretion through the acid–secretin mechanism.

Postoperative Pancreatitis. Pancreatitis can occur after operations on the biliary system, after common bile duct exploration or sphincteroplasty, after operations on the pancreas itself, after gastric resection, or after splenectomy.[33–36] It has also been described after distant and unrelated procedures, such as prostatectomy or cardiac surgery. It may be related to operative trauma to the pancreas, to vascular causes, to inspissation of pancreatic secretions and dehydration, or to circulating proteolytic enzymes in the blood stream. Postoperative pancreatitis, when it occurs, may be one of the most lethal forms of pancreatitis.

Vascular Conditions. Vascular causes of pancreatitis have been described. They include direct occlusion or spasm of the pancreatic arteries from dissecting aneurysms, and embolization of these arteries from spasm after translumbar aortography and from low-flow states as in prolonged shock or in mesenteric ischemia.[37] Vascular spasm or hypotension with inadequate perfusion of the pancreas may be a contributing factor in increasing the severity of edematous pancreatitis to hemorrhagic pancreatitis.[17,38–40]

Metabolic Conditions. Metabolic causes of pancreatitis include hyperparathyroidism, hyperlipemia, pancreatitis of pregnancy, and some heredi-

179

tary conditions of aminoaciduria, lysinuria, and cystinuria.[41-44] The mechanisms of these causes of pancreatitis are poorly understood. The role of calcium metabolism in activating pancreatic trypsinogen to trypsin has been studied by several investigators; elevated levels of serum calcium enhance this enzymatic reaction.[45,46] Serum hyperlipemia has been described both as a result of and as a cause of pancreatitis. Fat embolization of the pancreatic arterioles has been suggested by some authors.

Viral and Bacterial Infection.   These causes of pancreatitis are usually transient and mild. Pancreatitis (abdominal pain and hyperamylasemia) has been identified during mumps, infectious mononucleosis, and viral pneumonia.[47] Bacterial infection of the pancreatic duct system either by reflux of infected bile or by reflux of duodenal contents, when it occurs, may lead to severe pancreatitis.[48]

Congenital Pancreatitis.   Pancreatitis may be the result of congenital narrowing or stenosis of the pancreatic duct system in its midportion, where the ducts of Wirsung and Santorini join.[49] (Figure 9-2). This type of congenital lesion may explain many cases of pancreatitis in childhood.[4,50-53]

Drug-Induced Pancreatitis.   Pancreatitis occasionally follows prolonged usage of steroids, estrogens, azathioprine, or some chemotherapeutic agents, or it may be a result of the toxic effect of poisons such as methyl alcohol.[15,54,55] The causative mechanisms of these forms of pancreatitis are speculative.

Allergy.   Allergic causes of pancreatitis have been suggested by the experimental work of Thal, who created pancreatitis in animals through induction of both a Schwartzman and Arthus phenomenon.[7,8]

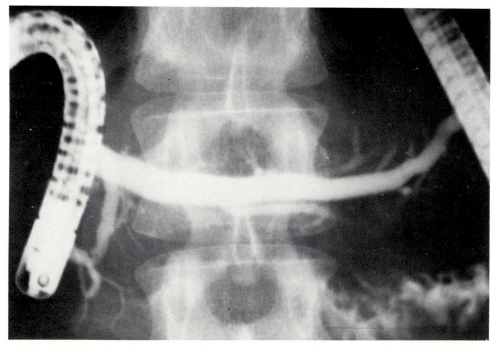

FIGURE 9-2.   ERCP demonstrating stenosis of the mid-pancreatic duct where the ducts of Wirsung and Santorini join. This patient had a history of several episodes of pancreatitis.

Emotional Problems. Emotional causes of pancreatitis are occasionally suggested by the frequent relationship of recurrent episodes of chronic pancreatitis to emotional upsets or times of tension in the lives of patients. These episodes of pancreatitis may be, in part, psychogenic in the same manner that peptic ulcer disease is related to emotional or psychogenic problems. Causative mechanisms may include acid–secretin stimulation or vagal–pancreozymin stimulation of the gland, or they may involve a more obscure metabolic change at the time of emotional stress or tension.

Idiopathic Pancreatitis. After all other causes of pancreatitis have been investigated and excluded, about 15% to 20% of patients remain with no identifiable cause for their pancreatitis.

Pathogenesis

From my observation and study of pancreatitis in its many forms, I believe that pancreatitis is most often an obstructive phenomenon in its earliest phases.[7,8,17,56–59] This obstruction is probably partial or incomplete and may occur anywhere in the pancreatic duct system, from the major ducts to the smallest ductules. In some patients with metabolic problems, the obstruction may be in the acinar cell and involve an inability to discharge zymogen granules from the cells. When pancreatic secretion is stimulated and there is ductal obstruction, pancreatic juice fills the pancreatic duct system and backs up into the interstitial or interlobular spaces of the gland. If cellular obstruction is the problem, pancreatic juice may rupture the cells and flood the pancreas. At this stage, edematous pancreatitis is seen.

As long as the proteolytic enzymes in the pancreatic juice remain in their inactive (zymogen) form, only edematous pancreatitis occurs; the edema will eventually reabsorb without permanent injury of the pancreas.

However, once any one of the following mechanisms occurs, increasingly severe pancreatitis may develop: activation of proteolytic enzymes, decrease in pancreatic trypsin inhibitor, hemorrhage from vascular injury, severe ischemia, increases in calcium concentration, hypoxemia and acidosis, reflux of enzymes (enterokinase) from the duodenum, reflux of bile into the pancreas, or bacterial infection of the edematous pancreas.[5,6,17,38,45,59–68] Any of these mechanisms can result in hemorrhagic pancreatitis or necrotizing pancreatitis with glandular destruction, necrosis of the pancreas, and massive fat necrosis in the peripancreatic tissue.

Pathology

Edematous Pancreatitis. This form is characterized by a bland watery edema of the pancreas confined within the capsule of the gland. There is no evidence of surrounding fat necrosis, inflammation, or hemorrhage. Histological studies confirm the bland nature of the edematous pancreas (Figure 9-3). There is minimal white cell response; principally lymphocytes are identified. The fluid is confined to distended ducts, intralobular and periacinar interstitial spaces.

Hemorrhagic Pancreatitis. With increasing severity of pancreatic inflammation, hemorrhagic pancreatitis may be seen in the area of the pancreas. It is characterized by hemorrhage seen grossly or microscopically in and around the pancreas (Figure 9-4). The hemorrhage may be confined to the capsule of the pancreas or may be extensive in the retroperitoneum. Vascular inflammatory changes of both thrombosis and hemorrhage may be seen in many small arteries, arterioles, and veins.

181

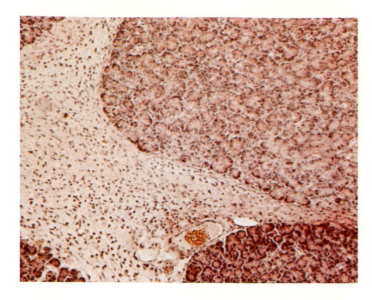

FIGURE 9-3. Edematous pancreatitis created experimentally by obstructing the pancreatic duct system.

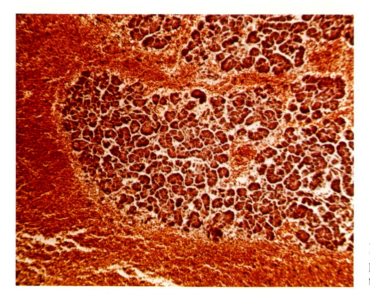

FIGURE 9-4. Hemorrhagic pancreatitis created experimentally by obstructing the pancreatic duct system and massively stimulating pancreatic secretion.

Necrotizing Pancreatitis. With severe pancreatitis, varying degrees of necrosis occur as well as hemorrhage; this stage may be termed *necrotizing pancreatitis,* especially when pancreatic necrosis predominates. Fat necrosis is also seen in and around the pancreas. Infection occurs and abscess formation, both intrapancreatic and peripancreatic, is common. An inflammatory mass or acute pseudocyst may be diagnosed clinically if there is significant swelling or entrapment of pancreatic juice in an area of pancreatic or peripancreatic necrosis. With resolution of the acute inflammatory process, depending on its severity, varying degrees of damage to the architecture of the pancreas will result. Resolution occurs with fibrosis.

Chronic Pancreatitis. This form develops with repeated episodes of inflammation. This stage of the disease is characterized by parenchymal fibrosis and scarring of the gland (Figure 9-5). Areas of stenosis and intermittent dilatation of the pancreatic ducts, interstitial calcification (calcium carbonate stones) in large and small ducts, and pancreatic juice trapped under pressure in saccular segments of pancreatic duct or in peripancreatic areas and walled off by fibrosis are commonly found.[69]

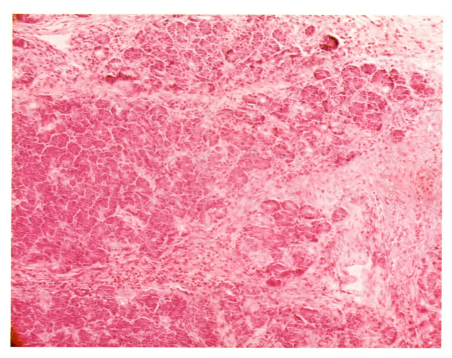

FIGURE 9-5. Repair by collagen deposition and fibrosis after acute pancreatitis.

Diagnosis

Clinical Features. Pancreatitis may have varying signs and symptoms. Most commonly, the patient has severe epigastric or central abdominal pain radiating into the back or encircling the upper abdomen like a belt. The pain may radiate to the shoulders and supraclavicular area or it may be in the left upper quadrant or right upper quadrant alone. Nausea, vomiting, and loss of appetite are common. The pain rapidly becomes constant. Abdominal distention is not usually present in mild, edematous pancreatitis but is apparent with severe pancreatitis from adynamic ileus.

Examination of the abdomen will identify mild to severe deep tenderness in the upper abdomen over the pancreas. In some patients with severe pancreatitis, an inflammatory mass may be palpated in the region of the pancreas. With severe hemorrhagic pancreatitis, peritoneal tenderness, guarding, and signs of peritonitis may be present. About 25% of patients are jaundiced. The temperature is frequently elevated. Respirations are increased and may be labored because of increased pain with diaphragmatic motion; mild hypotension to profound shock may be found. Retroperitoneal hemorrhage with flank tenderness and purplish discoloration of the skin of the flank (Grey Turner's sign) occasionally occurs.

Laboratory Studies. Since recognition by Elman et al.[70] in 1929, elevated serum amylase levels have been the classically recognized "hallmark" of pancreatitis. However, the serum amylase levels may rise only transiently and may return to normal 2 to 3 days after a mild attack of edematous pancreatitis; they may not rise at all in patients with chronic pancreatitis with a badly damaged, "burned out" pancreas; or the levels may rise in association with other acute intra-abdominal problems such as perforated duodenal ulcer, acute cholecystitis, acute cholangitis, small bowel obstruction, or mesenteric vascular occlusion.[71-73] Therefore, although the serum amylase determination is an essential study in a patient suspected of having pancreatitis, it is a finding that does not always correlate with the disease. Furthermore, the height of the amylase level does not correspond to the severity of the pancreatitis.

The urinary amylase level may be elevated for 2 to 3 days after the onset of acute pancreatitis since amylase is cleared from the serum through the kidneys and excreted in the urine. Warshaw and Lesser[74] and others[75] have emphasized the value of urinary amylase clearance studies in patients with pancreatitis. In patients with pancreatitis, the renal threshold for amylase is decreased and amylase excretion is increased. The normal amylase/creatinine ratio is 2% to 4% or less; in pancreatitis this ratio is elevated.

Paracentesis and measurement of amylase content in the peritoneal fluid may be the most valuable diagnostic study in a patient suspected of having pancreatitis. Peritoneal fluid levels of amylase are strikingly elevated in patients with pancreatitis.

The serum lipase level also rises and this is a valuable diagnostic study in patients with acute and chronic pancreatitis. Its rise is somewhat slower and more prolonged than the serum amylase level.

Serum calcium determinations are extremely important in any patient suspected of having pancreatitis. With severe, hemorrhagic, or necrotizing pancreatitis, serum calcium levels fall, often to very low levels (5.5 to 7.5 mg/dl). A significant decrease in serum calcium levels, shock, fever, and an elevated white blood cell count are prognostic signs that indicate severe and potentially lethal hemorrhagic pancreatitis.[76]

Blood glucose levels are frequently elevated in patients with pancreatitis and serum insulin levels may be decreased from pancreatic inflammation. Serum bilirubin levels may be elevated, as noted previously, and liver function tests may be deranged with elevation of the SGOT and alkaline phosphatase levels.

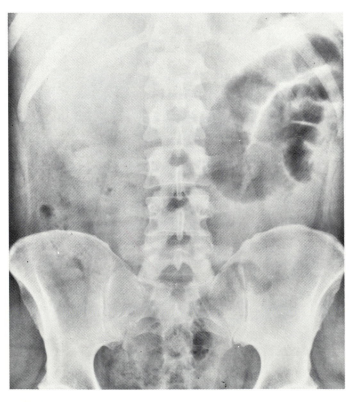

FIGURE 9-6. Dilated "sentinel" jejunal loop, occasionally seen in patients with acute pancreatitis.

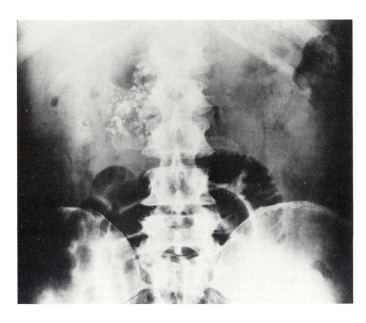

FIGURE 9-7. Calcification scattered throughout the pancreas. The calcific deposits are somewhat denser in the head but can also be seen in the body and tail of the gland.

Methemoglobin determinations have been reported to be elevated in patients with severe hemorrhagic pancreatitis.[77] We have not found them to be of value in diagnosis or in predicting the severity of the disease.

Roentgenographic Studies. A plain roentgenogram of the abdomen will frequently show a dilated, "sentinel" jejunal loop adjacent to the body or tail of the pancreas (Figure 9-6). In patients with recurrent chronic or chronic pancreatitis, calcification will be seen in the area of the pancreas (Figure 9-7). This is the hallmark of chronic alcoholic pancreatitis, but it may occasionally occur in patients with chronic pancreatitis due to other causes.

An oral cholecystogram usually shows no visualization of the gallbladder for 2 weeks to 1 month after an episode of pancreatitis. However, an intravenous cholangiogram frequently identifies the common bile duct and visualizes the gallbladder if there is no accompanying cholecystitis. It is thus a more valuable test to rule out biliary disease in a patient thought to have pancreatitis.[78,79]

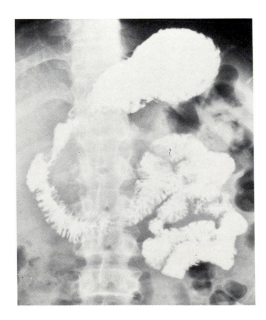

FIGURE 9-8. Upper gastrointestinal barium series showing edema and widening of the C-loop of the duodenum. This patient had resolving acute pancreatitis with an inflammatory mass suspected in the head of the pancreas.

185

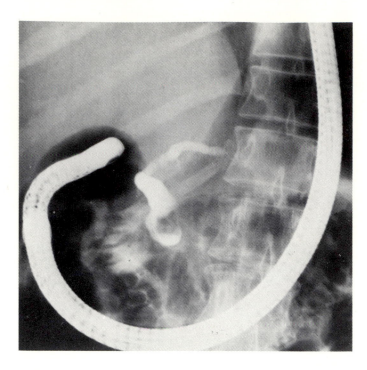

FIGURE 9-9. ERCP showing stenosis of the papilla of Vater with cystic dilatation of the pancreatic duct. (Some air has been introduced into the duct.) This obstruction was corrected by sphinteroplasty.

If an upper gastrointestinal series using barium is performed in a patient with subsiding acute or chronic pancreatitis, distortion of the stomach with elevation of the stomach anteriorly and forward, widening and straightening of the duodenal C-loop, and mucosal edema may be seen (Figure 9-8). This may be the best way to identify or clarify the presence of a pancreatic mass or a pseudocyst.

Pancreatic scans using selenomethionine[80] are of little or no value in pancreatic inflammatory disease.[78] They will usually show evidence of parenchymal disease with diffuse, deficient uptake of the radioisotope selenomethionine.

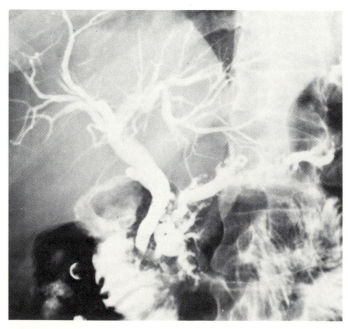

FIGURE 9-10. ERCP showing intermittent areas of stenosis and dilatation of the pancreatic ductal system.

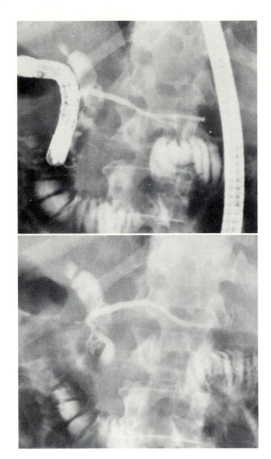

FIGURE 9-11. ERCP with multiple stones in the distal common bile duct, the probable cause of recurrent episodes of pancreatitis. The pancreatic duct is slightly dilated, possibly as a response to irritation and spasm of the sphincter of Oddi.

Endoscopic retrograde cholangiopancreatography (ERCP) should not be performed in the patient with acute pancreatitis during an episode of the disease. However, ERCP is of great value in identifying intrinsic biliary or pancreatic duct pathology in the patient with recurring episodes of pancreatitis or chronic pancreatitis when all signs of acute inflammation have subsided[81,82] (Figure 9-9). Areas of stenosis or dilatation of the pancreatic ducts can be seen, indicating a need for operative correction of these areas of pancreatic duct obstruction (Figure 9-10). In addition, stones in the common bile duct undetected by oral or intravenous cholangiography may be seen—thus the cause of the repeated episodes of pancreatitis may be identified (Figure 9-11).

Ultrasonography (echography) has recently been introduced and is becoming increasingly valuable in identifying pancreatic pseudocysts, stones in the biliary system, and inflammatory swelling of the pancreas or gallbladder[78] (Figure 9-12). Ultrasonograms, using the B-mode gray-scale unit, are being refined. Small cystic lesions larger than 2 cm can be seen, and larger lesions are readily apparent. The differentiation of a pseudocyst from a swollen, inflamed pancreas is possible.

Treatment

Acute Pancreatitis. The patient suspected of having acute pancreatitis should be hospitalized. During the first 12 hr of the episode it may not be possible to determine the potential severity of the attack. Thus all patients should be treated vigorously and careful observations should be made to determine whether the episode will be transient edematous pancreatitis or may progress to severe hemorrhagic or necrotizing pancreatitis.

187

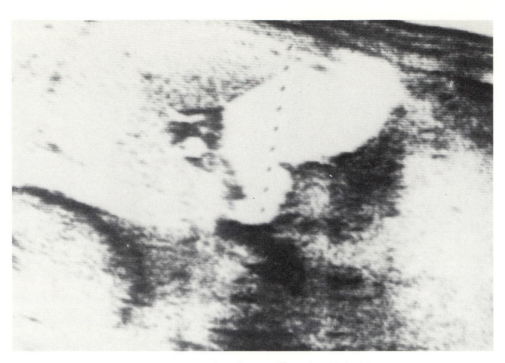

FIGURE 9-12.   Ultrasonogram showing a dilated gallbladder and bile duct with "swelling" of the pancreas.

MEDICAL THERAPY.   Initial therapy for pancreatitis should be medical. A nasogastric tube should be placed for nasogastric suction in order to block the acid–secretin stimulation of the pancreas. Fluid replacement therapy is essential to replace fluids lost by vomiting, gastrointestinal ileus, and intrapancreatic, intraperitoneal, and retroperitoneal transudation. Saline, plasma, and blood may be necessary, especially if pancreatic or gastrointestinal hemorrhage occurs. Calcium replacement with intravenous calcium gluconate may be necessary. Placement of a central venous catheter may be necessary to aid in the assessment of adequate fluid replacement therapy. Urinary output should be measured frequently.[83–85]

The use of anticholinergic drugs in the treatment of acute pancreatitis is controversial. I frequently use atropine or propantheline bromide, 15 mg q.i.d. intramuscularly, in young patients, as I believe these drugs offer some additional advantage in blocking parasympathetic (vagal) stimulation of the pancreas. I avoid their use in elderly patients because of the increased pulmonary complications and urinary retention associated with their use.

The use of antibiotics is also controversial; they should not be given routinely.[86] I prescribe them when the patient has a temperature over 100F and an elevated white blood cell count. My choice is usually cephalosporin, 500 mg q.i.d. intravenously, because of its broad-spectrum coverage. Blood cultures and sensitivities should be drawn for more specific antibiotic therapy after the first few days of broad-spectrum coverage.

Narcotics must be given liberally during an episode of acute pancreatitis as the pain can be intense. My choice is meperdine hydrochloride (Demerol), 100 mg intramuscularly every 3 to 4 hr. Supplementation with a tranquilizer such as hydroxyzine pamoate (Vistaril), 25 mg given concurrently, may be of value. Morphine is avoided because of its spasmodic effect on smooth muscle (sphincter of Oddi).[21] Other medications and drugs for the treatment of acute pancreatitis have been advised through the years

based on their effectiveness in experimental animals. However, none of these medications has been proven effective in acute pancreatitis in humans. These drugs include steroids, glucagon, acetazolamide (Diamox), low molecular weight dextran, propylthiouracil, and the proteinase inhibitor aprotinin (Trasylol).[87-98] As in patients with hemorrhagic shock, vasopressor agents should never be used to treat hypotension in patients with acute pancreatitis.[88] Peritoneal lavage has been effective in some patients.[99]

Most patients with acute pancreatitis respond to intensive medical therapy and all symptoms subside within 2 to 10 days. However, some patients do not improve and a complication of acute pancreatitis develops or they become progressively sicker with deteriorating vital signs.

INDICATIONS FOR OPERATION. In patients who have been treated intensively by medical therapy and initially respond, then deteriorate or get worse, operative exploration of the pancreas should be considered.[76,100,101] The indications for operation are (1) failure to improve with adequate, intensive medical therapy after 24 to 36 hr, (2) uncertainty about the diagnosis, and (3) treatment of a complication of pancreatitis (pancreatic abscess, pancreatic or retroperitoneal hemorrhage).

OPERATIVE STRATEGY. At operation, the surgeon should explore the entire abdomen to confirm the diagnosis of acute pancreatitis. As noted previously, a perforated duodenal ulcer, acute cholecystitis or cholangitis, small bowel obstruction, or a strangulated or infarcted mesenteric segment may be confused with acute pancreatitis by virtue of abdominal pain and hyperamylasemia. These conditions are potentially correctable by surgery. If nothing but severe pancreatitis is found, I irrigate the abdomen with saline, open the lesser peritoneal sac, drain and gently debride any areas of pancreatic necrosis, place a large tube (No 30) in the gallbladder (cholecystostomy) to decompress the biliary system, place two or three sump suction catheters in the upper and lower abdomen, and close the abdomen (Figure 9-13). I do not place a gastrostomy tube or feeding jejunostomy tube as advocated by Lawson and associates,[102] nor do I attempt to assess the biliary system for gallstones. If a large stone can be palpated or removed at the time of cholecystostomy, I remove it. I believe that in a critically ill patient with severe pancreatitis, cholecystectomy, operative cholangography, or common bile duct exploration should be left for another time.[103] The object of the operation is threefold: (1) to confirm the diagnosis of pancreatitis; (2) to decompress the biliary system (because of the incidence of biliary obstruction that accompanies acute pancreatitis and the frequency of common bile duct stones obstructing the biliary–pancreatic ducts); and (3) to remove necrotic tissue and peritoneal fluid in which toxic products of enzymes–blood–bacteria are accumulating.

Although the value of emergency subtotal or total pancreatectomy has been reported from time to time, our experience with this operation is poor.[104,105] We have performed it on three patients, with two post-operative fatalities. It is a serious and difficult operation for the patient because of the hemorrhagic necrosis of the pancreas and retroperitoneal area.

COMPLICATIONS. PANCREATIC ABSCESS. A pancreatic or peripancreatic abscess may occur during the course of acute pancreatitis in about 5% of patients.[106] Spiking fevers, ileus, abdominal tenderness, and a prolonged septic course from 10 days to 2 weeks after onset of the illness should make one consider a pancreatic abscess. An echogram or CT scan

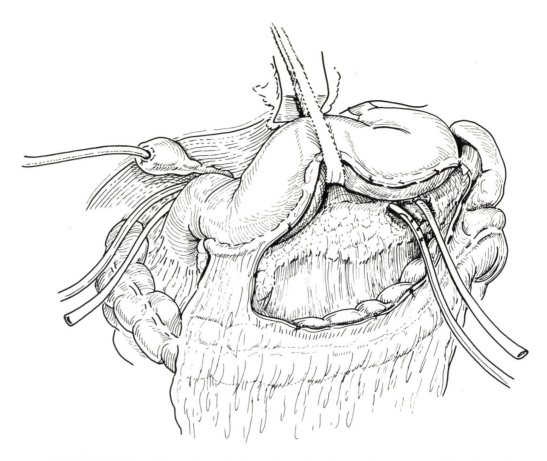

FIGURE 9-13.   After abdominal exploration for acute pancreatitis, the peritoneal cavity is drained with sump suction tubes and drains in the lesser peritoneal
sac, the areas around the pancreas, the subhepatic space, and the pelvis. A cholecystostomy tube is used to decompress the biliary system.

of the pancreas may help identify an abscess; a gallium scan may be helpful. A plain abdominal roentgenogram may show a "soap bubble" appearance of air–fluid level from gas-forming organisms in the abscess (Figure
9-14). Operative exploration and drainage is essential.[107–110]

INFLAMMATORY MASS (ACUTE PSEUDOCYST).   An area of pancreatic
or peripancreatic necrosis that remains sterile may become acutely swollen
and edematous with entrapped fluid and pancreatic juice. A tender abdominal mass may be noted. In the absence of fever, severe pain, or obvious
sepsis the correct treatment of this complication is observation. Over a
period of time (2 to 4 weeks) the inflammatory mass or acute pseudocyst
spontaneously subsides in 50% to 60% of patients. In 10% to 20% of patients, increasing symptoms may force an urgent operation, or the mass
matures into a chronic pseudocyst and persists, requiring a later operation
for drainage.[111]

If an acute pseudocyst or inflammatory mass requires operation, external drainage to outside the abdomen is the ideal treatment. The wall of
this type of inflammatory collection of fluid is not sufficiently mature or fibrotic to hold sutures for an internal drainage procedure to the stomach or
jejunum. A temporary pancreatic fistula may result but will usually close
spontaneously.

A full discussion of chronic pseudocyst as a complication of pancreatitis is presented in the section on Pseudocysts of the Pancreas.

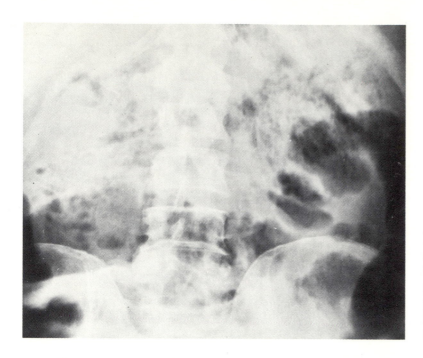

FIGURE 9-14. Plain roentgenogram of the abdomen showing a "soap bubble" appearance in the region of the pancreas from pancreatic and peripancreatic abscesses. From S. Kollins: *Surgery of the Pancreas,* 1978. Courtesy of Mosby.

HEMORRHAGE. A complication of acute pancreatitis can be hemorrhage into the pancreas, the retroperitoneum, or the intraperitoneal cavity. It may be from small pancreatic arteries or veins, or from erosion of a major vessel such as the splenic vein or artery. Its cause is an extension of the necrotizing process from the pancreas. Occasionally, massive bleeding into the gastrointestinal tract from a stress ulcer or erosive gastritis is the cause of the hemorrhage.[112,113] An operation may be necessary to stop the bleeding by ligation or oversewing of the bleeding vessels in the pancreas, by splenectomy and ligation of the splenic vessels, or by vagotomy and pyloroplasty and oversewing of stress erosions in the stomach or duodenum.

RESPIRATORY FAILURE. Acute respiratory failure has become an increasingly common complication of acute pancreatitis.[114,115] Whether this problem is being seen more frequently because of the overuse of fluids or because patients with acute pancreatitis are being increasingly saved from death caused by sepsis, only to develop pulmonary insufficiency, is not known. There has been speculation that circulating pancreatic enzymes affect the capillaries in the alveoli of the lungs, causing fluid loss into the interstitial spaces and alveoli. Respiratory support and treatment with mechanical, volume-controlled respirators may be necessary.

MORTALITY. It is difficult to obtain accurate mortality statistics for patients with acute pancreatitis since many patients with mild, edematous pancreatitis and pancreatitis secondary to acute cholecystitis may not be diagnosed. From all studies of patients with diagnosed acute pancreatitis, the overall mortality rate reported is probably less than 5%. If patients with mild, edematous pancreatitis are excluded, however, the mortality rate is approximately 15%. In patients who have severe hemorrhagic or necrotizing pancreatitis (shock, decreased serum calcium levels, fever, elevated white blood count), the mortality rate is between 40% and 50%. The mortality rate of patients operated on for pancreatic abscess is approximately 35%.[10,80,116–119]

From studies we have reported, the most common cause of death in the first 4 days of the episode is shock and inadequate fluid replacement.[90]

The most common cause of death from the fifth day to the second week is sepsis and respiratory failure. The most common cause of death from the second to the fourth week after onset is hemorrhage, although continuing sepsis or infection still accounts for many deaths.

Interval Period.   After an episode of acute pancreatitis has subsided, careful studies should be performed to ascertain the cause of the pancreatitis. These studies should include oral or intravenous cholangiograms, upper gastrointestinal roentgenograms with barium (to identify a peptic ulcer), tests of parathyroid function, blood lipid studies, and careful questioning of the patient and his family in regard to the use of alcohol.

If no cause can be determined, further tests of biliary or pancreatic function, or both should be considered. A duodenal drainage study using cholecystokinin stimulation of the gallbladder and inspection of the duodenal aspirate for cholesterol crystals should be considered. The morphine evocative test has been advocated by Nardi and Acosta[21] as a test for "papillitis" or stenosis of the sphincter of Oddi. Serum amylase levels are obtained after morphine sulfate, 10 mg, and prostigmine, 1 mg, are given intramuscularly. A positive test is an elevated serum amylase, above 400 Somogyi units, after morphine–prostigmine stimulation.

If biliary disease, peptic ulcer, or hyperparathyroidism is diagnosed, these problems should be corrected surgically. If no surgical problem is identified, the patient is kept on a low-fat, bland diet and a mild antispasmodic such as Donnatal tablets, 1 t.i.d. before meals, is prescribed. Alcohol in all forms must be avoided.

Recurrent Pancreatitis.   Repeated episodes of acute pancreatitis are again treated as described previously. With recurring episodes of the inflammatory process, the seriousness of the episodes often decreases. However,

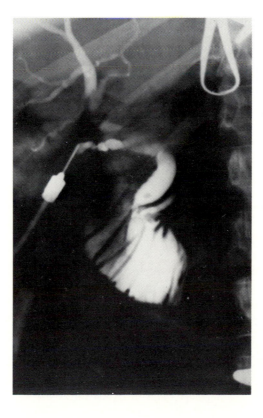

FIGURE 9-15.   Operative cholangiogram in a patient with recurrent pancreatitis. A stone is seen in the distal bile duct.

lethal episodes of acute hemorrhagic pancreatitis occasionally have been described during a second, third, or fourth episode.

With repeated episodes of pancreatitis, if no cause can be identified for the disease, and if the patient has tried to follow a reasonably low-fat, bland diet and has avoided alcohol, an ERCP study should be advised. This study should be performed during an interval period, at least 2 weeks after an attack of recurrent pancreatitis has subsided. Frequently, hidden biliary pathology, stenosis of the papilla of Vater, or stenosis of the intra pancreatic ducts may be found[81,120–123] (Figures 9-9 and 9-10).

OPERATIVE STRATEGY. If a patient has had more than three episodes of recurrent pancreatitis in the absence of a history of alcoholism or any other obvious cause for the pancreatitis, I advise biliary and pancreatic exploration.[124] At operation, an operative cholangiogram and operative pancreatogram are performed (Figures 9-15 and 9-16). Depending on the findings of these studies, I do one or more of the following procedures: cholecystectomy, common bile duct exploration, sphinteroplasty and pancreatic duct exploration, pancreatic duct drainage (longitudinal pancreatojejunostomy), or partial pancreatectomy and drainage of the distal pancreas with a Roux-Y jejunal segment. The decision as to which operative procedure or which combination of procedures to perform requires surgical judgment based on the course and severity of the disease and the pathological anatomy of the pancreas and pancreatic duct seen at operation.[125] The operative pancreatogram or endoscopic pancreatogram done pre-operatively

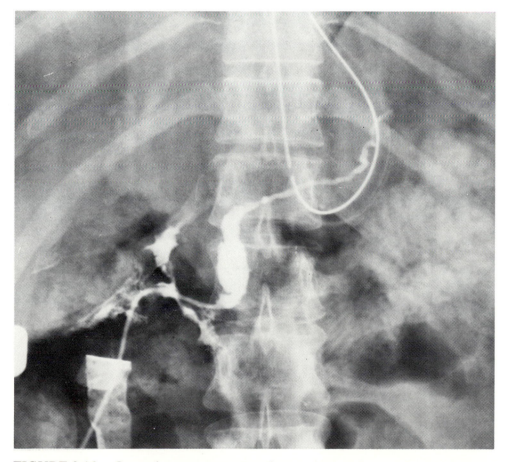

FIGURE 9-16. Operative pancreatogram in a patient with recurring episodes of pancreatitis showing distention of the pancreatic duct. A transduodenal sphincteroplasty was performed.

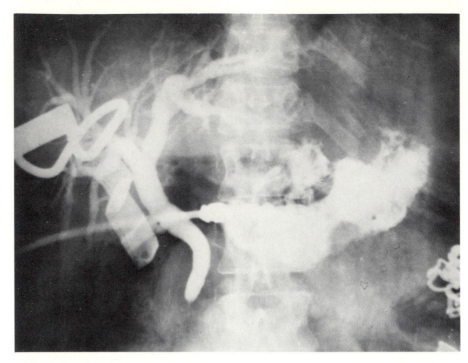

FIGURE 9-17.   Operative pancreatogram showing a massively dilated pancreatic duct. A longitudinal pancreatojejunostomy was performed.

provides the key to rational operative judgment as to whether there is enough evidence of pancreatic duct obstruction to correct with a ductal drainage operation alone or whether a distal pancreatic resection may be necessary.[10,126–140] (Figures 9-17 and 9-18). My philosophy for most pa-

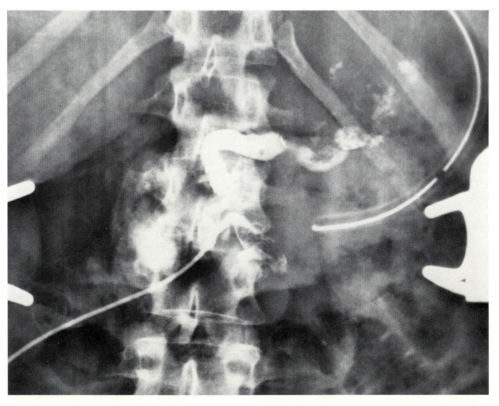

FIGURE 9-18.   Operative pancreatogram showing a dilated duct with severe distal ductal deformity. A distal pancreatectomy was performed; the proximal duct was drained by a Roux-Y jejunal segment.

tients with recurrent pancreatitis is to be conservative; I prefer a ductal drainage procedure to a major pancreatic resection whenever possible at this stage of the disease.

RESULTS. Approximately 70% to 75% of patients with recurring episodes of pancreatitis have had good or excellent control of their disease after one or more of the conservative operative procedures described. If biliary disease was the cause of the pancreatitis, the results of operation have been much better—in the range of 80% to 85% successful control of the disease —than if alcoholism or an idiopathic, undetected problem was the cause of the pancreatitis.[10,133,140]

Chronic Pancreatitis. When further episodes of pancreatitis lead to pancreatic fibrosis, calcifications in the pancreas, steatorrhea and weight loss, early or mild diabetes, and recurring or constant episodes of pain requiring narcotics, the diagnosis of chronic pancreatitis can be made.[141] Alcoholism is a cause in most but not all patients whose disease progresses to this stage. We have had patients with biliary disease and idiopathic pancreatitis in whom the disease progressed to chronic pancreatitis, identical to alcoholic pancreatitis.

OPERATIVE STRATEGY. At this stage of the disease treatment must be directed at the pancreas. It can be drained if areas of ductal stenosis remain with segmental pancreatic duct dilatation, or the pancreas can be resected.[27,142-149] Finally, if nothing further can be done, a bilateral splanchnic resection can be performed for relief of pain.[150] In our experience, this procedure is less effective in relieving pain in patients with chronic pancreatitis than in relieving pain in patients with carcinoma of the pancreas.

The decision as to operative therapy must again be based on the remaining function of the pancreas and the pathological anatomy found at operation, especially that of the pancreatic duct system as shown by an operative pancreatogram (Figures 9-19 and 9-20) If the patient is not diabetic, or is only mildly so, and has remaining useful pancreatic function with mild

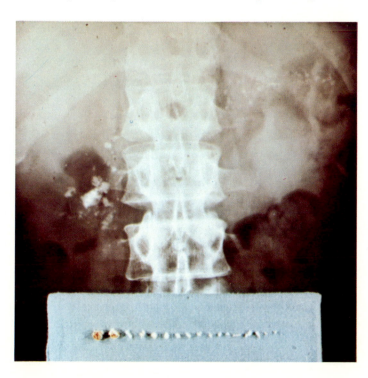

FIGURE 9-19. Patient with chronic pancreatitis. A sphincteroplasty and pancreatic duct exploration was performed with curettage and removal of pancreatic duct stones. The operative pancreatogram showed predominant obstruction at the sphincter of Oddi.

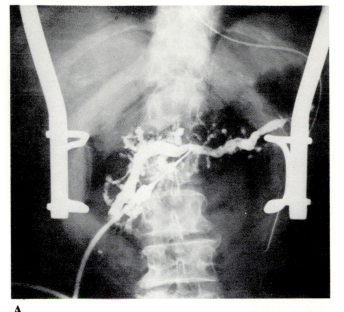

A

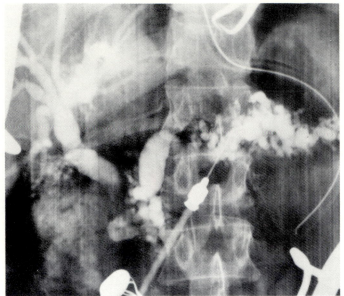

B

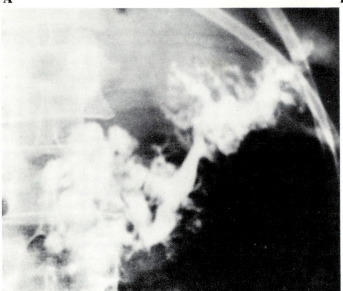

C

FIGURE 9-20. Operative pancreatograms showing varying stages of chronic pancreatitis. The classical findings of "chain of lakes" deformity, intermittent stenosis and dilatation of the obstructed pancreatic duct, are demonstrated (**B** and **C**).

steatorrhea and weight loss, I am conservative in regard to pancreatic resection. I would prefer a partial pancreatectomy of the most fibrotic segment of the pancreas (Figure 9-21), up to an 85%, resection, with longitudinal pancreatojejunostomy of the remaining gland to adequately drain the pancreatic duct into a Roux-Y jejunal segment. In patients with end-stage, chronic pancreatitis with little or no remaining pancreatic function and severe chronic pain, a radical subtotal pancreatectomy would be performed, as advocated by Child and associates.[151-153]

RESULTS. Table 9-2 lists 140 operations Dr. Stanley O. Hoerr and I have performed for recurrent chronic and chronic pancreatitis in 99 patients from 1961 to 1973. We achieved good results after surgery in approximately 65% of patients; 35% had further episodes of pancreatitis or pain, or required other operative procedures. The mortality rate for operations on the pancreas in patients with recurrent chronic or chronic pancreatitis was 5%. If alcoholism is the cause of the chronic pancreatitis and cannot be controlled, the long-term prospects for control of the disease are discouraging.

1 CM

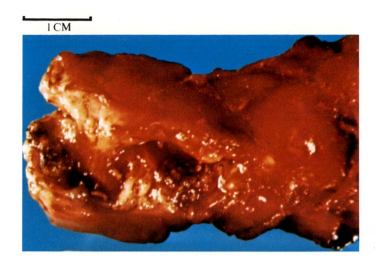

FIGURE 9-21. Operative specimen of resected pancreas with chronic pancreatitis.

TABLE 9-2   Operations for Recurrent Chronic and Chronic Pancreatitis[a] (1961–1973)

Procedure	No.
Cholecystectomy, common bile duct exploration	37
Biliary bypass	23
Sphincteroplasty and pancreatic duct exploration	21
Drainage of pseudocyst	19
Pancreatojejunostomy	9
Subtotal pancreatectomy, with or without pancreatojejunostomy	11
Others: exploration, biopsy, drainage of abscess, vagotomy, and pyloroplasty	20
Total	140

[a] Operations were performed by S. O. Hoerr and R. E. Hermann.

197

Pseudocysts of the Pancreas

Pseudocysts must be distinguished from true cysts and neoplastic cysts of the pancreas. Approximately 90% of all pancreatic cysts are pseudocysts; 10% are primary or true cysts, cystadenomas, or cystadenocarcinoma.[159] Pseudocysts are fibrous-lined cystic collections of pancreatic juice and necrotic pancreatic tissue that develop after pancreatitis, carcinoma, or trauma. They result from pancreatic secretions that collect in damaged areas of the pancreas, in the lesser peritoneal cavity, or in areas adjacent to the pancreas. They may be classified as *acute,* i.e., those transient cystic collections that occur during or after an episode of acute pancreatitis, or *chronic,* i.e., those that gradually develop over a period of weeks or months after an episode of pancreatitis or pancreatic injury.[160,161]

Pseudocysts are caused by pancreatitis in the majority (75%) of patients.[162] In 15% to 20% of patients they are the result of trauma to the pancreas; in 5% to 10% of patients they are caused by pancreatic duct obstruction from cancer of the pancreas, or they are idiopathic.[163–165] In children, trauma to the pancreas is the leading cause of pseudocyst.[166,167]

The frequency and incidence of pseudocysts are unknown. In patients with severe, acute pancreatitis, acute pseudocysts can be diagnosed in up to 50% of patients by ultrasonography.[160,168–170] The incidence in recurrent or chronic pancreatitis is estimated at between 5% and 10%.[159,169,171]

Pathology

Pseudocysts are characterized histopathologically by the absence of glandular or ductal epithelium in the wall of the cyst. The cyst wall consists of fibrous tissue, usually with evidence of recent or subsiding inflammation (Figure 9-22). The presence of an epithelial lining establishes the diagnosis of a primary or true cyst of the pancreas or a neoplastic cyst (cystadenoma or cystadenocarcinoma), as opposed to a pseudocyst. The interior of the pseudocyst frequently contains necrotic pancreatic tissue. The cyst fluid is

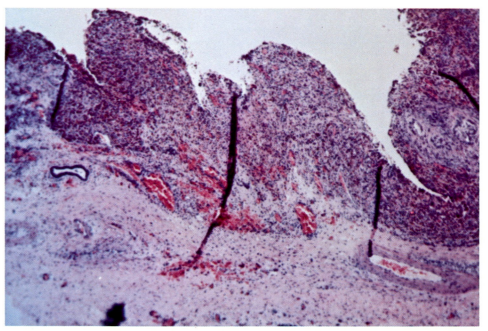

FIGURE 9-22. Photomicrograph of the wall of a pseudocyst. The wall consists of fibrous connective tissue with evidence of chronic inflammation.

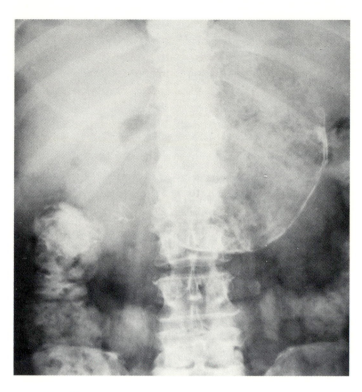

FIGURE 9-23. Plain abdominal roentgenogram showing a calcified pseudocyst.

usually clear pancreatic juice, rich in amylase; occasionally it may be dark or colored by old hemorrhage. Areas of fat necrosis around a pseudocyst are frequently seen. The walls of old, chronic pseudocysts may occasionally be calcified (Figure 9-23).

Diagnosis

Clinical Features of Acute Pseudocysts. An acute pseudocyst may be termed an *inflammatory mass* of the pancreas. As noted, such an inflammatory mass may be found by ultrasonography or other careful diagnostic studies in up to 50% of patients. This type of acute pseudocyst consists of pancreatic tissue and pancreatic juice in various stages of injury, inflammation, necrosis, or repair. Hemorrhage may be a prominent feature. The patient has signs and symptoms of acute pancreatitis, usually in the subsiding phase. Epigastric pain, fullness, anorexia, nausea and vomiting, and weight loss are common.[160,162,169,172–175] The history of onset of the pancreatitis or of trauma is that of a recent episode, perhaps several days or weeks. An acute pseudocyst will usually be seen on follow-up evaluation to subside gradually over the next 2 to 4 weeks.[160,161]

Clinical Features of Chronic Pseudocysts. The patient with a chronic pseudocyst of the pancreas has a history of trauma or pancreatitis several weeks or months preceding development of the abdominal mass. The pancreatitis has subsided and there is usually a disease-free interval in which the patient has returned to varying degrees of good health. Gradually, epigastric discomfort, a sense of heaviness or fullness, nausea, anorexia, and weight loss are noted. Most prominently, the patient notes an enlargement of the upper abdomen or development of a tender mass.[159,162,169,174,176]

On physical examination, the main finding is a mass with varying degrees of tenderness in the upper abdomen in the region of the pancreas. In approximately 10% of patients, atypical features or complications may exist, such as jaundice, hemorrhage, perforation, or pancreatic ascites.[170,172,175,177–183]

Laboratory Studies. Routine laboratory tests should be obtained in all patients. Liver function studies may show some degree of abnormality, especially the alkaline phosphatase and SGOT levels, or occasionally an elevated bilirubin level. The serum amylase levels are usually elevated to three to four times normal, occasionally to even higher levels, in at least two-thirds of all patients.[184] Serum amylase levels are rarely as high as in patients with acute pancreatitis. Urinary amylase levels are also frequently elevated.

Roentgenographic Studies. A plain roentgenogram of the abdomen may show a homogeneous density in the upper abdomen or the region of the lesser peritoneal sac. Occasionally calcification is seen in a chronic pseudocyst (Figure 9-23). An upper gastrointestinal roentgenographic series using barium should be performed in all patients. This usually reveals extrinsic compression deformity of the antrum or body of the stomach and widening of the duodenal C-loop (Figure 9-24). Barium studies of the colon may show downward displacement of the transverse colon. An ultrasonogram or CT scan is helpful in diagnosing pseudocysts larger than 2 cm and is helpful in indicating, by density determination, whether a pancreatic mass is solid or cystic.[168]

Complications. The principal complications associated with pseudocysts are infection of the cyst, jaundice, perforation of the cyst into the peritoneal cavity with the development of pancreatic ascites, erosion of the pseudocyst into an adjacent organ such as the stomach or colon, and erosion of the pseudocyst into the splenic artery or vein, with massive hemorrhage into the cyst.[170,172,175,177-183] Of these complications, massive hemorrhage into the cyst is the most critical, requiring immediate operative exploration to control the bleeding; it has the highest mortality rate. Pre-operatively a selective celiac–superior mesenteric arteriogram is helpful in identifying the site of bleeding. Cogbill[179] reported a mortality rate of 50% associated with hemorrhage into a pseudocyst. Occasionally a pseudocyst erodes into an adjacent organ and massive hemorrhage occurs, with the additional complication of massive gastrointestinal bleeding from the splenic vessels through the pseudocyst into the stomach or colon.

The next most critical complication of a pseudocyst is infection of the cyst. This complication may result from undue delay in operative exploration and drainage of the cyst. Spontaneous rupture of a pseudocyst into the peritoneal cavity with the development of pancreatic ascites is discussed in the section on Pancreatic Ascites. Unless the pseudocyst fluid is infected, rupture of the pseudocyst may go unnoticed until ascites develops. The development of jaundice in patients with pancreatic pseudocysts is usually caused by obstruction and narrowing of the distal pancreatic duct by compression distortion of the common bile duct as it passes through the head of the pancreas (Figure 9-25).

Treatment

The treatment of pseudocysts of the pancreas must be individualized. Treatment of an acute pseudocyst differs from that of a chronic pseudocyst.

Acute Pseudocysts. At least 50% or more of all acute pseudocysts resolve spontaneously, usually within 6 weeks after detection. All acute pseudocysts or inflammatory masses that develop during an episode of acute pan-

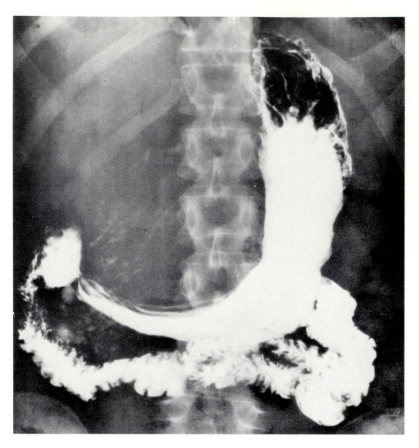

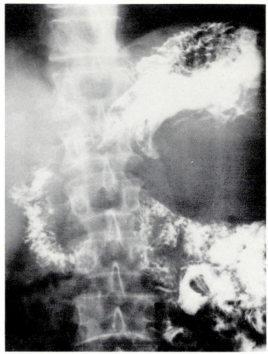

FIGURE 9-24. Gastrointestinal series with barium showing displacement of the antrum and body of the stomach, typical of a pseudocyst of the pancreas.

creatitis should be initially treated medically and observed for up to 6 weeks. Small (less than 5-cm) asymptomatic pseudocysts, especially those diagnosed by ultrasonography, may be observed for 2 or 3 months before surgery is decided upon. If the pseudocyst is enlarging or becomes symptomatic, operative exploration should be performed.

If a patient with an acute pseudocyst has evidence of infection of the cyst, pain increases, or hemorrhage develops, immediate operative exploration should be performed.[160] An acute pseudocyst or inflammatory mass should be drained externally, any necrotic pancreatic tissue debrided, the fluid and pancreatic tissue cultured, and the bleeding from peripancreatic vessels carefully controlled. Because an acute pseudocyst lacks

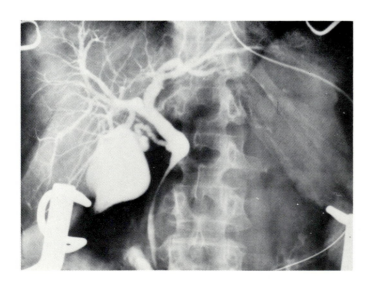

FIGURE 9-25. Pseudocyst in the head of the pancreas may distort the distal common bile duct, occasionally leading to obstruction of the biliary system.

201

a firm, fibrous wall, it is hazardous to attempt internal anastomosis of this type of pseudocyst with the stomach or other intra-abdominal organs.

Chronic Pseudocysts. A pseudocyst that gradually develops after an episode of pancreatitis or pancreatic injury, or a pseudocyst that persists after an episode of acute pancreatitis and gradually enlarges, develops a firm, thick, fibrous wall lining. An acute pseudocyst matures in approximately 6 weeks. Chronic pseudocysts are usually large—frequently 6 to 12 cm or larger in diameter. Operative exploration should be advised for internal drainage or excision of the pseudocyst.

At operative exploration, a pseudocystogram should be obtained. This is performed by direct needling of the cyst cavity, directly into an area to be used for drainage. (Figures 9-26 and 9-27). This will demonstrate whether the pseudocyst communicates with the main pancreatic duct or whether it is multilocular. Although the former reason is academic, the latter is of practical importance; if the cyst is multilocular, an opening into both adjoining pseudocyst cavities must be made to provide effective drainage.

An operative cholangiogram is also of great value in showing the presence or absence of stones in the common bile duct, distortion of the duct, or its anatomical location in case cystoduodenal drainage is contemplated. A cholangiogram is essential if there has been a history of jaundice associated with the cyst.

Most pseudocysts are intimately adherent to the posterior wall of the stomach and can be drained most effectively by cystogastrostomy.[171,173,185–190] A biopsy specimen of the pseudocyst wall should always be submitted for examination. The cyst fluid should be cultured and submitted for cytological study and amylase determination.

Although cystogastrostomy is most commonly performed, internal drainage into other intra-abdominal organs is also effective. Cystojejunostomy with a Roux-Y jejunal segment and cystoduodenostomy are also performed. Table 9-3 shows the method of drainage of 46 pseudocysts of the

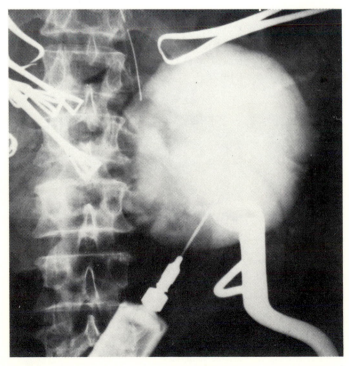

FIGURE 9-26. Pseudocystogram showing a large, unilocular cystic collection in the head and neck of the pancreas.

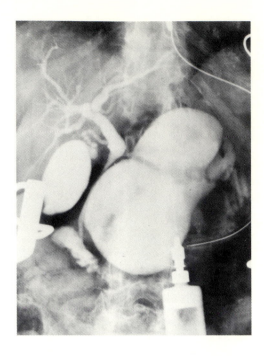

FIGURE 9-27. Pseudocystogram showing a multilocular cyst cavity in the body of the pancreas.

pancreas in patients operated upon at the Cleveland Clinic during 1962 to 1973.[187]

After internal drainage of a pseudocyst, the pseudocyst wall collapses and the anastomotic opening between the pseudocyst and the organ of internal drainage becomes obliterated; in most patients this occurs 1 to 3 weeks after internal drainage.[185,186,190] Barium or food can rarely be demonstrated to reflux into the pseudocyst cavity after internal drainage procedures.

Small pseudocysts of the tail of the pancreas may occasionally be excised (Figure 9-28). Excision of a pseudocyst has been performed by most surgeons in less than 10% of cases. Excision should probably be confined to pseudocysts of the tail of the pancreas.

When a pseudocyst has eroded into the splenic vessels and hemorrhage occurs, wide opening of the pseudocyst, ligation of the splenic artery and vein with suture ligatures of 2-0 silk, and splenectomy are necessary.[172,177,179,180,182] The remaining cyst cavity should be drained externally.

The most common complication of internal and external drainage of pseudocysts is post-operative bleeding from the wall of the cyst, from the splenic vessels, or from the anastomotic margin. This complication occurs in about 5% of patients and is slightly more common after cystogastrostomy

TABLE 9-3 Operations for Pseudocyst (Cleveland Clinic, 1962–1973)

	No.
Internal drainage	
Cystogastrostomy	21
Cystojejunostomy (Roux-Y)	6
Cystoduodenostomy	1
External drainage	11
Excision of cyst	3
Total	42

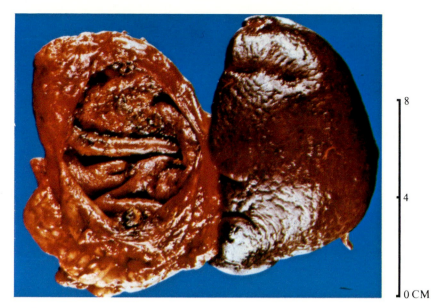

8

4

0 CM

FIGURE 9-28. Operative specimen of a pseudocyst of the tail of the pancreas. The thick cyst wall lining can be seen with necrotic pancreatic tissue inside the cyst.

than after cystoduodenostomy, cystojejunostomy, or external drainage. Occasionally, after cystogastrostomy, hemorrhagic gastritis may be the cause of bleeding. A bland diet should be given to patients after cystogastrostomy.

Results. The operative mortality of cystogastrostomy, cystojejunostomy, or cystoduodenostomy is approximately 5%[159,187] The recurrence rate of pseudocysts has been reported to be 10% to 15%.[159,191] A pancreatic fistula develops in up to 25% of patients who have had external drainage. This external fistula usually closes spontaneously but may require subsequent operative closure.

Pancreatic Ascites and External Pancreatic Fistulas

Pancreatic ascites and external pancreatic fistulas both represent leakage of pancreatic juice out of the pancreatic duct system, into the peritoneal cavity in patients with pancreatic ascites and outside the abdominal cavity through a fistulous tract in patients with an external pancreatic fistula. Although the exact site of leakage of pancreatic juice has not been conclusively demonstrated in all patients reported with pancreatic ascites, in the majority of the cases reported a pancreatic ductal or pseudocyst leakage point has been identified.

Pancreatic Ascites

Pancreatic ascites has been described as a complication of pancreatitis or of pancreatic pseudocysts only during the past 25 years.[192,193] The incidence seems to be increasing as case reports are reviewed and added to the surgical literature. Jordan[194] has stated the pancreatic ascites occurred in 6% of his patients with pseudocysts of the pancreas. Although malignant ascites may be a late complication of carcinoma of the pancreas and ascites may occur in association with alcoholic cirrhosis or with advanced chronic pancreatitis, the type of pancreatic ascites that has increased so dramatically is that caused by rupture of the pancreatic duct system with leakage of pancreatic juice into the abdominal cavity.[192,195−197]

Pathology. Most patients with pancreatic acites have a pseudocyst of the pancreas that ruptures and leaks pancreatic juice into the peritoneal cavity with a resultant internal pancreatic fistula. Less commonly, pancreatic ascites may be present in a patient with chronic pancreatitis without a pseudocyst. The duct leakage point may be difficult to identify. In addition, ascites may transiently accompany acute hemorrhagic pancreatitis. This type of hemorrhagic ascites is temporary and clears spontaneously with treatment of the pancreatitis. Rarely, chronic pancreatitis may cause ascites by massive inflammatory or cicatricial obstruction of the retroperitoneal lymphatics without direct leakage of pancreatic juice into the peritoneal cavity.

Diagnosis. Pancreatic ascites is usually a painless, gradual accumulation of ascites in a patient with a history of chronic (usually alcoholic) pancreatitis, a recent history of pancreatic injury or blunt abdominal injury, or an episode of recurrent pancreatitis within the past 4 to 6 months. The diagnosis is made by performing paracentesis, obtaining an amylase determination of the ascitic fluid, and comparing it to the serum amylase.[193,195] Cytological examination of the fluid and cultures for routine organisms and tuberculosis should always be performed. Although the serum amylase is moderately elevated (300 to 800 Somogyi units), the amylase level in the ascitic fluid is usually very high, in the range of 3000 to 8000 Somogyi units. In addition, protein levels in the ascitic fluid are elevated, in the range of 2.5 to 4.0 g/dl. When ascitic fluid amylase levels are significantly higher than serum amylase levels, the diagnosis of pancreatic ascites is secure.[193−196] Results of liver function studies are usually normal.

Occasionally pleural effusion accompanies pancreatic ascites. Pleural fluid amylase and protein levels are also elevated and the diagnosis is made by thoracentesis and examination of the pleural fluid.

205

Identification of the site of pancreatic duct leakage can often be made pre-operatively by ERCP (Figure 9-29). Pseudocysts may occasionally be seen.

At operation, operative pancreatography may be a diagnostic aid in identifying the point of pancreatic duct leakage, as well as the anatomy of the pancreatic duct system and the presence of pseudocysts (Figure 9-30).

Treatment. MEDICAL TREATMENT. A trial of medical therapy should be attempted initially in the treatment of pancreatic ascites. It has been successful in clearing the ascites in 30% to 45% of patients.[193,195,196] Nasogastric suction, Diamox, atropine, multiple paracenteses, total parenteral nutrition, and peritoneal lavage have all been effective in patients with acute pancreatic ascites.[195] It is probably worthwhile to attempt a trial of medical therapy for 2 to 3 weeks in asymptomatic patients without significant pancreatic duct leakage demonstrated on ERCP.

When a significant pancreatic duct leak is demonstrated, if the ascites is massive, a large pseudocyst is demonstrated, or medical therapy is unsuccessful, operative correction of the pancreatic ascites is indicated.

OPERATIVE THERAPY. At operation, every effort should be made to identify the pancreatic duct leak. It usually can be seen grossly, if not found by pre-operative endoscopic pancreatography or operative pancreatography. When it is found, a defunctionalized Roux-Y jejunal segment is used to reintroduce the pancreatic juice back into the intestinal tract by pancreatojejunostomy. If a pseudocyst is found, a cystojejunostomy (Roux-Y) should be performed to decompress and internally drain the pseudocyst. Occasionally, a distal pancreatectomy may be considered, which involves resection of the area of pancreatic leakage and the use of a Roux-Y jejunal segment to drain the pancreatic duct and the divided distal pancreas.

RESULTS. The operative mortality in good risk patients should be less than 5%. Long-term results are usually good; the pseudocyst or pancreatic ascites recurs in only 3% to 5% of patients.

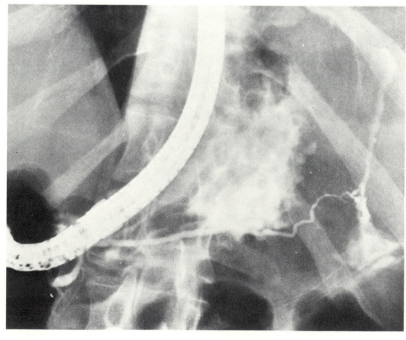

FIGURE 9-29. ERCP showing leakage of dye through the tail of the pancreas into the peritoneal cavity.

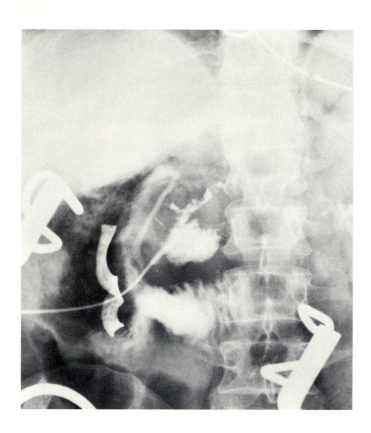

FIGURE 9-30. Operative pancreatogram showing a pseudocyst of the head of the pancreas. The pseudocyst was ruptured and was leaking into the abdominal cavity.

External Pancreatic Fistula

Pancreatic cutaneous fistulas most often occur as a late result of trauma to the pancreas, somewhat more commonly from blunt than from penetrating trauma.[198] Approximately 20% of pancreatic injuries are complicated by the development of a pancreatic fistula. Less often, an external fistula may follow the marsupialization or external drainage of a pancreatic pseudocyst. Finally, pancreatic cutaneous fistulas may occur as a late complication of operations on the pancreas, such as partial pancreatic resection or pancreatic biopsy. The overall incidence of pancreatic fistula after operations on the pancreas ranges from 10% to 20%.[199] External fistulas rarely occur spontaneously from pancreatitis, rupture of a pseudocyst, or spontaneous rupture of the pancreatic duct system.

Pathology. The basis of external pancreatic fistula is injury to the pancreatic duct or division by trauma or operation, inadequate closure of the injured or divided duct, leakage of a pancreatointestinal anastomosis, or continued external drainage through a drain tract after external drainage of a pseudocyst of the pancreas.[199]

Most pancreatic fistulas discharge small to moderate amounts of pancreatic juice, from 100 to 300 ml/day. When a high-volume fistula occurs or persists, with discharge of 500 ml or more of pancreatic juice daily, one must consider partial or complete obstruction of the pancreatic duct system in the head of the pancreas.

Pure pancreatic duct fistulas discharge clear, colorless pancreatic juice. There is minimal or no skin excoriation at the site of the fistula because the proteolytic enzymes in the juice are inactive. When the pancreatic fistula discharge is bile stained, greenish, or of a dark color, or causes moderate or severe skin excoriation, one must consider the presence of a combined pancreatic–biliary or pancreatic–intestinal fistula, with activation of the proteolytic enzymes in the pancreatic juice.

207

Diagnosis. A pancreatic fistula may be defined as any pancreatic drainage that persists for longer than 2 weeks. The diagnosis can easily be made from the type of fluid discharged (clear, colorless, or bile stained), from analysis of the amylase or lipase level in the fluid, or from an injection fistulogram study of the tract that demonstrates its origin in or near the pancreas (Figure 9-31). ERCP may demonstrate the fistula and its site of origin from the pancreatic duct.

A fistulogram roentgenographic study should be obtained on all established fistulas to assess fistula size and site of origin in the pancreas and to determine the presence of a peripancreatic fluid or pseudocyst collection. The fistulogram should be repeated periodically while awaiting spontaneous closure to assess changes in the size of the fistulous tract or adjacent collections. In addition, as noted before, ERCP may be useful in determining patency of the pancreatic duct and in helping to assess whether spontaneous closure is likely or unlikely.

Treatment. MEDICAL THERAPY. Most pure pancreatic fistulas close spontaneously 3 weeks to 3 months after onset of the fistula; approximately 80% of pancreatic fistulas close spontaneously.[199] Combined fistulas (pancreatic–biliary or pancreatic–intestinal), especially those with high output losses (500 to 2000 ml/day), are less likely to close spontaneously.

While waiting for spontaneous closure of the fistula, treatment of the patient should include the following measures: adequate replacement of fluid and electrolyte (principally sodium bicarbonate) losses; protection of the skin from excoriation or infection; antibiotics, after appropriate cultures, if there is evidence of infection; and limitation of oral intake, with maintenance of nutrition by means of total parenteral nutrition or elemental diet, to decrease pancreatic stimulation.[198,199]

OPERATIVE THERAPY. Any fistula that continues to put out pancreatic juice in amounts greater than 300 to 500 ml/day for longer than 4 to 6 weeks

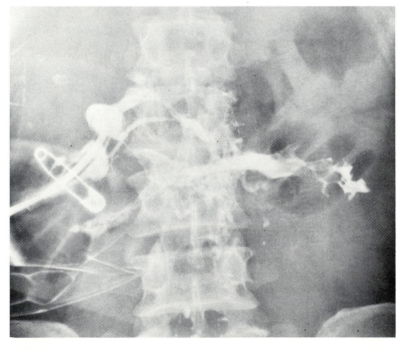

FIGURE 9-31. Fistulogram of a fistula originating in the distal pancreas.

should be considered for operative closure. About 20% of external pancreatic fistulas require operative closure.

Operations performed for external pancreatic fistulas are essentially the same as those for internal fistulas (pancreatic ascites). The site of the fistula must be identified and a defunctionalized jejunal segment (Roux-Y) brought up to cover the fistula to reroute the pancreatic juice into the intestine. This is the safest effective operative procedure. With some selected fistulas of the tail or distal pancreas, resection of the distal gland and pancreatojejunostomy are performed, joining the divided distal gland to a Roux-Y jejunal segment.

RESULTS. The overall mortality of patients with pancreatic fistulas is approximately 10%. Complications of the fistula or of the underlying condition which led to fistula formation (trauma, pseudocyst, or pancreatic resection) include sepsis, hemorrhage, or erosion into adjacent viscera. These complications are the major causes of death in patients with pancreatic fistula.

With fistula closure, either spontaneously or by operation, recurrence of the fistula is rare. Long-term results depend on the status of the pancreas and the degree of pancreatitis or ductal fibrosis in the remaining gland.

References

Pancreatitis
 1. Sarles, H., and Camatte, R.: Pancreatitis signs. In, *Conceptions et Therapeutiques Recentes*. Paris, Masson et Cie, 1963.
 2. White, T. T.: Inflammatory diseases of the pancreas. *Adv. Surg.,* **9,** 247, 1975.
 3. Anderson, M. C.: Review of pancreatic disease. *Surgery,* **66,** 434, 1969.
 4. Batson, J. M., and Law, D. H.: Chronic calcific pancreatitis in a child. *Gastroenterology,* **43,** 95, 1962.
 5. Dreiling, D. A., and Richman, A.: Pancreatitis: a review. *J. Mt. Sinai Hosp.,* **21,** 122, 1954.
 6. Dreiling, D. A., and Richman, A.: Pancreatitis: a review (Part II). *J. Mt. Sinai Hosp.,* **21,** 176, 1954.
 7. Hermann, R. E.: Basic factors in the pathogenesis of pancreatitis. *Cleve. Clin. Q.,* **30,** 1, 1963.
 8. Schiller, W. R., Suriyapa, C., and Anderson, M. C.: A review of experimental pancreatitis. *J. Surg. Res.,* **16,** 69, 1974.
 9. White, T. T., Murat, J., and Morgan, A.: Pancreatitis. I. Review of 733 cases of pancreatitis from three Seattle hospitals. *Northwest Med.,* **67,** 374, 470, 557, 643, 731, 1968.
10. Hermann, R. E., Al-Jurf, A. S., and Hoerr, S. O.: Pancreatitis. Surgical management. *Arch. Surg.,* **109,** 298, 1974.
11. Howard, J. M., and James, P. M.: Pancreatitis: a survey of its current status. *Rev. Surg.,* **19,** 301, 1962.
12. Howard, J. M., and Ehrlich, E. W.: Gallstone pancreatitis: a clinical entity. *Surgery,* **51,** 177, 1962.
13. Hurvitz, S. A., Ayerbrook, B. D., and Hurvitz, R. J.: Pancreatitis with biliary disease. *Arch. Surg.,* **86,** 168, 1963.
14. Anderson, M. C., Mehn, W. H., and Method, H. L.: An evaluation of the common channel as a factor in pancreatic or biliary disease. *Ann. Surg.,* **151,** 379, 1960.
15. Bartlett, M. K.: Might gallstones and recurrent pancreatitis have a common cause? *Arch. Surg.,* **95,** 887, 1967.

16. Blumenberg, R. M., and Powers, S. R., Jr.: Acute biliary pancreatis. An experimental reappraisal of factors governing biliary reflux into the pancreas. *Ann. Surg.,* **158,** 1058, 1963.

17. Dreiling, D. A., Kirschner, P. A., and Nemser, H.: Chronic duodenal obstruction: a mechano-vascular etiology of pancreatitis. *Am. J. Dig. Dis.,* **5,** 991, 1960.

18. Glenn, F., and Frey, C.: Re-evaluation of the treatment of pancreatitis associated with biliary tract disease. *Ann. Surg.,* **160,** 723, 1964.

19. Howard, J. M., and Jordan, G. L., Jr.: Relapsing pancreatitis secondary to choledocholithiasis. *Arch. Surg.,* **73,** 960, 1956.

20. Maingot, R.: Observations on pancreatitis. *R. Free Hosp. J.,* **88,** 169, 1969.

21. Nardi, G. L., and Acosta, J. M.: Papillitis as a cause of pancreatitis and abdominal pain: role of evocative test, operative pancreatography and histologic evaluation. *Ann. Surg.,* **164,** 611, 1966.

22. Schapiro, H., Britt, L. G., Blackwell, C. F., et al.: Acute hemorrhagic pancreatitis in the dog. I. The action of bile. *Arch. Surg.,* **107,** 608, 1973.

23. White, T. T., and Magee, D. F.: Perfusion of the dog pancreas with bile without production of pancreatitis. *Ann. Surg.,* **151,** 245, 1960.

24. Acosta, J. M., and Ledsesma, C. L.: Gallstone migration as a cause of acute pancreatitis. *N. Engl. J. Med.,* **290,** 484, 1974.

25. Kelly, T. R.: Gallstone pancreatitis: pathophysiology. *Surgery,* **80,** 488, 1976.

26. Fitzgerald, O., Fitzgerald, P., and McMullin, J. P.: Chronic pancreatitis. A review. *Rev. Surg.,* **21,** 77, 1964.

27. Warren, K. W., and Veidenheimer, M.: Pathological considerations in the choice of operation for chronic relapsing pancreatitis. *N. Engl. J. Med.,* **266,** 323, 1962.

28. Webster, P. D., III: Secretory and metabolic effects of alcohol on the pancreas. *Ann. N.Y. Acad. Sci.,* **252,** 183, 1975.

29. Lowenfels, A. B., Masih, B., Lee, T. C. Y., et al.: Effect of intravenous alcohol on the pancreas. *Arch. Surg.,* **96,** 440, 1968.

30. Cueto, J., Tajen, N., and Zimmermann, B.: Studies of experimental alcoholic pancreatitis in the dog. *Surgery,* **62,** 159, 1967.

31. Llanos, O. L., Swierczek, J. S., Teichmann, R. K., et al.: Effect of alcohol on the release of secretin and pancreatic secretion. *Surgery,* **81,** 661, 1977.

32. Anderson, M. C., and Bergan, J. J.: An experimental study of pancreatic inflammation. *Arch. Surg.,* **86,** 186, 1963.

33. Bardenheier, J. A., III, Kaminski, D. L., and Willman, V. L.: Pancreatitis after biliary tract surgery. *Am. J. Surg.,* **116,** 773, 1968.

34. Burnett, W. E., Rosemond, G. P., Caswell, H. T., et al.: Studies on so-called postgastrectomy pancreatitis. *Ann. Surg.,* **149,** 737, 1959.

35. Peterson, L. M., Collins, J. J., and Wilson, R. E.: Acute pancreatitis occurring after operation. *Surg. Gynecol. Obstet.,* **127,** 23, 1968.

36. White, T. T., Morgan, A., and Hopton, D.: Postoperative pancreatitis. A study of seventy cases. *Am. J. Surg.,* **120,** 132, 1970.

37. Goodhead, B.: Acute pancreatitis and pancreatic blood flow. *Surg. Gynecol. Obstet.,* **129,** 331, 1969.

38. Anderson, M. C., and Bergan, J. J.: Significance of vascular injury as a factor in the pathogenesis of pancreatitis. *Ann. Surg.,* **154,** 58, 1961.

39. Menguy, R. B., Hallenbeck, G. A., Bollman, J. L., et al.: Ductal and vascular factors in etiology of experimentally induced acute pancreatitis. *A.M.A. Arch. Surg.,* **74,** 881, 1957.

40. Pfeffer, R. B., Lazzarini-Robertson, A., Jr., Safadi, D., et al.: Gradations of pancreatitis, edematous through hemorrhagic, experimentally produced by controlled injection of microspheres into blood vessels in dogs. *Surgery,* **51,** 764, 1962.

41. Cameron, J. L., Crisler, C., Margolis, S., et al.: Acute pancreatitis with hyperlipemia. *Surgery,* **70,** 53, 1971.

42. Farmer, R. G., Winkelman, E. I., Brown, H. B., et al.: Hyperlipoproteinemia and pancreatitis. *Am. J. Med.,* **54,** 161, 1973.

43. Hernandez, I. A., Powers, S. R., and Frawley, T. F.: The role of the parathyroid glands in calcium and magnesium metabolism in acute hemorrhagic pancreatitis. *Surgery,* **50,** 143, 1961.

44. Kelly, T. R.: Relationship of hyperparathyroidism to pancreatitis. *Arch. Surg.,* **97,** 267, 1968.

45. Anderson, M. C., Hays, R. J., and Thornton, F. H.: Role of calcium in necrotizing pancreatitis produced with enzyme-digested blood. *J. A. M. A.,* **186,** 999, 1964.

46. Manson, R. R.: Acute pancreatitis secondary to iatrogenic hypercalcemia, implications of hyperalimentation. *Arch. Surg.,* **108,** 213, 1974.

47. Witte, C. L., and Schanzer, B.: Pancreatitis due to mumps. *J. A. M. A.,* **203,** 1068, 1968.

48. Byrne, J. J., and Joison, J.: Bacterial regurgitation in experimental pancreatitis. *Am. J. Surg.,* **107,** 317, 1964.

49. Gerber, B. C., and Aberdeen, S. D.: Hereditary pancreatitis, the role of surgical intervention. *Arch. Surg.,* **87,** 86, 1963.

50. Dean, R. H., Scott, H. W., Jr., and Law, D. H.: Chronic relapsing pancreatitis in childhood: case report and review of the literature. *Ann. Surg.,* **173,** 443, 1971.

51. Fonkalsrud, E. W., Henney, R. P., Riemenschneider, T. A., et al.: Management of pancreatitis in infants and children. *Am. J. Surg.,* **116,** 198, 1968.

52. Logan, A., Jr., Schlicke, C. P., and Manning, G. B.: Familial pancreatitis. *Am. J. Surg.,* **115,** 112, 1968.

53. Robechek, P. J.: Hereditary chronic relapsing pancreatitis. A clue to pancreatitis in general? *Am. J. Surg.,* **113,** 819, 1967.

54. Cortese, A. F., and Glenn, F.: Hypocalcemia and tetany with steroid-induced acute pancreatitis. *Arch. Surg.,* **96,** 119, 1975.

55. Schrier, R. W., and Bulger, R. J.: Steroid-induced pancreatitis. *J. A. M. A.,* **194,** 564, 1965.

56. Carey, L. C., and Rodgers, R. E.: Pathophysiologic alterations in experimental pancreatitis. *Surgery,* **60,** 171, 1966.

57. Dumont, A. E., and Martelli, A. B.: Pathogenesis of pancreatic edema following exocrine duct obstruction. *Ann. Surg.,* **168,** 302, 1968.

58. Hermann, R. E., and Davis, J. H.: The role of incomplete pancreatic duct obstruction in the etiology of pancreatitis. *Surgery,* **48,** 318, 1960.

59. Hermann, R. E., and Knowles, R. E.: The production of experimental bile-reflux pancreatitis in a pathophysiologic system. *Surgery,* **116,** 422, 1963.

60. Anderson, M. C., Needleman, S. B., Gramatica, L., et al.: Further inquiry into the pathogenesis of acute pancreatitis. *Arch. Surg.,* **99,** 185, 1969.

61. Hermann, R. E., Mitve, A., and Knowles, R. C.: Unpublished data.

62. Konok, G. P., and Thompson, A. G.: Pancreatic ductal mucosa as a protective barrier in the pathogenesis of pancreatitis. *Am. J. Surg.,* **117,** 18, 1969.

63. McHardy, G., Craighead, C. C., Balart, L., et al.: Pancreatitis—intrapancreatic proteolytic trypsin activity. *J. A. M. A.* **183,** 527, 1963.

64. Nemir, P., Jr., Hoferichter, J., and Drabkin, D. L.: The protective effect of proteinase inhibitor in acute necrotizing pancreatitis: an experimental study. *Ann. Surg.,* **158,** 655, 1963.

65. Poncelet, P., and Thompson, A. G.: Action of bile phospholipids on the pancreas. *Am. J. Surg.,* **123,** 196, 1972.

66. Sim, D. N., Duprez, A., and Anderson, M. C.: Alterations of the lymphatic circulation during acute experimental pancreatitis. *Surgery,* **60,** 1175, 1966.

67. Thal, A. P., Kobold, E. E., and Hollenberg, M. J.: The release of vasoactive substances in acute pancreatitis. *Am. J. Surg.,* **105,** 708, 1963.

68. Wickbom, G., Bushkin, F. L., Linares, C., et al.: On the corrosive properties of bile and pancreatic juice on living tissue in dogs. *Arch. Surg.,* **108,** 680, 1974.

69. Thal, A. P., Goott, B., and Margulis, A. R.: Sites of pancreatic duct obstruction in chronic pancreatitis. *Ann. Surg.,* **150,** 49, 1959.

70. Elman, R., Ameson, N., and Graham, G. A.: Value of blood amylase estima-

211

tion in the diagnosis of pancreatic disease. *Arch. Surg.*, **19**, 443, 1929.

71. Abruzzo, J. L., Homa, M., Houck, J. C., et al.: Significance of the serum amylase determination. *Ann. Surg.*, **147**, 921, 1958.

72. Boyd, T. F., Perez, J. L., and Byrne, J. J.: Serum amylase levels in experimental intestinal obstruction: does small bowel necrosis cause a rise in serum amylase? *Ann. Surg.*, **154**, 85, 1961.

73. Rogers, F. A.: Elevated serum amylase: a review and an analysis of findings in 1000 cases of perforated peptic ulcer. *Ann. Surg.*, **153**, 228, 1961.

74. Warshaw, A. L., and Lesser, P. N.: Amylase clearance in differentiating acute pancreatitis from peptic ulcer with hyperamylasemia. *Ann. Surg.*, **181**, 314, 1975.

75. Johnson, S. G., Ellis, C. J., and Levitt, M. D.: Mechanism of increased renal clearance of amylase/creatinine in acute pancreatitis. *N. Engl. J. Med.*, **295**, 1214, 1976.

76. Ranson, J. H. C., Rifkind, K. M., and Roses, D. F.: Prognostic signs and the role of operative management in acute pancreatitis. *Surg. Gynecol. Obstet.*, **139**, 69, 1974.

77. Goodhead, B.: Significance of methemalbuminemia in acute abdominal emergencies. *Arch. Surg.*, **101**, 376, 1970.

78. Ferrucci, J. T., Jr., and Eaton, S. B.: Radiology of the pancreas. *N. Engl. J. Med.*, **288**, 506, 1973.

79. Rubaum, N. J., and Shohl, T.: X-ray visualization of the pancreas. *Ann. Surg.*, **153**, 246, 1961.

80. Jacobs, M. L., Daggett, W. M., Civette, J. M., et al.: Acute pancreatitis: analysis of factors influencing survival. *Ann. Surg.*, **185**, 43, 1977.

81. Cooperman, A. M. Sivak, M. V., Sullivan, B. H., Jr., et al.: Endoscopic pancreatography: its value in preoperative and postoperative assessment of pancreatic disease. *Am. J. Surg.*, **129**, 38, 1975.

82. Sugawa, C., Raouf, R., Bradley, V., et al.: Peroral endoscopic cholangiography and pancreatography. The surgeon's helper. *Arch. Surg.*, **109**, 231, 1974.

83. Anderson, M. C., and Schiller, W. R.: Acute pancreatitis. *Surg. Annu.*, **5**, 335, 1973.

84. Banks, P. A.: Acute pancreatitis. *Gastroenterology*, **61**, 382, 1971.

85. Cogbill, C. L., and Song, K. T.: Acute pancreatitis. *Arch. Surg.*, **100**, 673, 1970.

86. Finch, W. T., Sawyers, J. L., and Schenker, S.: A prospective study to determine the efficacy of antibiotics in acute pancreatitis. *Ann. Surg.*, **183**, 667, 1976.

87. Carey, L. C.: Low molecular weight dextran in experimental pancreatitis. *Am. J. Surg.*, **119**, 197, 1970.

88. Facey, F. L., Weil, M. H., and Rosoff, L.: Mechanism and treatment of shock associated with acute pancreatitis. *Am. J. Surg.*, **111**, 374, 1966.

89. Grozinger, K. H., Artz, C. P., Hollis, A. U., et al.: Evaluation of Trasylol in experimental acute pancreatitis. *Surgery*, **56**, 400, 1964.

90. Hermann, R. E., and Knowles, R. C.: Lethal factors and response to therapy in experimental bile-reflux pancreatitis. *Ann. Surg.*, **161**, 456, 1965.

91. Kneisel, J. J.: A clinical trial of an enzyme inhibitor in pancreatitis: reflux pancreatitis in a pathophysiologic system. *Surgery*, **116**, 422, 1963.

92. McCutcheon, A. D., and Race, D.: Experimental pancreatitis: use of a new antiproteolytic substance, Trasylol. *Ann. Surg.*, **158**, 233, 1963.

93. Morgan, A., Robinson, L. A., and White, T. T.: Postoperative changes in the trypsin inhibitor activities of human pancreatic juice and the influence of infusion of Trasylol on the inhibitor activity. *Am. J. Surg.*, **115**, 131, 1968.

94. Popieraitis, A. S., and Thompson, A. G.: The site of bradykinin release in acute experimental pancreatitis. *Arch. Surg.*, **98**, 73, 1969.

95. Schiller, W. R., Duprez, A., Iams, W. B., et al.: Experimental pancreatitis. Treatment by colloid replacement and adenocorticosteroid therapy combined with thoracic duct drainage. *Arch. Surg.*, **98**, 698, 1969.

96. Skinner, D. B., Corson, J. G., and Nardi, G. L.: Aprotinin therapy as prophylaxis against postoperative pancreatitis in humans. *J. A. M. A.,* **204,** 945, 1968.

97. Smith, R. B., III, Orahood, R. C., Wangensteen, S. L., et al.: Effect of a trypsin-inhibitor on experimentally induced pancreatitis in the dog. *Surgery,* **54,** 922, 1963.

98. Trapnell, J. E., Chir, T. M., and Capper, W. M.: Trasylol in acute pancreatitis. *Am. J. Dig. Dis.,* **12,** 409, 1967.

99. Ranson, J. H. C., Rifkind, K. M., and Turner, J. W.: Prognostic signs and nonoperative peritoneal lavage in acute pancreatitis. *Surg. Gynecol. Obstet.,* **143,** 209, 1976.

100. Trapnell, J. E., and Anderson, M. C.: Role of early laparotomy in acute pancreatitis. *Ann. Surg.,* **165,** 49, 1967.

101. Warshaw, A. L., Imbembo, A. L., Civetta, J. M., et al.: Surgical intervention in acute necrotizing pancreatitis. *Am. J. Surg.,* **127,** 484, 1974.

102. Lawson, D. W., Daggett, W. M., Civetta, J. M., et al.: Surgical treatment of acute necrotizing pancreatitis. *Ann. Surg.,* **172,** 605, 1970.

103. Salzman, E. W., and Bartlett, M. K.: Pancreatic duct exploration in selected cases of acute pancreatitis. *Ann. Surg.,* **158,** 859, 1963.

104. Norton, L., and Eiseman, B.: Near total pancreatectomy for hemorrhagic pancreatitis. *Am. J. Surg.,* **127,** 191, 1974.

105. Watts, G. T.: Total pancreatectomy for fulminant pancreatitis. *Lancet,* **2,** 384, 1963.

106. Holden, J. L., Berne, T. V., and Rosoff, L.: Pancreatic abscess following acute pancreatitis. *Arch. Surg.,* **111,** 858, 1976.

107. Camer, S. J., Tan, E. G., Warren, K. W., et al.: Pancreatic abscess—a clinical analysis of 113 cases. *Am. J. Surg.,* **129,** 426, 1975.

108. Miller, T. A., Lindenauer, S. M., Frey, C. F., et al.: Pancreatic abscess. *Arch. Surg.,* **108,** 545, 1974.

109. Steedman, R. A., Doering, R., and Carter, R.: Surgical aspects of pancreatic abscess. *Surg. Gynecol. Obstet.,* **125,** 757, 1967.

110. Warshaw, A. L.: Pancreatic abscesses. *N. Engl. J. Med.,* **287,** 1234, 1972.

111. Bradley, E. L., III, Gonzalez, A. C., and Clements, J. L.: Acute pancreatic pseudocysts: incidence and implications. *Ann. Surg.,* **184,** 734, 1976.

112. Haller, J. D., Pena, C., and Dargan, E. L.: Massive upper gastrointestinal hemorrhage due to pancreatitis. *Arch. Surg.,* **93,** 567, 1966.

113. Kisken, W. A.: Gastrointestinal bleeding secondary to pancreatitis. *J.A.M.A.,* **202,** 287, 1967.

114. Interiano, B., Stuard, I. D., and Hyde, R. W.: Acute respiratory distress syndrome in pancreatitis. *Ann. Intern. Med.,* **77,** 923, 1972.

115. Ranson, J. H. C., Turner, J. W., Roses, D. F., et al.: Respiratory complications in acute pancreatitis. *Ann. Surg.,* **179,** 557, 1974.

116. Norback, Y. E., and Risholm, L.: Acute pancreatitis, etiology and prevention of recurrence. Follow-up study of 188 patients. *Rev. Surg.,* **25,** 153, 1968.

117. Shader, A. E., and Paxton, J. R.: Fatal pancreatitis. *Am. J. Surg.,* **111,** 369, 1966.

118. Storck, G., Pettersson, G., and Edlund, Y.: A study of autopsies upon 116 patients with acute pancreatitis. *Surg. Gynecol. Obstet.,* **143,** 241, 1976.

119. Whalen, J., Rush, B., Albano, E., et al.: Fatal acute pancreatitis. A clinicopathologic analysis. *Am. J. Surg.,* **121,** 16, 1971.

120. Dixon, J. A., and Englert, J. R.: Growing role of early surgery in chronic pancreatitis: a practical clinical approach. *Gastroenterology,* **61,** 375, 1971.

121. Egdahl, R. H., and Hume, D. M.: Surgery in pancreatitis. *Am. J. Surg.,* **106,** 471, 1963.

122. Nardi, G. L.: Pancreatitis. *N. Engl. J. Med.,* **268,** 1065, 1963.

123. Nardi, G. L.: Remediable chronic pancreatitis. *Surg. Clin. North Am.,* **54,** 613, 1974.

124. Bartlett, M. K., and Nardi, G. L.: Treatment of recurrent pancreatitis by

213

transduodenal sphincterotomy and exploration of the pancreatic duct. *N. Engl. J. Med.,* **262,** 643, 1960.

125. Howard, J. M., and Nedwich, A.: Correlation of the histologic observations and operative findings in patients with chronic pancreatitis. *Surg. Gynecol. Obstet.,* **132,** 387, 1971.

126. Bartlett, M. K., and Carter, E. L.: The technic of pancreatic duct exploration for recurrent pancreatitis. *Am. J. Surg.,* **105,** 755, 1963.

127. Bartlett, M. K., and Nardi, G. L.: Treatment of recurrent pancreatitis by resection inhibition and retrograde drainage of the pancreas. *Ann. Surg.,* **152,** 861, 1960.

128. DuVal, M. K., Jr., and Enquist, I. F.: The surgical treatment of chronic pancreatitis by pancreatojejunostomy: an 8-year reappraisal. *Surgery,* **50,** 965, 1961.

129. Gillesby, W., and Puestow, C. B.: Pancreatojejunostomy for chronic relapsing pancreatitis: an evaluation. *Surgery,* **50,** 859, 1961.

130. Grodsinsky, C., Schuman, B. M., and Block, M. A.: Absence of pancreatic duct dilatation in chronic pancreatitis. *Arch. Surg.,* **112,** 444, 1977.

131. Hermann, R. E.: Clinical aspects of pancreatitis. *Postgrad. Med.,* **36,** 135, 1964.

132. Howard, J. M., and Short, W. F.: An evaluation of pancreatography in suspected pancreatic disease. *Surg. Gynecol. Obstet.,* **129,** 319, 1969.

133. Jordan, G. L., Jr., Strug, B. S., and Crowder, W. E.: Current status of pancreatojejunostomy in the management of chronic pancreatitis. *Am. J. Surg.,* **133,** 46, 1977.

134. Partington, P. F., and Rochelle, R. E. L.: Modified Puestow procedure for retrograde drainage of the pancreatic duct. *Ann. Surg.,* **152,** 1037, 1960.

135. Thal, A. P.: A technique for drainage of the obstructed pancreatic duct. *Surgery,* **51,** 313, 1962.

136. Trapnell, J. E., Howard, J. M., and Brewster, J.: Transduodenal pancreatography: an improved technique. *Surgery,* **60,** 1112, 1966.

137. White, T. T., and Murat, J. E.: Treatment of the common bile duct in pancreatitis. *Am. Surg.,* **33,** 524, 1967.

138. White, T. T.: Results of pancreatojejunostomy for pancreatitis and cancer of the pancreas. *Am. Surg.,* **34,** 514, 1968.

139. White, T. T.: Results of 89 operations for pancreatitis: a personal experience. *Surgery,* **58,** 1061, 1965.

140. White, T. T., and Keith, R. G.: Long-term followup study of fifty patients with pancreatojejunostomy. *Surgery,* **136,** 353, 1973.

141. Stobbe, K. C., ReMine, W. H., and Baggenstoss, A. H.: Pancreatic lithiasis. *Surg. Gynecol. Obstet.,* **131,** 1090, 1970.

142. Guillemin, G., Cuilleret, J., Michel, A., et al.: Chronic relapsing pancreatitis. Surgical management including sixty-three cases of pancreaticoduodenectomy. *Am. J. Surg.,* **122,** 802, 1971.

143. Leger, L., Lenriot, J. P., and Lemaigre, G.: Five to twenty year followup after surgery for chronic pancreatitis in 148 patients. *Ann. Surg.,* **180,** 185, 1974.

144. Priestley, J. T., ReMine, W. H., Barber, K. W., Jr., et al.: Chronic relapsing pancreatitis: treatment by surgical drainage of pancreas. *Ann. Surg.,* **161,** 838, 1965.

145. Rignault, D., Mine, J., and Moine, D.: Splenoportographic changes in chronic pancreatitis. *Surgery,* **63,** 571, 1968.

146. Sato, T., Saitoh, Y., Noto, N., et al.: Appraisal of operative treatment of chronic pancreatitis. With special reference to side-to-side pancreaticojejunostomy. *Am. J. Surg.,* **129,** 621, 1975.

147. Warren, K. W.: Surgical management of chronic relapsing pancreatitis. *Am. J. Surg.,* **117,** 24, 1969.

148. Way, L. W., Gadacz, T., and Goldman, L.: Surgical treatment of chronic pancreatitis. *Am. J. Surg.,* **127,** 202, 1974.

149. Weiland, D. E., Kuntz, D. J., and Kimball, H. W.: Subtotal pancreatectomy for chronic pancreatitis. *Am. J. Surg.,* **118,** 973, 1969.

150. White, T. T., Lawinski, M., Stacher, G., et al.: Treatment of pancreatitis by left splanchnicectomy and celiac ganglionectomy. Analysis of 146 cases. *Am. J. Surg.*, **112**, 195, 1966.

151. Child, C. G., III, Frey, C. F., and Fry, W. J.: A reappraisal of removal of ninety-five percent of the distal portion of the pancreas. *Surg. Gynecol. Obstet.*, **129**, 49, 1969.

152. Frey, C. F., Child, C. G., and Fry, W.: Pancreatectomy for chronic pancreatitis. *Ann. Surg.*, **184**, 403, 1976.

153. Fry, W. J., and Child, C. G., III: Ninety-five percent distal pancreatectomy for chronic pancreatitis. *Ann. Surg.*, **162**, 543, 1965.

154. Brooks, F. P.: Testing pancreatic function. *N. Engl. J. Med.*, **286**, 300, 1972.

155. Farrell, J. J., Richmond, K. C., and Morgan, M. M.: Transduodenal pancreatic duct dilatation and curettage in chronic relapsing pancreatitis. *Am. J. Surg.*, **105**, 30, 1963.

156. Madding, G. F., and Kennedy, P. A.: Chronic alcoholic pancreatitis. Treatment by ductal obstruction. *Am. J. Surg.*, **125**, 538, 1973.

157. Williams, L. F., and Byrne, J. J.: Natural variation in experimental hemorrhagic pancreatitis. *Surg. Gynecol. Obstet.*, **124**, 531, 1967.

158. Yacoub, R. S., Appert, H. E., Pairent, F. W., et al.: Systemic manifestations of acute pancreatitis. Effects of the intravenous infusion of pancreatic juice in dogs. *Arch. Surg.*, **99**, 47, 1969.

Pseudocysts of the Pancreas

159. Becker, W. F., Pratt, H. S., and Gans, H.: Pseudocysts of the pancreas. *Surg. Gynecol. Obstet.*, **127**, 744, 1968.

160. Bradley, E. L., III, Gonzalez, A. C., and Clements, J. L.: Acute pancreatic pseudocysts. *Ann. Surg.*, **184**, 734, 1976.

161. Polk, H. C., Jr., Zeppa, R., and Warren, W. D.: Surgical significance of differentiation between acute and chronic pancreatic collections. *Ann. Surg.*, **169**, 444, 1969.

162. Jordan, G. L., Jr., and Howard, J. M.: Pancreatic pseudocysts. *Am. J. Gastroenterol.*, **45**, 444, 1966.

163. Fox, N. M., Jr., Ferris, D. O., Moertel, C. G., et al.: Pseudocyst co-existent with pancreatic carcinoma. *Ann. Surg.*, **158**, 971, 1963.

164. Howard, J. M., Trapnell, J. E., and Pairent, F. W.: Distinction between pseudocysts of the head of the pancreas and carcinoma of the pancreas. *Ann. Surg.*, **165**, 293, 1967.

165. Shafer, R. B., and Silvis, S. E.: Pancreatic pseudo-pseudocysts. *Am. J. Surg.*, **127**, 320, 1974.

166. Kilman, J. W., Kaiser, G. C., King, R. D., et al.: Pancreatic pseudocysts in infancy and childhood. *Surgery*, **55**, 455, 1964.

167. Stone, H. H., and Whitehurst, J. O.: Pseudocysts of the pancreas in children. *Am. J. Surg.*, **114**, 448, 1967.

168. Goldberg, B. B., and Lehman, L. S.: Some observations on the practical uses of a-mode ultrasound. *Am. J. Roentgenol. Radium Ther. Nucl. Med.*, **107**, 198, 1969.

169. Rosenberg, I. K., Kahn, J. A., and Walt, A. J.: Surgical experience with pancreatic pseudocysts. *Am. J. Surg.*, **117**, 11, 1969.

170. Sidel, V. W., Wilson, R. E., and Shipp, J. C.: Pseudocyst formation in chronic pancreatitis: a cause of obstructive jaundice. *Arch. Surg.*, **77**, 933, 1958.

171. VanHeerden, J. A., and ReMine, W. H.: Pseudocysts of the pancreas. *Arch. Surg.*, **110**, 500, 1975.

172. Dardik, I., and Dardik, H.: Patterns of hemorrhage into pancreatic pseudocysts. *Am. J. Surg.*, **115**, 774, 1968.

173. Parshall, W. A., and ReMine, W. H.: Internal drainage of pseudocysts of the pancreas. *Arch. Surg.*, **91**, 480, 1965.

174. Scharplatz, D., and White, T. T.: A review of 64 patients with pancreatic cysts. *Ann. Surg.*, **176**, 638, 1972.

175. Shatney, C. H., and Sosin, H.: Spontaneous perforation of a pancreatic

pseudocyst into the colon and duodenum. *Am. J. Surg.*, **126**, 433, 1973.

176. Thomford, N. R., and Jesseph, J. E.: Pseudocyst of the pancreas; a review of fifty cases. *Am. J. Surg.*, **118**, 86, 1969.

177. Bucknam, C. A.: Arterial hemorrhage in pseudocyst of pancreas. *Arch. Surg.*, **92**, 405, 1966.

178. Christensen, N. M., Demling, R., and Mathewson, C., Jr.: Unusual manifestations of pancreatic pseudocysts and their surgical management. *Am. J. Surg.*, **130**, 199, 1975.

179. Cogbill, C. L.: Hemorrhage in pancreatic pseudocysts. Review of literature and report of two cases. *Ann. Surg.*, **167**, 112, 1968.

180. Cordero, O. C., Khademi, M., Lazaro, E., and Swaminathan, A. P.: Intracystic hemorrhage: a complication of pseudocyst of the pancreas. *Br. J. Radiol.*, **48**, 602, 1975.

181. Gonzalez, L. L., Jaffe, M. S., Wiot, J. F., et al.: Pancreatic pseudocyst: a cause of obstructive jaundice. *Ann. Surg.*, **161**, 569, 1965.

182. Greenstein, A., DeMaio, E. F., and Nabseth, D. C.: Acute hemorrhage associated with pancreatic pseudocysts. *Surgery*, **69**, 56, 1971.

183. Weinstein, B. R., Korn, R. J., and Zimmerman, H. J.: Obstructive jaundice as a complication of pancreatitis. *Ann. Intern. Med.*, **58**, 245, 1963.

184. Vajcner, A., and Nicoloff, D. M.: Pseudocysts of the pancreas: value of urine and serum amylase levels. *Surgery*, **66**, 842, 1969.

185. Brewer, W. A., and Shumway, O. L.: Transgastric catheter drainage of pancreatic pseudocysts. *Arch. Surg.*, **78**, 79, 1959.

186. Ehrlich, E. W., and Gonzales-Lavin, L.: Pseudocysts treated by cystogastrostomy: assessment by catheter contrast visualization. *Arch. Surg.*, **93**, 996, 1966.

187. Hermann, R. E., Al-Jurf, A. S., and Hoerr, S. O.: Pancreatitis; surgical management. *Arch. Surg.*, **109**, 298, 1974.

188. Hillson, R. F., and Taube, R. R.: Surgical management of pancreatic pseudocysts. *Am. Surg.*, **41**, 492, 1975.

189. Warren, K. W., Athanassiades, S., Frederick, P., et al.: Surgical treatment of pancreatic cysts: review of 183 cases. *Ann. Surg.*, **163**, 886, 1966.

190. Warren, W. D., Marsh, W. H., and Muller, W. H., Jr.: Experimental production of pseudocysts of the pancreas with preliminary observations of internal drainage. *Surg. Gynecol. Obstet.*, **105**, 385, 1957.

191. Folk, F. A., and Freeark, R. J.: Reoperation for pancreatic pseudocyst. *Arch. Surg.*, **100**, 430, 1970.

Pancreatic Ascites and External Pancreatic Fistulas

192. MacLaren, L. F., Howard, J. M., and Jordan, G. L., Jr.: Ascites associated with a pseudocyst of the pancreas. *Arch. Surg.*, **93**, 301, 1966.

193. Smith, R. B., III, Warren, W. D., Rivard, A. A., et al.: Pancreatic ascites: diagnosis and management with particular reference to surgical technics. *Ann. Surg.*, **177**, 538, 1973.

194. Jordan, G. L.: Discussion of Cameron, J. L., et al.: The treatment of pancreatic ascites. *Ann. Surg.*, **170**, 675, 1969.

195. Cameron, J. L., Kieffer, R. S., Anderson, W. J., and Zuidema, G. D.: Internal pancreatic fistulas: pancreatic ascites and pleural effusions. *Ann. Surg.*, **184**, 587, 1976.

196. Cameron, J. L., Brawley, R. K., Bender, H. W., et al.: The treatment of pancreatic ascites. *Ann. Surg.*, **170**, 668, 1969.

197. Paloyan, D., and Skinner, D. B.: Clinical significance of pancreatic ascites. *Am. J. Surg.*, **132**, 114, 1976.

198. Jordan, G. L., Jr.: Pancreatic fistula. *Am. J. Surg.*, **119**, 200, 1970.

199. Zinner, M. J., Baker, R. R., and Cameron, J. L.: Pancreatic cutaneous fistulas. *Surg. Gynecol. Obstet.*, **138**, 710, 1974.

Cysts and Neoplasms

10

True Pancreatic Cysts

Primary or true cystic lesions of the pancreas are unusual. Howard and Jordan[1] have classified pancreatic cysts into two types: *true* cysts, which have a thin-walled epithelial lining; and *false* or *pseudocysts,* secondary to inflammation or trauma, which have a thick-walled, fibrous lining. Among the true cysts are congenital, retention (acquired), and neoplastic cysts (cystadenomas and cystadenocarcinomas).

Of the true cysts of the pancreas, neoplastic cysts are the most common. According to Becker et al.[2] at least 10% of all pancreatic cysts, including pseudocysts, are neoplastic. My experience is that neoplastic and other true cysts of the pancreas are much less common; they account for only 3% to 5% of all cysts of the pancreas we have seen.

Congenital Cysts

Congenital simple cysts of the pancreas are probably the rarest of all. Only isolated case reports of this type of true cyst of the pancreas have been documented.[3]

Pathology. Congenital pancreatic cysts are thin walled, epithelial-lined, and usually unilocular but occasionally multilocular. The lining of the cyst wall is that of ductal epithelium (Figure 10-1). They may arise in any area of the pancreas and are usually large when diagnosed. The surrounding pancreas is usually normal, without evidence of inflammatory changes or significant fibrosis. The etiology of this type of cyst is probably congenital, segmental pancreatic duct obstruction, with secretion of pancreatic juice into the obstructed duct segment and gradual "ballooning" of this segment with cyst formation.

Diagnosis. CLINICAL FEATURES. Most congenital pancreatic cysts, like mesenteric cysts or lymphangiomatous cysts, are asymptomatic. The presenting symptom is an upper abdominal mass. Occasionally, they may cause upper abdominal pain, a feeling of fullness, nausea, vomiting, or bloating because of their size and compression effects on adjacent viscera. Most importantly, there is no history of pancreatitis.

217

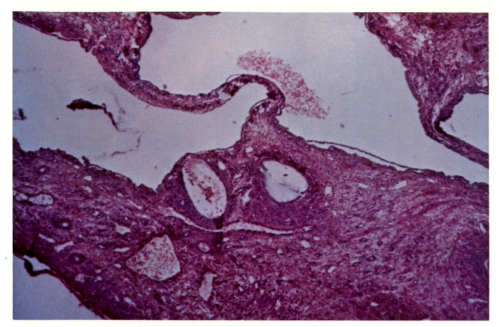

FIGURE 10-1.   Photomicrograph of the lining epithelium of a congenital pancreatic cyst.

ROENTGENOGRAPHIC STUDIES.   An upper gastrointestinal series using barium will outline the mass displacing the stomach cephalad and anteriorly, widening the duodenal C-loop, or displacing the transverse colon down. Abdominal ultrasonography will identify the cystic lesion (Figure 10-2), as will CT. Selective celiac and superior mesenteric arteriograms will show an avascular (cystic) mass in the pancreas. An arteriogram, although not necessary or advisable for the pre-operative evaluation of a suspected pseudocyst of the pancreas (a cystic mass with an antecedent history of pancreatitis), may be advisable when studying a patient with a pancreatic mass who has no previous history of pancreatitis. The arteriogram may be helpful in distinguishing between a simple cyst, a retention cyst secondary to malignancy, and a neoplastic cyst of the pancreas[4] (Figure 10-3).

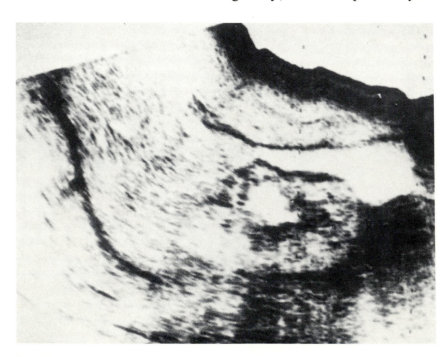

FIGURE 10-2. Ultrasonogram of the abdomen showing a small cystic mass in the pancreas.

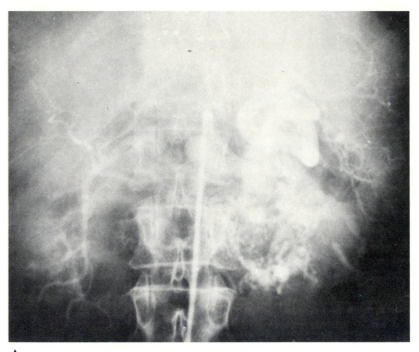

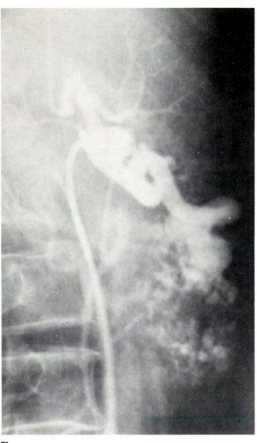

A

FIGURE 10-3. Arteriograms of a neoplastic cyst of the pancreas identified by the presence of abnormal tumor vessels in the region of the cystic mass. (A) Anteroposterior view. (B) Lateral view.

B

Treatment. Operative exploration should be undertaken for all cystic masses of the pancreas that do not resolve spontaneously. At operation it is essential to explore and expose the entire pancreas to look for evidence of prior pancreatitis or a neoplasm. If a congenital, simple cyst of the pancreas is found and excision is possible by partial (distal) pancreatectomy, this is the treatment of choice. If excision of the entire cyst cannot safely be performed, the anterior wall of the cyst should be resected both for biopsy and to remove the cystic mass. A Roux-Y jejunal segment should then be used to cover the remaining cyst wall left in or on the pancreas. Internal drainage alone should not be performed, since the cyst wall is too thin and fragile for a secure anastomosis. A pancreatoduodenectomy (Whipple operation) is rarely advisable for a congenital cyst of the pancreas unless there is a strong suspicion that the cyst is neoplastic.

Retention Cysts

Retention cysts have been reported more frequently than congenital, simple cysts. They are acquired, true (epithelial-lined) cysts of the pancreas, secondary to pancreatic duct obstruction from a carcinoma of the pancreas or from chronic pancreatitis.[5,6]

Pathology. Retention cysts are usually smaller than pseudocysts or congenital cysts of the pancreas. At times, it may be difficult to distinguish them from pseudocysts when the patient has a history of pancreatitis and the cyst forms as a result of chronic pancreatitis. However, when the cause of the pancreatic duct obstruction is carcinoma of the pancreas, it is obviously important to determine the cause of the cyst and to distinguish it from a pseudocyst or from a neoplastic cyst (cystadenoma or cystadenocarcinoma) of the pancreas.[5-8]

219

These cysts are true cysts of the pancreas, with thin, epithelial-lined walls. The diagnosis is made by biopsy of the cyst wall. The surrounding pancreas is not normal; there is evidence of either chronic pancreatitis or a carcinoma of the pancreas with pancreatic duct obstruction. In addition to biopsy of the cyst wall, biopsy of the pancreas in an area of its greatest induration or mass formation should be performed.

Diagnosis. CLINICAL FEATURES. Two groups of patients have retention cysts of the pancreas: those with chronic pancreatitis and those with carcinoma. Symptoms in patients with chronic pancreatitis are recurrent episodes of pancreatitis, abdominal pain, nausea, vomiting, weight loss, steatorrhea, and the development of a pancreatic mass. Symptoms in patients with carcinoma of the pancreas, not previously diagnosed, are the progressive development of vague, steady abdominal and back pain, loss of appetite, depression or a feeling of uneasiness, and gradual weight loss. The development of a mass in the pancreas is usually less noticeable in this group of patients and may not be identified until operative exploration.

ROENTGENOGRAPHIC STUDIES. Helpful pre-operative studies, as noted before, include an upper gastrointestinal roentgenogram series, echograms or CT scans of the abdomen, and selective celiac and superior mesenteric arteriography. The presence of a pancreatic mass or cystic mass on these studies is an indication for operative exploration of the pancreas.

Treatment. At operation, thorough exposure and exploration of the pancreas is essential. If the pancreas is indurated, thickened, or fibrotic, or there is evidence of a pancreatic mass, and the pancreatic cyst is not a typical thick-walled pseudocyst, then biopsy should be performed on both the cyst wall and the most indurated area of the pancreas. If a retention cyst is found in association with chronic pancreatitis, it can be treated in one of several ways: (1) if the wall is thick enough to hold sutures, an internal drainage procedure can be performed, usually a cystojejunostomy to a Roux-Y jejunal segment; (2) if the wall is thin and too fragile for an internal anastomosis, the anterior wall of the cyst can be excised back to fibrotic pancreas and the residual cyst area on the pancreas covered with a Roux-Y jejunal segment, as in treatment of a congenital cyst; or (3) if the cyst is in the body or tail of the pancreas, and distal pancreatectomy appears safe, this can be accomplished with removal of the cyst and distal pancreas. A Roux-Y jejunal segment should probably be used to cover the divided distal gland.

If, however, carcinoma of the pancreas is identified as the underlying cause of a retention cyst, then the location of the carcinoma, its size, evidence of local or regional invasion, or metastases will determine the operative procedure. In this situation it is rare to find a resectable lesion; advanced carcinoma in the pancreas is much more likely. Internal drainage of the cyst, partial resection of the cyst wall and internal drainage, or partial pancreatectomy should all be considered. If the cyst is small or not significant in relationship to the newly diagnosed malignancy, then no therapy of the cyst may be necessary. The treatment is that of the carcinoma, which, in this setting, is unlikely to be cured by operative resection.

Neoplastic Cysts: Cystadenoma and Cystadenocarcinoma

Of all the true cysts of the pancreas, neoplastic cysts are the most common. As noted previously, Becker and associates[2] have stated that at least 10% of pancreatic cysts are neoplastic cysts. Approximately 400 cases have been reported in the surgical literature. From these reports, it appears that benign cystadenomas are approximately twice as common as cystadenocarcinomas.[2,9-13] There have been several reports of the malignant transformation of cystadenomas into cystadenocarcinomas.[10,14] Indeed, some authors believe that all cystadenocarcinomas develop from benign cystadenomas.[2,10,15-17] Rarely, other cystic neoplasms such as cystic leiomyosarcoma, cystic rhabdomyosarcoma, and cystic islet cell adenomas of the pancreas have been reported.[16,18]

Neoplastic cysts are diagnosed most frequently in patients between the ages of 40 and 60 years. There is a striking predominance in women; they have a 9:1 incidence over men for both cystadenoma and cystadenocarcinoma.[2,9-11]

Pathology. Neoplastic cysts may be large, solitary cysts, but more frequently they are multiloculated or multicystic (Figure 10-4). They may become large, often large enough to fill much of the abdominal cavity. Occasionally, however, relatively small cysts are encountered. When evaluated at operation, the lesion is usually discrete or localized, more often found in the body or tail than in the head of the pancreas. The remainder of the pancreas usually appears fairly normal when inspected and palpated. The contents of the cyst may be serous or mucoid material.

Microscopically, the diagnosis of a neoplastic cyst is made by identifying neoplastic tissue in the base or wall of the cyst. This tissue may be of two types: a lining of flat, cuboidal or tall, columnar cells; or papillary

1 CM

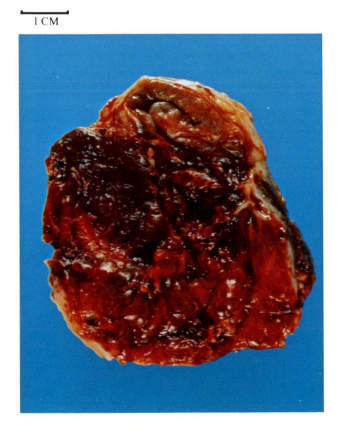

FIGURE 10-4. Operative specimen of a cystadenoma of the pancreas.

221

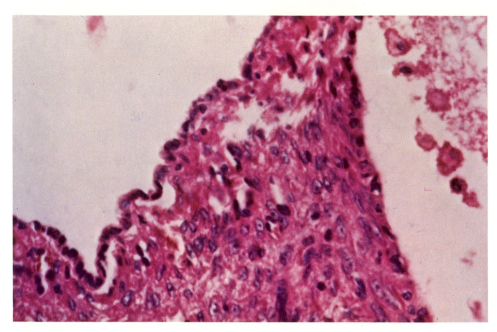

FIGURE 10-5.   Photomicrograph showing the lining of a cystadenoma of the pancreas.

projections recognized grossly or microscopically in many areas (Figure 10-5). Frequently, with enlargement and growth of the cyst, the walls of the cyst may become so compressed and fibrotic that differentiation from a pseudocyst on a purely histological basis may be difficult. Occasionally the wall of the cyst may be calcified.

Differentiation of a cystadenoma and a cystadenocarcinoma may be difficult. Cystadenocarcinomas are usually slowly growing tumors with a low degree of malignancy (Figure 10-6). The diagnosis of carcinoma is made by histological evidence of invasion of blood vessels or contiguous structures, by perineural invasion, or by lymph node or other metastases.[2,8,12,14,15]

Diagnosis. CLINICAL FEATURES.   A principal characteristic of neoplastic cysts is that they are usually painless masses in their early stages. There is

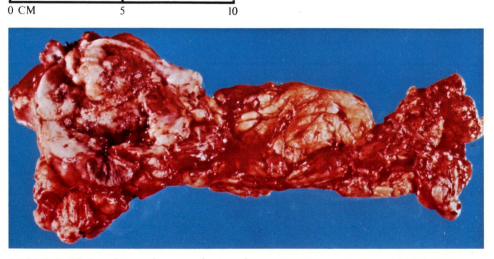

FIGURE 10-6.   Operative specimen of a cystadenocarcinoma of the pancreas.

usually no history of pancreatitis or abdominal injury. As the mass in the upper abdomen becomes larger, most patients have a sensation of gradual abdominal fullness and discomfort. About 50% of patients experience pain, especially when the cystic lesion becomes large. The pain is usually epigastric or left upper abdominal, often radiating to the back.

Examination of the abdomen usually discloses the presence of a mass in the upper abdomen. Serum amylase levels may be mildly elevated but are usually normal.

ROENTGENOGRAPHIC STUDIES. An upper gastrointestinal series using barium usually shows displacement of the stomach anteriorly or widening of the duodenal C-loop. The transverse colon is usually displaced downward. Echography or sonography will usually identify the cystic mass. Selective celiac and superior mesenteric arteriography should be performed whenever a neoplastic cyst is suspected, so that the relationship to major arteries can be identified in assessing the lesion for resection[4] (Figure 10-3).

Treatment. BIOPSY. At operation, whenever a cystic mass of the pancreas is found, especially in the absence of a history of pancreatitis or trauma, or when a multiloculated cyst is found, a cystic neoplasm should be considered. The cyst should be opened and some of its contents submitted for cytological studies. Biopsies of the cyst wall should be obtained in several areas and tissue within the cyst cavity should be gently removed for histological study.

Total surgical excision of the entire lesion and a margin of normal pancreas is the treatment of choice for both cystadenoma and cystadenocarcinoma of the pancreas.[2,6,17,19–22] Since it is difficult to identify malignancy in many such lesions, it is essential that the entire cystic tumor be excised if at all possible. For tumors of the body and tail of the pancreas, distal pancreatectomy and splenectomy is the operation of choice. For tumors of the head of the pancreas, a pancreatoduodenectomy (Whipple operation) should be performed. Rarely, a total pancreatectomy may be necessary.

In those patients in whom the entire cystic tumor mass cannot be totally excised, most of the tumor should be removed, leaving only that posterior remnant of cyst wall attached to vital structures such as the mesenteric vessels or portal vein. A Roux-Y jejunal segment may be sewn to this remaining cystic structure for internal drainage of the remnant if necessary.

Simple drainage alone, either by internal drainage into a loop of intestine or by tube drainage to the exterior, should be avoided except as a last resort. Neoplastic tissue usually grows into the anastomotic opening and occludes it with recurrence of the cyst. However, several cases have been reported in which significant palliation has been achieved for several years with only biopsy or drainage of a cystic neoplasm.[2,12]

RADIATION THERAPY. We have had experience with one patient in whom only biopsy and drainage of a cystadenocarcinoma could be performed; the tumor mass was marked with silver clips and a course of intensive cobalt-60 therapy was given to the lesion. All evidence of a mass has disappeared and the patient has been asymptomatic for 4 years. Thus, although radiation therapy is not generally believed to be of great value in treating cystadenocarcinomas of the pancreas, it should be considered when a lesion is unresectable. There have been no reports indicating that chemotherapy is of any value in treating these lesions.

223

RESULTS. Survival results after total excision of cystadenomas and cystadenocarcinomas of the pancreas have been good when the tumor has been completely removed. ReMine[21] has reported a 63% 5-year survival in a series of patients with cystadenocarcinoma of the pancreas in whom the lesions were completely excised.

Carcinoma of the Pancreas and Periampullary Region

The incidence of cancer of the pancreas and the region surrounding the pancreas has steadily increased in the United States, by approximately 20% in the past 20 years. The increase has been second only to the expanding incidence of cancer of the lung. At the present time, cancer of the pancreas is the fourth or fifth commonest fatal carcinoma, exceeded only by cancers of the lung, colon–rectum, prostate (in males), and breast and ovary (in females). It accounts for approximately 4% of all malignant diseases in the general population.[23–28]

Despite its frequency, cancer of the pancreas continues to be one of the most difficult carcinomas to diagnose early and one of the most discouraging to treat. Cures are rare because of our inability to diagnose the disease before it has extended beyond the limits of curative resection. Because of the infrequency of long-term survival after resection of a carcinoma of the pancreas and because of the high operative mortality associated with resections, controversy abounds as to whether the use of resective procedures for cancer of the pancreas should be continued, abandoned and replaced by palliative operations, limited to major surgical centers, or expanded to total or regional pancreatectomy.

In discussing cancer of the pancreas, it is important to distinguish between carcinomas of the head and uncinate process and those that arise in the body or tail of the gland. Cancers of the head and uncinate process cause symptoms different from those of the body and tail, are diagnosed slightly earlier, and are therefore somewhat more favorable in terms of potential for long-term survival. Similarly, it is important to differentiate between carcinomas of the periampullary region, ampulla of Vater, distal common bile duct, and periampullary duodenum, which cause symptoms almost identical to cancer of the head of the pancreas but have a much more favorable long-term survival after resection. There is little argument about the value of pancreatoduodenal resection for periampullary carcinomas.[29–34]

Pathology

Cancer of the pancreas arises from ductal cells in about 90% of patients and from acinar cells in about 10%. The lesion is an adenocarcinoma with an extensive fibrous or scirrhous component (Figure 10-7). The histological type is usually columnar cell carcinoma with tubular or acinar formation in a fibrous stoma. Occasionally squamoid, pleomorphic, or undifferentiated cells predominate. It is an infiltrating tumor with no identifiable gross margins.

The active tumor component is often small in relation to the bulk mass of the lesion, being surrounded by a zone of pancreatitis which may account for up to two-thirds of the mass. Early histological features include hyperplasia of the pancreatic ducts, dilatation of the ducts as they become obstructed, and varying degrees of pancreatitis in the obstructed pancreas.

About two-thirds of all carcinomas of the pancreas arise in the head and uncinate process; about one-third arise in the body and tail of the pancreas.[25,27,28,35]

With progressive growth of the tumor, invasion and obstruction of the distal bile duct occur in 75% to 90% of patients. Lymph node metastases are present in 80% to 90% of patients. Approximately 70% of patients have identifiable liver metastases at operative exploration. The tumor spreads

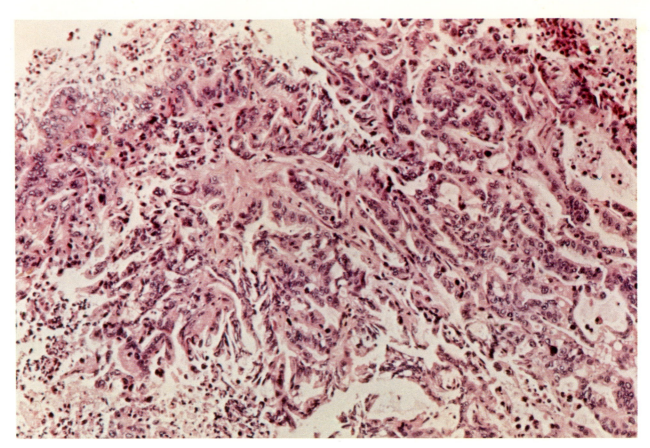

FIGURE 10-7. Photomicrograph of an adenocarcinoma of the head of the pancreas, ductal type.

progressively into the duodenum, along the portal and superior mesenteric veins, and into the nerves of the retroperitoneum.

Diagnosis

Cancer of the Head of the Pancreas and Periampullary Region.

SYMPTOMS. The onset of symptoms of cancer of the head and uncinate process of the pancreas and of the periampullary region is insidious and progressive. At the earliest stages, patients are aware of mild discomfort or pain, some weight loss or anorexia, or a vague feeling of unrest or depression. Most patients have had some symptoms for 1 to 3 months prior to seeking medical attention. Unfortunately, at the time of *initial* medical examination, all studies prove to be negative in a high percentage of patients, the disease is misdiagnosed, and patients are sent home with a placebo or made to believe they have functional distress. There may thus be another delay of 2 to 4 months before symptoms worsen, the results of tests become suspicious or positive, or the diagnosis is suspected.

The most common symptoms of carcinoma of the head of the pancreas, weight loss and pain, occur in 80% to 90% of patients (Table 10-1). The pain is characteristically dull, vague, and constant, often described as "like a toothache;" it is epigastric or central abdominal in location and radiates into the back. The patient may sit up, lean forward, or sleep on his side to gain relief.

Jaundice occurs in approximately 75% of patients and is probably the most common indication of organic or serious disease, leading to further

226

diagnostic studies and eventual operation in most patients. The jaundice is rarely painless, except in patients with carcinoma of the ampulla of Vater, distal common bile duct, or duodenum. It is constant, rarely fluctuates, and becomes progressively worse. Anorexia, nausea, diarrhea, constipation, weakness, lack of energy, and mental depression are other symptoms.

PHYSICAL FINDINGS. The most frequent physical finding on examination is an enlarged liver. Jaundice is apparent in about 75% of patients. An abdominal mass, usually a distended gallbladder (Courvoisier's sign) can be palpated in about 25% of patients; abdominal tenderness to deep palpation is found in about 25%. Occasionally liver tenderness is apparent. Patients with advanced disease may have ascites, muscular wasting, or palpable Virchow's nodes in the supraclavicular region of the neck.

Cancer of the Body and Tail of the Pancreas.

SYMPTOMS. Cancer of the body and tail of the pancreas is diagnosed even later in its course than is cancer of the head or uncinate process, with an average delay in diagnosis from onset of symptoms of approximately 6 to 8 months. Weight loss and pain are again the most common symptoms (Table 10-1).

The weight loss associated with carcinoma of the body of the pancreas may be profound; a loss of 20 to 30 pounds (9 to 13.5 kg) is not uncommon. Nausea, anorexia, loss of pancreatic enzymes, food intolerance, and mental depression all contribute to the profound weight loss.

The pain is more often in the central abdomen or left upper quadrant with pronounced radiation into the back. Occasionally band-like pain around the upper abdomen is described. Sitting up, assuming a knee–chest position, or lying on the side may gain relief from pain; the pain is worse when patients lie down and it frequently keeps them awake at night.

Jaundice is not a frequent symptom with carcinoma of the body and tail of the pancreas. It is present in only about 10% of patients, usually when the tumor has become advanced or metastatic to the liver.

Mental depression is more common, probably because of the delay in diagnosis, the patients' continuing distressing symptoms, and the subconscious knowledge that they are seriously ill. The incidence of thrombophlebitis has been overemphasized.[35]

TABLE 10-1   Clinical Features of Carcinoma
of the Pancreas

Symptoms	Head (%)	Body and Tail (%)
Weight loss	90	90
Abdominal pain	80	90
Back pain	20	70
Anorexia and nausea	50	50
Jaundice	75	10
Diarrhea	20	10
Constipation	10	25
Weakness	15	20
Depression	10	30
Thrombophlebitis	5	15

SOURCE   Data from Brown et al.,[25] Rastogi et al.,[28] and Howard and Jordan.[35]

PHYSICAL FINDINGS. Physical evidence of weight loss and malnutrition may be the most common finding. An enlarged liver is palpable in about one-third of patients. Deep abdominal tenderness and a vague or definite abdominal mass may be found in 20% to 30% of patients; diabetes mellitus is present in 10% to 20%. Evidence of advanced disease, ascites, Virchow's nodes, a rectal shelf, duodenal or colonic obstruction, and jaundice is found in 10% to 20% of patients.

Diagnostic Studies. A comparative wealth of diagnostic studies are available for the study of patients suspected of having carcinoma of the pancreas. Despite the many studies available, a high percentage of lesions diagnosed are still unresectable or incurable at operative exploration. The following studies are presently in use, with varying degrees of success.

BASIC LABORATORY TESTS. Routine or basic laboratory studies should be obtained on all patients. These should include a complete blood count, urinalysis, stool examination for guaiac, liver function tests, and blood glucose, prothrombin, and serum amylase determinations. Evidence of occult blood in the stool or anemia is present in 15% to 20% of patients. Liver enzyme changes, high levels of the alkaline phosphatase, and mild elevation of SGOT are common. The bilirubin is elevated in about 75% of patients with carcinoma of the head of the pancreas and in 85% to 90% of patients with carcinoma of the periampullary region. Prothrombin levels are decreased in patients with obstructive jaundice. Serum amylase levels may be mildly elevated at 200 to 400 Somogyi units (normal is less than 200 Somogyi units).

UPPER GASTROINTESTINAL SERIES. An upper gastrointestinal series using barium should be obtained in all patients suspected of having carcinoma of the pancreas, whether in the head or body and tail, or carcinoma of the periampullary region. The characteristic findings are widening and straightening of the C-loop of the duodenum, mucosal irregularities of the duodenum, the Frostberg "reversed 3" sign, distortion of the antrum of the stomach, or narrowing or compression of the third part of the duodenum (Figure 10-8).

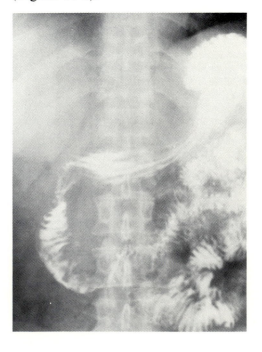

FIGURE 10-8. Upper gastrointestinal series in a patient with carcinoma of the head of the pancreas. The duodenum is widened and the mucosa is irregular.

ORAL CHOLECYSTOGRAPHY OR INTRAVENOUS CHOLANGIOGRAPHY. These indirect methods of visualizing the biliary system are of no value in the patient with clinical evidence of jaundice or with a serum bilirubin level higher than 3.0 mg/dl. In patients without jaundice, in whom the carcinoma may be in the body or tail of the pancreas, the biliary system should visualize and will probably be normal.

ENDOSCOPY—BIOPSY AND CYTOLOGY. Endoscopic examination of the stomach, duodenum, and periampullary region is extremely important in the evaluation of a patient with suspected carcinoma of the pancreas, ampulla of Vater, distal common bile duct, or duodenum. Biopsy of any polypoid lesion or mucosal irregularity should be obtained (Figure 10-9). If the pre-operative diagnosis of carcinoma can be made by biopsy and histological study, immediate plans for operation to determine resectability can be made. At operation, additional biopsy attempts can be avoided, thereby shortening operative time and lessening the risk of spreading tumor.

If a direct biopsy of a visible lesion cannot be made, cytological studies of the duodenum or pancreatic duct can be attempted. These have proved somewhat discouraging in providing a diagnosis of carcinoma, but many endoscopists are continuing attempts at improving the accuracy of cytological studies.

ENDOSCOPIC RETROGRADE CHOLANGIOPANCREATOGRAPHY. Direct visualization of the bile duct and pancreatic duct may be obtained in some patients with cancer of the pancreas or common bile duct. If the tumor is obstructing the papilla of Vater or is immediately inside the papillary orifice, then ERCP may not be possible. However, tumors of the bile duct at a higher level may be found with a normal bile duct below (see the section on Carcinoma of the Bile Ducts, Chapter 4) or cancers of the body and tail of the pancreas may be diagnosed (Figure 10-10). The finding of a localized

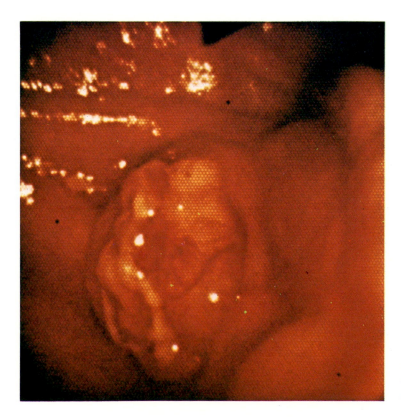

FIGURE 10-9. Endoscopic view of a carcinoma of the ampulla of Vater. A biopsy confirmed the diagnosis pre-operatively.

229

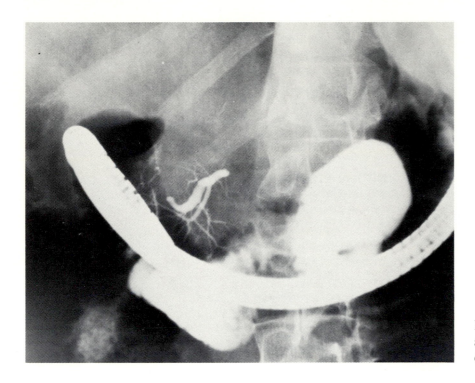

FIGURE 10-10. ERCP showing an abrupt obstruction of the pancreatic duct due to carcinoma.

obstruction in the pancreatic duct is good evidence for the presence of carcinoma.[36]

PERCUTANEOUS TRANSHEPATIC CHOLANGIOGRAPHY. In patients with jaundice suspected of having carcinoma of the head of the pancreas or periampullary region, percutaneous transhepatic cholangiography should be performed for direct visualization of the obstructed biliary system. Examples of typical findings are shown in Figure 10-11. We have usually performed this study pre-operatively, on the morning of operation immediately before surgery. The procedure is done in the Radiology Department under local anesthesia and the patient is then sent to the operating room. Recently, with the introduction of the skinny Chiba needle, some radiologists have performed the study several days pre-operatively, with little or no leakage of bile out of the needle tract into the abdomen.

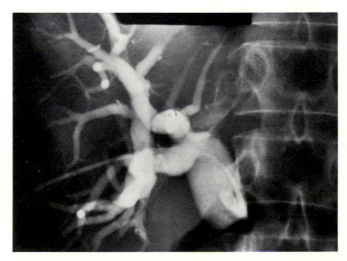
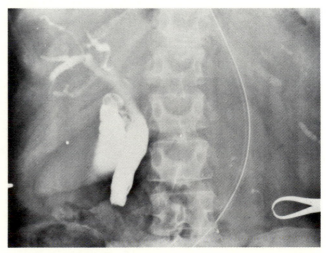

FIGURE 10-11. Transhepatic cholangiograms showing obstruction of the distal common bile duct from carcinoma of the head of the pancreas or periampullary region.

In some patients with obstructive jaundice of several weeks' duration, it may be wise to perform percutaneous transhepatic cholangiography 7 to 10 days pre-operatively and place a small polyethylene catheter into the biliary system for decompression of the jaundice to allow improvement in liver function. A period of time may be spent improving the patient's nutrition, prothrombin time, and overall operative risk prior to operation. We have done this in a few selected patients with obstructive jaundice of greater than 2 to 3 weeks and a bilirubin level higher than 10 to 12 mg/dl.

RADIOISOTOPE SCANS. Isotopic scans using selenomethionine-75 have been disappointing in the diagnosis of early lesions of the pancreas: small tumors are easily missed; false-positive results are seen in patients with pancreatitis or poor absorption of the isotope; the liver obscures the identification of pancreas; and resolution of the image has been disappointing (Figure 10-12). We rarely perform isotopic scans of the pancreas at the present time.

COMPUTED TOMOGRAPHY. CT technics are new methods of scanning solid organs of the body utilizing a 130-KV x-ray scanning gantry which scans the abdomen axially through an arc of 180 degrees. CT has proved to be of diagnostic value in patients with hidden tumors of the pancreas, liver, and other retroperitoneal structures. Tumor masses 2 cm or larger can be visualized and obstructive jaundice can be identified by visualization of obstructed bile ducts in the liver (Figure 10-13). Our experience with CT is still developing;[37] we are enthusiastic about its potential value.

ULTRASONIC SCANS—ECHOGRAPHY. Ultrasonic scans using a B-mode scanner, gray-scale, 2.25-MH transducer are being utilized and studied by many groups to ascertain their value in the diagnosis of early cancers of the pancreas. Lesions larger than 2 cm can be detected. Similarly, obstructive jaundice can be diagnosed based on the identification of dilated bile ducts seen on scans of the liver. Our experience with sonography is developing. We believe that it holds promise but is, at present, less accurate in the

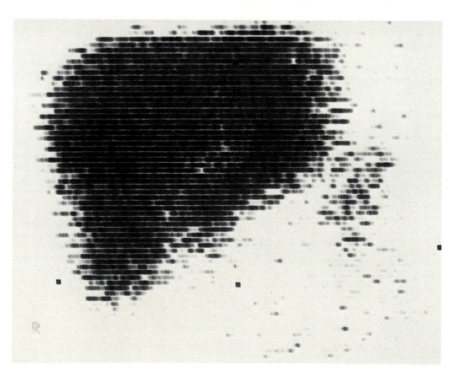

FIGURE 10-12. Selenomethionine-75 scan of the pancreas in a patient with carcinoma of the pancreas. Radioactivity in the pancreas is decreased.

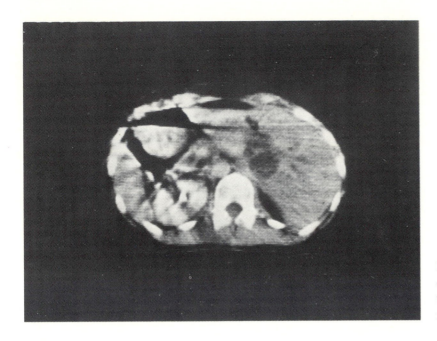

FIGURE 10-13. CT scan of the abdomen showing a dilated biliary system in the liver of a patient with carcinoma of the head of the pancreas.

diagnosis of small lesions than is CT. It has the advantage of being less expensive.

SELECTIVE CELIAC–SUPERIOR MESENTERIC ANGIOGRAPHY. Selective celiac and superior mesenteric arteriography has been available for almost 15 years.[39] During this time, it has become apparent that arteriography will not identify small carcinomas in the pancreas or periampullary region because of the avascularity of most of these tumors. Angiograms have their greatest value in the identification of benign and malignant islet cell tumors which are vascular. Advanced carcinomas of the pancreas can be identified because of their encasement and narrowing of the splenic, hepatic, or superior mesenteric arteries (Figure 10-14). Identification of this degree of involvement of any of the major vessels indicates unresectable disease.

Occasionally liver metastases may be seen by a vascular blush on the venous or late phase of the angiographic study in the liver.

TUMOR-RELATED ANTIGEN. Recent interest has centered on the use of blood or serum tests for tumor-related antigens. One of these is the carcinoembryonic antigen (CEA), which is markedly elevated in colon cancer, a variety of other neoplasms, and some inflammatory diseases. Martin and associates[40] have recently reported on the initial phase of an ongoing study utilizing CEA levels in the serum of patients with suspected carcinoma of the pancreas to determine its accuracy in helping make the diagnosis. These studies indicate that CEA levels are positive (above 2.5 ng/dl) in 75% of patients with large carcinomas of the pancreas or metastatic disease. CEA levels are not as yet helpful in the diagnosis of small or early tumors otherwise unsuspected. It is hoped that further studies of this and other tumor-related antigens, such as pancreatic oncofetal antigen, will help improve this method of diagnosis.[40a]

ACCURACY OF DIAGNOSTIC STUDIES. Several reports have focused on the usefulness and accuracy of the newer diagnostic studies in patients suspected of having cancer of the pancreas or periampullary region. Recent

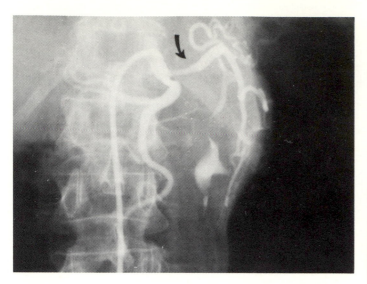
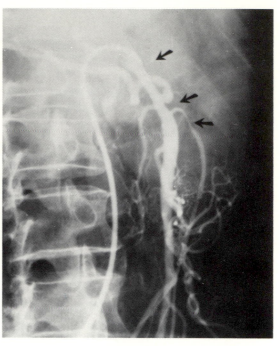

FIGURE 10-14. Arteriograms showing encasement of the splenic and superior mesenteric arteries in a patient with carcinoma of the pancreas. Arterial encasement is evidence that the lesion is not resectable.

reports indicate that CT, ultrasonography, and ERCP are 70% to 80% accurate.[41] Angiography, isotopic scans of the pancreas, and duodenoscopy with cytological studies or biopsy of any visible lesion have great value in selected patients but are not applicable to all patients. At the present time, two important questions in regard to the many new and expensive diagnostic studies now available are (1) how to use them cost effectively, and (2) whether they will diagnose small cancers potentially resectable for cure of this difficult disease.

Treatment

Operative Exploration and Biopsy. All patients in whom carcinoma of the pancreas or periampullary area is suspected should be explored for possible resection of the tumor. The operative exploration should be performed in a hospital that treats cancer of the pancreas with some frequency and by a surgeon familiar with operations on the pancreas who is capable of performing a pancreatic resection with an overall operative mortality of less than 10%.

After assessment of a mass in the pancreas, the pancreas should be mobilized and carefully evaluated as to (1) the size and location of the primary mass lesion, (2) invasion of a contiguous structure such as portal vein, superior mesenteric vein, or common hepatic artery, and (3) the presence of lymph node, liver, peritoneal, omental, or other metastases.

At this point, biopsy of the primary lesion and of any lymph node or other metastases should be performed. Biopsy can be obtained by (1) sharp scalpel biopsy of any superficial lesion on the surface of the pancreas, (2) Tru-cut needle biopsy into the pancreatic mass, preferably going through the duodenum (Figures 10-15 and 10-16), or (3) needle aspiration cytology of the lesion, going directly into the mass with a 21-gauge needle (Figure 10-17).[42-45] Biopsy of any suspicious area in the liver should also be performed.

Controversy surrounds the value of pancreatic biopsy, its accuracy, and the risk of the procedure.[43,46,47] I have recently reviewed the surgical literature on this subject. The accuracy of pancreatic biopsy is approxi-

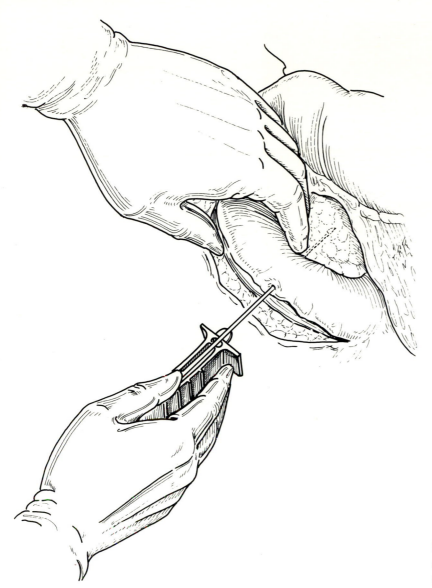

FIGURE 10-15. Transduodenal needle biopsy into a mass in the head of the pancreas.

mately 85%, with a 15% incidence of false negatives (misdiagnosis of pancreatitis). Biopsy of the pancreas is relatively safe, with a morbidity of about 5% and a mortality attributed to the biopsy alone of less than 1%. Obviously, the biopsy must be done with caution, avoiding biopsy into a palpable vessel or into the pancreatic duct system. If pancreatic duct leakage occurs after transduodenal Tru-cut needle biopsy, the leaking pancreatic juice will go into the duodenum. Small leaks into the peritoneal cavity can usually be controlled by silk sutures.

IS BIOPSY NECESSARY PRIOR TO RESECTION? How long should one persist in biopsy attempts? Is it necessary to have histological proof of the diagnosis in a small lesion prior to embarking on a pancratic resection for possible cure?

At the Cleveland Clinic, we believe that biopsy proof of the diagnosis is preferable, but not essential in patients with potentially curable carcinomas. If one insists on biopsy proof of all lesions prior to curative resection, then an excessive amount of time will be spent performing repeated biopsies on the pancreas and waiting for frozen-section reports in patients

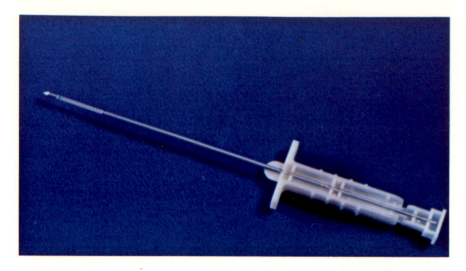

FIGURE 10-16.
Tru-cut biopsy needle.

with the *smallest* tumors which are most likely to be cured. The highest
incidence of false-negative histological reports on frozen section will also
be found in this group of patients with the most favorable lesions. In addition, repeated biopsies of a tumor mass can massage tumor cells into the
venous or lymphatic system.

We therefore make at least *two* good biopsy attempts of the lesion,
then make a decision for or against pancreatic resection based on clinical
and operative findings. These factors include (1) history (absence of a history of pancreatitis), (2) diagnostic studies, especially the type of cut-off of
the distal bile duct on percutaneous transhepatic cholangiography; and (3)
operative findings of localized disease (Table 10-2). In addition, if one is to
make this important operative decision for resection of a pancreatic mass
lesion based solely on clinical grounds, unsupported by biopsy proof of
malignancy, we believe intraoperative consultation with another senior
surgeon is advisable. If he agrees in the decision for resection, then we
proceed with the operation.

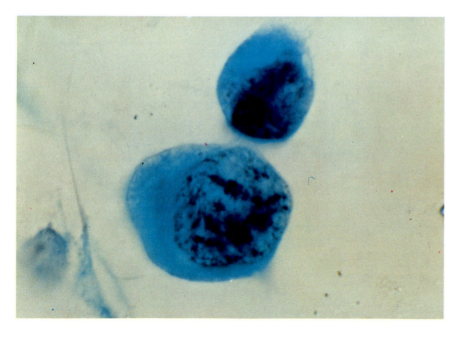

FIGURE 10-17. Cytological examination of cells obtained from needle
aspiration of a pancreatic mass showing atypical cells compatible with malignancy. Needle aspiration cytology
is the safest and may become the most
effective way to biopsy a mass in the
pancreas.

235

TABLE 10-2   Determination of Resectability of Carcinoma of the Pancreas

1. Tumor is localized in pancreas, no larger than 4 cm
2. No invasion of portal, superior mesenteric vein, or hepatic artery
3. No evidence of lymph node, liver, or other metastases beyond the field of resection

IS BIOPSY NECESSARY IF RESECTION IS NOT POSSIBLE?   If resection is not possible because of extensive or advanced disease and a palliative procedure or biopsy alone is to be performed, then I believe it is more necessary to prove the diagnosis before closing the abdomen. In such a patient we persist longer in attempting to obtain histological proof of the diagnosis of cancer since future treatment with chemotherapy or radiation therapy and the prognosis for the patient hinge on the accuracy of the diagnosis of carcinoma. Even with persistence, however, in about 5% of patients the diagnosis will be made on clinical evidence not supported by biopsy or histological proof of the malignancy.

STAGING.   At operation, patients with carcinoma of the pancreas or periampullary region may be usefully staged using the criteria of Hermreck et al.:[48] stage I indicates localized disease; stage II, extension into surrounding tissues (duodenum, portal vein, or mesenteric vein); stage III, metastases to regional lymph nodes; and stage IV, distant metastases.

Operative Procedures for Carcinoma of the Head of the Pancreas and Periampullary Region.   Great controversy continues among surgeons as to the "best" operative procedure for a patient with a cancer of the head of the pancreas.

It is important to assess carefully the potential resectability of any tumor when considering possible resection. Our criteria for resectability have been given in Table 10-2. Multiple biopsies of lymph nodes adjacent to the lesion, as well as a biopsy of any suspicious area in the liver should be performed when determining resectability.

PANCREATODUODENAL RESECTION.   Pancreatoduodenal resection was introduced by Whipple and associates[49] in 1935 as a technic of regional resection of a carcinoma of the ampulla of Vater, applicable also to carcinoma of the head of the pancreas (Figure 10-18). The Whipple operation has now had extensive use in the United States and throughout the world. Unfortunately, 5-year survival results for carcinoma of the pancreas are poor.[27,30,50–71] Table 10-3 lists reports from 18 major institutions in the United States, England, Scandinavia, and Japan, giving the results of over 1000 patients on whom the Whipple operation was performed for cancer of the pancreas. These results indicate the low resectability rate encountered with this disease, the variable mortality, and the low percentage (4%) of 5-year survivors. In a survey of operative mortalities by the Commission on Professional and Hospital Activities, Ann Arbor, Mich., of 271 Whipple operations performed in *community hospitals* in the United States in 1969, the average operative mortality was 32%[72]

Although the results of pancreatoduodenal resection for cancer of the head of the pancreas are discouraging, it is important to state that cancers arising in the ampulla of Vater, the distal common bile duct, and the duodenum have a much more favorable prognosis. Their resectability rates range from 50% to 80% (ampullary cancers being the most favorable since they

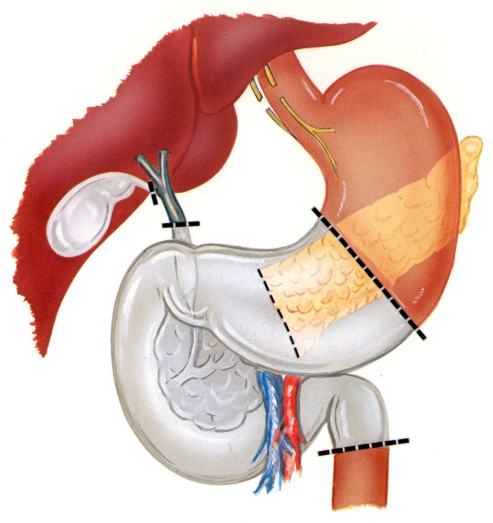

FIGURE 10-18. Extent of resection of a pancreatoduodenal resection (Whipple procedure).

are most often localized), and their 5-year survivals range from approximately 20% to 45%.[29,31–34,58,62,73,74] Table 10-4 lists 5-year results in a compilation of series collected from the surgical literature.

PALLIATIVE BYPASS PROCEDURES. When a carcinoma of the head of the pancreas or uncinate process cannot be resected, a bypass procedure of the obstructed common bile duct provides decompression and relief of the jaundice. This may be obtained either by a side-to-side choledochoduodenostomy or by cholecystojejunostomy, if the cystic duct is patent and joins the common bile duct well above the area of obstruction. In addition, if there is significant narrowing or obstruction of the duodenum from the cancer, a gastrojejunostomy should also be performed. Although some surgeons have urged that *both* bypass procedures always be performed when an operation for palliation is done, I believe that one can perform biliary bypass and/or gastrointestinal bypass selectively, based on pre-operative symptoms, diagnostic studies, and the operative evidence of obstruction of the distal bile duct and duodenum.

Because of the discouraging results of the Whipple operation for cancer of the pancreas (not periampullary cancer), several surgeons, most notably Crile, have advocated that it be abandoned and have suggested pal-

TABLE 10-3   Results of Pancreatoduodenal Resection for Carcinoma of the Pancreas

Report	Patients Resected	Resectability Rate (%)	Mortality Rate (%)	5-Year Survivors
Mayo Clinic[61]	119	10	25	8
Columbia-Presbyterian Hospital[63]	17	9	11	0
Massachusetts General Hospital[70]	26	21	34	2
Cornell University[27]	25	9	24	1
Baylor University[58]	36	—	22	1
University of Minnesota[67]	38	18	33	1
Ochsner Clinic[59]	22	—	27	3
University of Pennsylvania	51	27	31	0
University of Louisiana[65]	43	26	—	2
Vermont[60]	6	21	0	2
Texas[31]	16	—	31	0
Ellis Fischel Hospital[56]	13	—	24	0
Lahey Clinic[71]	138	—	15	10
UCLA	39	26	10	1
Cleveland Clinic[75]	28	4	10	0
Smith[68]	44	—	20	2
Norway[55]	12	6	8	0
Japan[62]	332	18	25	6
Total	1005	15	20	39 (4%)

liative bypass of the obstructed biliary and/or gastrointestinal system alone. Crile[75] Hertzberg,[55] and Shapiro[76] have compared the mortality rates, mean survival, and longest survival of patients with potentially resectable cancer of the pancreas after pancreatoduodenal resection and bypass procedures. In addition, Shapiro has compared the results of a collected series of 17 authors performing pancreatoduodenal resection and bypass procedures at Presbyterian–St. Luke's Hospital in Chicago. These results are given in Table 10-5.

TOTAL PANCREATECTOMY. Because long-term survival results after pancreatoduodenal resection are discouraging and because much of the postoperative morbidity and mortality relate to complications of the pancreatojejunal anastomosis, several surgeons, notably ReMine et al.[77,78] and Brooks and Culebras,[79] have begun to perform total pancreatectomy for cancer of the head of the pancreas. Other reports of total pancreatectomy collected from published reports over the past 15 to 20 years are given in Table 10-6, including the most recent results reported by ReMine and

TABLE 10-4   Periampullary Cancer 5-Year Survivals (Collected Series)

Site	Percent
Ampulla of Vater	30 − 45
Duodenum	35 − 40
Common bile duct (distal)	15 − 25
Average	26

TABLE 10-5 Comparison of Pancreatoduodenal Resection (PDR) and Biliary Bypass for Carcinoma of the Pancreas (in Potentially Resectable Patients)

Report	No. of Patients	Mortality Rate (1%)	Survival (months) Mean	Survival (months) Longest
Crile[75]				
PDR	28	10	6	22
Bypass	28	8	12	41
Hertzberg[55]				
PDR	12	8	17	36
Bypass	12	12.8	24	50
Monge et al.[61]				
PDR	94	25	12	60+
Bypass	23	—	12	42
Shapiro[76]				
PDR	24	8	10.6	22
Bypass	24	4	8.1	24
Collected series (Shapiro) of 17 authors				
PDR	496	21	13.9	60+

Brooks and their associates. At present, these operative procedures are competitive as far as operative mortality and 5-year survival are concerned. However, the post-operative morbidity after total pancreatectomy from the altered nutrition and brittle diabetes of total loss of the pancreas[80] exceeds that of pancreatoduodenal resection and for this reason many surgeons hesitate to advocate total pancreatectomy.

REGIONAL PANCREATECTOMY. Fortner et al.,[81] at Memorial Hospital, New York, are investigating a radical, regional pancreatectomy in which segments of the portal and superior mesenteric veins, celiac axis, and hepatic artery are removed along with the entire pancreas. This difficult and long operative procedure has not been proved applicable for the average surgeon as yet and cannot be recommended.

LOCAL RESECTION OF AMPULLARY CARCINOMA. In highly selected, elderly patients with polypoid carcinomas of the ampulla of Vater, local resection of the tumor has been performed through a duodenotomy incision. This procedure can be done with a low operative mortality and has resulted in several long-term survivals. It is not applicable to cancer of the head of the pancreas, distal bile duct, or duodenum, or to most cancers of the ampulla of Vater.

SUMMARY. From this discussion, the following points are clear: (1) Operations that resect cancer of the pancreas have a high operative mortality rate of 5% to 35%. (2) The resectability rate varies greatly. (3) The 5-year survival rate for cancer of the pancreas after any operative procedure is poor, but (4) the 5-year survival rate for cancer of the ampulla of Vater, distal common bile duct, and duodenum is significantly better. (5) Operations that bypass the obstructed biliary system have a lower operative mortality rate with a mean survival rate similar to the mean survival rate of patients after a pancreatic resection, but (6) the only chance to "cure" cancer of the

TABLE 10-6. Comparison of Pancreatoduodenal Resection (PDR) and Total Pancreatectomy for Carcinoma of the Pancreas

Report	Patients Resected	Mortality Rate (%)	5-Year Survivors
Porter[63]			
PDR	27	11	0
Total	18	28	0
Warren et al.[71]			
PDR	138	15	10 (7%)
Total	11	10	0
Jordan[58]			
PDR	36	22	1
Total	113	36	0
Brooks and Culebras[79]			
PDR	11	21	0
Total	16	12.5	3
Nakase[62]			
PDR	308	25	6
Total	45	20	
ReMine et al.[78] and Monge et al.[61]			
PDR	119	25	8 (7%)
Total	33	21	2 (6%)

pancreas, at the present time, lies in early diagnosis and complete resection of the carcinoma.

Operative Procedures for Carcinoma of the Body and Tail of the Pancreas. Cancer of the body and tail of the pancreas is rarely resectable for cure when encountered by the surgeon. At operative exploration, the tumor is almost always found to have involved or surrounded the celiac axis, hepatic artery, or superior mesenteric artery and vein. This can often be appreciated on the pre-operative arteriogram if one has been obtained. If the tumor has extended to or invaded these contiguous vital vascular structures, a biopsy should be obtained; needle aspiration cytology study may be the safest technic.[42,44,45] If there is no obstruction of the biliary system, duodenum, or other digestive organs, then the abdomen should be closed without a palliative bypass procedure.

In this situation, thought should be given to relief of the severe visceral and back pain experienced by these patients. Injection of the celiac ganglion or the para-aortic splanchnic nerve trunks with concentrated alchol solutions or diluted phenol solutions has been advocated by some authors.[49,82] At the Cleveland Clinic, we have had success with bilateral splanchnic resection, dividing the greater, lesser, and least splanchnic nerves through separate incisions performed through the back.[83]

Pre-operatively, if cancer of the body or tail of the pancreas is suspected in a patient with characteristic, severe back pain, a neurosurgeon examines the patient. Splanchnic blocks are rarely performed. At operation, if an unresectable tumor is found after biopsy has been performed, the abdomen is closed and, under the same anesthetic, the patient is turned into the prone position. The neurosurgical team then performs a bilateral splanchnicectomy through separate back incisions. Postoperative pain relief is obtained in about 80% of patients and is most gratifying to them.

Rarely, a small localized carcinoma may be encountered in the body or tail of the pancreas of a patient being explored for biliary disease or a peptic ulcer. (In my experience, it is not unusual for patients to have had an operation on the biliary system or on a longstanding duodenal ulcer, 6 or 8 months prior to discovery of a cancer of the body and tail of the pancreas. One wonders if the cancer might not have been the cause of the initial symptoms.) If, at the time of biliary or other surgery, a small tumor is discovered on palpation of the pancreas, this early lesion may be potentially resectable for cure. A distal pancreatectomy, 60% to 80% resection, and splenectomy should be performed. The only 5-year survival we have had at the Cleveland Clinic for a cancer of the body of the pancreas is a patient in whom the cancer was discovered incidentally by S. O. Hoerr while he was performing another operative procedure. A distal pancreatic resection was performed with excellent results.

Radiation Therapy. Postoperative cobalt or radiation therapy has proved to be of little benefit in most patients with cancer of the pancreas. Intensive radiation therapy with high-voltage units such as a 45-MV Betatron generator, cyclotron, or neutron accelerator unit is under trial.[84] The use of intraoperative radiation therapy directed into the open abdomen aimed specifically at the tumor is being investigated by some groups.

Chemotherapy. Chemotherapy given postoperatively has also been discouraging in the palliative treatment of cancer of the pancreas.[40,85,86] The use of 5-fluorouracil, either singly or in combination with other agents, has been studied the most thoroughly with objective remissions in 5% to 15% of patients. Recent studies have focused on the use of combination drugs. Intensive investigative efforts are proceeding under the auspices of the National Pancreatic Cancer Project[87] in the hope that greater success can eventually be achieved in controlling this discouraging disease.

References

True Cysts
1. Howard, J. M., and Jordan, G. L.: *Surgical Diseases of the Pancreas.* Philadelphia, Lippincott, 1960.
2. Becker, W. F., Welsh, R. A., and Pratt, H. S.: Cystadenoma and cystadenocarcinoma of the pancreas. *Ann. Surg.,* **161,** 845, 1965.
3. Rosato, F. E., and Mackie, J. A.: Pancreatic cysts and pseudocysts. *Arch. Surg.,* **86,** 551, 1963.
4. Swanson, G. E.: A case of cystadenoma of the pancreas studied by selective angiography. *Radiology,* **81,** 592, 1963.
5. Harbrecht, P. J.: Cystic disease of the pancreas. *Am. J. Surg.,* **124,** 607, 1972.
6. Warren, K. W., Athanassiades, S., Frederick, P., et al.: Surgical treatment of pancreatic cysts: review of 183 cases. *Ann. Surg.,* **163,** 886, 1966.
7. Buck, B. A., and Fletcher, W. S.: Carcinoma associated with pancreatic cyst. *Surg. Gynecol. Obstet.,* **134,** 44, 1972.
8. Priestly, J. T., and ReMine, W. H.: Problems in the surgical treatment of pancreatic cysts. *Surg. Clin. North Am.,* **38,** 1313, 1958.
9. Didolkar, M. S., Malhotra, Y., Holyoke, E. D., et al.: Cystadenoma of the pancreas. *Surg. Gyncecol. Obstet.,* **140,** 925, 1975.
10. Glenner, G. G., and Mallory, G. K.: The cystadenoma and related nonfunctional tumors of the pancreas. *Cancer,* **9,** 980, 1956.
11. Palm, E. T., and Scott, H. C.: Cystadenoma of the pancreas. *Minn. Med.,* **48,** 909, 1965.

12. Piper, C. E., Jr., ReMine, W. H., and Priestley, J. T.: Pancreatic cystadenomata; report of 20 cases. *J. A. M. A.,* **180,** 648, 1962.

13. Zintel, H. A., Enterline, H. T., and Rhoads, J. E.: Benign cystadenoma of pancreas. *Surgery,* **35,** 612, 1954.

14. Probstein, J. G., and Blumenthal, H. T.: Progressive malignant degeneration of a cystadenoma of the pancreas. *Arch. Surg.,* **81,** 683, 1960.

15. Cullen, P. K., Jr., ReMine, W. H., and Dahlin, D. C.: A clinicopathological study of cystadenocarcinoma of the pancreas. *Surg. Gynecol. Obstet.,* **117,** 189, 1963.

16. Sawyer, R. B., Sawyer, K. C., and Spencer, J. R.: Proliferative cysts of the pancreas. *Am. J. Surg.,* **116,** 763, 1968.

17. Warren, K. W., and Hardy, K, J.: Cystadencarcinoma of the pancreas. *Surg. Gynecol. Obstet.,* **127,** 734, 1968.

18. Winston, J. H., Jr.: Malignant islet cell adenoma in a pancreatic cyst. Report of a case. *J. Natl. Med. Assoc.,* **57,** 203, 1965.

19. Doubilet, H., and Mulholland, J. H.: Pancreatic cysts: principles of treatment. *Surg. Gynecol. Obstet.,* **96,** 683, 1953.

20. Iversen, H. G., and Johansen, A.: Cystadenocarcinoma of the pancreas. *Acta Chir. Scand.,* **131,** 381, 1966.

21. ReMine, W. H.: Discussion of Becker, W.F., et al.: *Ann. Surg.,* **161,** 862, 1965.

22. Burk, L. B., Jr., and Hill, R. P.: Papillary cystadenocarcinoma of the pancreas. *Ann. Surg.,* **136,** 883, 1952.

Carcinoma of the Pancreas and Periampullary Region

23. *Facts and Figures.* New York, American Cancer Society, 1977.

24. Bowden, L., and Pack, G. T.: Cancer of the head of the pancreas. *G.E.N.,* **23,** 339, 1969.

25. Brown, C. H., Rastogi, H., Alfidi, R., et al.: Diagnostic studies in carcinoma of the pancreas: a review of 100 patients. *J. L. Med. Soc.,* **120,** 375, 1968.

26. Cohn, I., Jr.: Surgical decisions in pancreatic disease. *Am. J. Dig. Dis.* [New Series] **9,** 918, 1964.

27. Glenn, F., and Thorbjarnarson, B.: Carcinoma of the pancreas. *Ann. Surg.,* **159,** 945, 1964.

28. Rastogi, H., and Brown, C. H.: Carcinoma of the pancreas. A review of one hundred cases. *Cleve. Clin. Q.,* **34,** 243, 1967.

29. Akwari, O. E., vanHeerden, J. A., Adson, M. A., et al: Radical pancreatoduodenectomy for cancer of the papilla of Vater. *Arch. Surg.,* **112,** 451, 1977.

30. Douglass, H. O., Jr.: Carcinoma of the head of the pancreas and periampullary region. *Surg. Annu.,* **6,** 161, 1974.

31. Fish, J. C., and Cleveland, B. R.: Pancreaticoduodenectomy for periampullary carcinoma. Analysis of 38 cases. *Ann. Surg.,* **159,** 469, 1964.

32. Stephenson, L. W., Blackstone, E. H., and Aldrete, J. S.: Radical resection for periampullary carcinomas. *Arch. Surg.,* **112,** 245, 1977.

33. Warren, K. W., Choe, D. S., Plaza, J., et al.: Results of radical resection for periampullary cancer. *Ann. Surg.,* **181,** 534, 1975.

34. Warren, K. W., Cattell, R. B., Blackburn, J. P., et al.: A long-term appraisal of pancreaticoduodenal resection for periampullary carcinoma. *Ann. Surg.,* **155,** 653, 1962.

35. Howard and Jordan: Malignancies of pancreas. In, *Surgical Diseases of Pancreas.* Philadelphia, Lippincott, 1960, p. 451.

36. Cooperman, A. M., Sivak, M. V., Sullivan, B. H., et al: Endoscopic pancreatography. Its value in preoperative and postoperative assessment of pancreatic disease. *Am. J. Surg.,* **129,** 38, 1975.

37. Cooperman, A. M., Haaga, J., Alfidi, R., et al.: Computed tomography: a valuable aid to the abdominal surgeon. *Am. J. Surg.,* **133,** 121, 1977.

38. McCormack, L. R., Seat, S. G., and Strum, W. R.: Pancreatic carcinoma. Survival following detection by ultrasonic scanning. *J. A. M. A.,* **238,** 240, 1977.

39. Meaney, T. F., Winkelman, E. I., Sullivan, B. H., et al.: Selective splanchnic

arteriography in the diagnosis of pancreatic tumors. *Cleve. Clin. Q., 30,* 193, 1963.

40. Martin, E. W., Jr., Kibbey, W. E., and Minton, J. P.: Carcinoembryonic antigen (CEA): a new diagnostic tool. *Ohio State Med. J., 71,* 300, 1975.

40a. Levin, B., Re Mine, W. H., Hermann, R. E., et al.: Cancer of the pancreas. *Am. J. Surg., 135,* 185, 1978.

41. Wood, R. A. B., Moosa, A. R., Blackstone, M. O., et al.: Comparative value of four methods of investigating the pancreas. *Surgery. 80,* 518, 1976.

42. Forsgren, L., and Orell, S.: Aspiration cytology in carcinoma of the pancreas. *Surgery, 73,* 38, 1973.

43. Isaacson, R., Weiland, L. H., and McIlrath, D. C.: Biopsy of the pancreas. *Arch. Surg. 109,* 227, 1974.

44. Kline, T. S., and Neal, H. S.: Needle aspiration biopsy: a safe diagnostic procedure for lesions of the pancreas. *Am. J. Clin. Pathol.,* 1975.

45. Tylen, U., Arnesjo, B., Lindberg, L. G., et al.: Percutaneous biopsy of carcinoma of the pancreas guided by angiography. *Surg. Gynecol. Obstet., 142,* 737, 1976.

46. Lightwood, R., Reber, H. A., and Way, L. W.: The risk and accuracy of pancreatic biopsy. *Am. J. Surg., 132,* 189, 1976.

47. Winegarner, F. G., Hague, W. H., and Elliott, D. W.: Tissue diagnosis and surgical management of malignant jaundice. *Am. J. Surg., 111,* 5, 1966.

48. Hermreck, A. S., Thomas, C. Y., IV, and Friesen, S. R.: Importance of pathologic staging in the surgical management of adenocarcinoma of the exocrine pancreas. *Am. J. Surg., 127,* 653, 1974.

49. Whipple, O. A., Parson, W. B., and Mullins, C. R.: Treatment of carcinoma of ampulla of Vater. *Ann. Surg., 102,* 763, 1935.

50. Aston, S. J., and Longmire, W. P., Jr.: Pancreaticoduodenal resection. Twenty years' experience. *Arch. Surg., 106,* 813, 1973.

51. Aston, S. J., and Longmire, W. P., Jr.: Management of the pancreas after pancreaticoduodenectomy. *Ann. Surg., 179,* 322, 1974.

52. Braasch, J. W., and Gray B. N.: Considerations that lower pancreatoduodenectomy mortality. *Am. J. Surg., 133,* 480, 1977.

53. Buckwalter, J. A., Lawton, R. L., and Tidrick, R. T.: Pancreatoduodenectomy. *Arch. Surg., 89,* 331, 1964.

54. Gilsdorf, R. B., and Spanos, P.: Factors influencing morbidity and mortality in pancreaticoduodenectomy. *Ann. Surg., 177,* 332, 1973.

55. Hertzberg, J.: Pancreaticoduodenal resection and bypass operation in patients with carcinoma of the head of the pancreas, ampulla, and distal end of the common duct. *Acta Chir. Scand., 140,* 523, 1974.

56. Hoffman, R. E., and Donegan, W. L.: Experience with pancreatoduodenectomy in a cancer hospital. *Am. J. Surg., 129,* 292, 1975.

57. Jordan, G. L., Jr.: The current status of pancreatoduodenectomy for malignant lesions of the pancreas. *Surg. Gynecol. Obstet., 127,* 598, 1968.

58. Jordan, G. L.: Surgical management of carcinoma of the pancreas and periampullary region. *Am. J. Surg., 107,* 313, 1964.

59. Lansing, P. B., Blalock, J. B., and Ochsner, J. L.: Pancreatoduodenectomy: a retrospective review 1949 to 1969. *Am. Surg., 38,* 79, 1972.

60. Leadbetter, A., Foster, R. S., Jr., and Haines, C. R.: Carcinoma of the pancreas. Results from the Vermont Tumor Registry. *Am. J. Surg., 129,* 356, 1975.

61. Monge, J. J., Judd, E. S., and Gage, R. P.: Radical pancreatoduodenectomy: a 22 year experience with the complications, mortality rate, and survival rate. *Ann. Surg., 160,* 711, 1964.

62. Nakase, A.: Surgical treatment of cancer of the pancreas and the periampullary region: cumulative results in 57 institutions in Japan. *Ann. Surg., 185,* 52, 1977.

63. Porter, M. R.: Carcinoma of the pancreatico-duodenal area operability and choice of procedure. *Ann. Surg., 148,* 711, 1958.

64. Richards, A. B., and Sosin, H.: Cancer of the pancreas: the value of radical and palliative surgery. *Ann. Surg., 177,* 325, 1973.

65. Richard, L., Jr., and Cohn, I., Jr.: Cancer of the pancreas. *Am. Surg.*, **35**, 95, 1969.

66. Ruilova, L. A., and Hershey, C. D.: Experience with 21 pancreaticoduodenectomies. *Arch. Surg.*, **111**, 27, 1976.

67. Salmon, P. A.: Carcinoma of the pancreas and extrahepatic biliary system. *Surgery*, **60**, 554, 1966.

68. Smith, R.: Progress in the surgical treatment of pancreatic disease. *Am. J. Surg.*, **125**, 143, 1973.

69. Smith, P. E., Krementz, E. T., Reed, R. J., and Bufkin, W. J.: An analysis of 600 patients with carcinoma of the pancreas. *Surg. Gynecol. Obstet.*, **124**, 1288, 1967.

70. Tepper, J., Nardi, G., and Suit, H.: Carcinoma of the pancreas: review of MGH experience from 1963 to 1973; analysis of surgical failure and implications for radiation therapy. *Cancer*, **37**, 1519, 1976.

71. Warren, K. W., Braasch, J. W., and Thum, C. W.: Carcinoma of the pancreas. *Surg. Clin. North Am.*, **48**, 601, 1968.

72. Commission on Profession and Hospital Activities. Personal communication, January 1972.

73. Beall, M. S., Dyer, G. A., and Stephenson, H. E., Jr.: Disappointments in the management of patients with malignancy of pancreas, duodenum, and common bile duct. *Arch. Surg.*, **101**, 461, 1970.

74. Crile, G., Jr., Isbister, W. H., and Hawk, W. A.: Carcinoma of the ampulla of Vater and the terminal bile and pancreatic ducts. *Surg. Gynecol. Obstet.*, **131**, 1052, 1970.

75. Crile, G., Jr.: The advantages of bypass operations over radical pancreatoduodenectomy in the treatment of pancreatic carcinoma. *Surg. Gynecol. Obstet.*, **131**, 1049, 1970.

76. Shapiro, T. M.: Adenocarcinoma of the pancreas: a statistical analysis of biliary bypass vs Whipple resection in good risk patients. *Ann. Surg.*, **182**, 715, 1975.

77. Pliam, M. B., and ReMine, W. H.: Further evaluation of total pancreatectomy. *Arch. Surg.*, **110**, 506, 1975.

78. ReMine, W. H., Priestley, J. T., Judd, E. S., et al.: Total pancreatectomy. *Ann. Surg.*, **172**, 595, 1970.

79. Brooks, J. R., and Culebras, J. M.: Cancer of the pancreas. Palliative operation, Whipple procedure, or total pancreatectomy? *Am. J. Surg.*, **131**, 516, 1976.

80. Waugh, J. M., Dixon, C. F., Clagett, O. T., et al.: Total pancreatectomy: a symposium presenting four successful cases and a report on metabolic observations. *Proc. Staff Meet. Mayo Clin.*, **21**, 25, 1946.

81. Fortner, J. G., Kim, D. K., Cubilla, A., et al.: Regional pancreatectomy: in bloc pancreatic, portal vein and lymph node resection. *Ann. Surg.*, **186**, 42, 1977.

82. Tank, T. M., Dohn, D. F., and Gardner, W. J.: Intrathecal injections of alcohol or Phenol for relief of intractable pain. *Cleve. Clin. Q.*, **30**, 111, 1963.

83. Sadar, E. S., and Cooperman, A. M.: Bilateral thoracic sympathectomy–splanchnicectomy in the treatment of intractable pain due to pancreatic carcinoma. *Cleve. Clin. Q.*, **41**, 185, 1974.

84. Haslam, J. B., Cavanaugh, P. J., and Stroup, S. L.: Radiation therapy in the treatment of irresectable adenocarcinoma of the pancreas. *Cancer*, **32**, 1341, 1973.

85. Moertel, C. G., Douglass, H. O., Hanley, J., et al.: Phase II study of Methyl-CCNU in the treatment of advanced pancreatic carcinoma. *Cancer. Treat. Rep.*, **60**, 1659, 1976.

86. Moertel, C. G.: Chemotherapy of gastrointestinal cancer. *Clin. Gastroenterol.*, **5**, 777, 1976.

87. National Pancreatic Cancer Project. Newsletter. (Isidore Cohn, Jr., Chairman. Louisiana State University).

Injuries of the Pancreas

11

Introduction

Pancreatic injuries are relatively uncommon because of the high intra-abdominal position of the pancreas and its deep retroperitoneal location, which protects it from all but the most forceful abdominal trauma. In addition, because of its relationship to the aorta, inferior vena cava, and portal, splenic, and superior mesenteric veins, many patients with major injuries of the pancreas do not survive the lethal effect of massive hemorrhage long enough to reach the hospital alive. Pancreatic injuries account for only about 2% of all abdominal injuries.[1,2]

Blunt trauma as a mechanism of injury to the pancreas, from steering wheels, bicycle handlebars, or forceful blows to the abdomen, is now somewhat more common than penetrating injuries from knife, gunshot, or shotgun wounds. This increasing frequency of blunt over penetrating injuries is a result of the greater number of high-speed automobile, motorcycle, and bicycle injuries seen in civilian practice.[3,4] In the past, however, from reviews of cases reported in the surgical literature and of cases reported from wartime experiences, penetrating injuries were roughly twice as common as blunt injuries.[5-8] Injuries to the pancreas during operative procedures on the stomach still occasionally occur.[9]

The pancreas is fixed and immobile in its retroperitoneal position and therefore is easily compressed against the spine. Three distinct types of injuries occur: injuries of the head, injuries of the midpancreas, and injuries of the distal pancreas. Injuries to the head of the pancreas also commonly injure the common bile duct, duodenum, portal vein, liver, gastroduodenal artery, right kidney, and right colon. These injuries frequently disrupt or crush the gland and are the most difficult to treat. They carry the highest mortality rate of all pancreatic injuries (28%).[6,10]

Injuries to the central pancreas commonly cause transection of the gland and may also injure the superior mesenteric vessels, splenic vein, liver, stomach, or transverse colon.[11] With blunt injuries to the mid-upper abdomen, no other injury except the injury of the pancreas may occur.

Injuries of the distal pancreas are the least serious and the least difficult to manage. Injuries of the distal gland frequently are associated with injuries of the spleen, splenic vessels, left diaphragm, left kidney, stomach, and splenic flexure of the colon. The mortality rate of injuries of the central and distal pancreas (16%) is roughly one-half that of injuries to the head.

The overall mortality of pancreatic injuries in 734 patients collected from the literature and reviewed by Northrup and Simmons was 20%.[6] Blunt injuries of a high-impact force, such as injuries from steering wheels, were extremely lethal, causing death in almost 50% of patients. Knife wounds had the lowest mortality (8%). Gunshot wounds had a mortality rate of 25% and shotgun wounds had a mortality rate of 60%. The mortality rate was dependent, to a great extent, on the associated injuries encountered. Pancreatic injury alone appeared to cause a mortality rate of only about 3% to 6%. Associated injuries, especially vascular injuries, increased the mortality precipitously. The more organs injured, the higher the overall mortality. Death appeared to be related predominantly to injuries of the major blood vessels, duodenum, and colon. The major cause of death was hemorrhage in 50% of patients, renal failure in 16%, and sepsis in 12%.

The late complications of pancreatic injury are pancreatic fistulas, pseudocysts, and abscesses. These have been discussed in detail in Chapter 9. Pancreatic fistulas occur in about 20% of patients after treatment of injuries to the pancreas. They are more common after injuries to the head of the pancreas (43%) than after injuries of the midgland (35%) or distal pancreas (10%).

Pseudocysts occur after approximately 10% of all pancreatic injuries. They are much more common in patients who have had blunt trauma (30%) than in those whose injury was penetrating. The development of a pancreatic pseudocyst after pancreatic injury is not a benign complication; this type of pseudocyst has a high frequency of further complications such as infection, perforation, hemorrhage, and erosion into adjacent viscera, with a mortality rate of 20%.

Pancreatic or peripancreatic abscesses, like pseudocysts (they are, in essence, infected pseudocysts), are much more common in patients who have had blunt or crushing injuries to the pancreas. They are the least frequent major late complication of pancreatic injuries and occur in about 5% of patients. Associated bowel or duodenal injuries are not common. They carry a mortality rate of 10% to 15%.[1,2,6]

Pathology

The pathology encountered in the injured pancreas is of three general types: (1) crush injury with necrosis and dissolution of pancreatic substance; (2) localized penetrating injury or missile tract into or through the pancreas; or (3) transection of the gland with complete division of its substance. It is important at operative exploration to fully assess the extent of the injury of the entire pancreas, exposing the entire organ to operative view. In addition, the duodenum, major vessels, common bile duct, spleen, kidneys, and other adjacent organs must all be carefully inspected.

Diagnosis

The history of the injury to the abdomen, especially that of blunt injuries, may initially appear to be insignificant. A careful history of the type of injury, the probable force of the injury, and its location is exceedingly important. The appearance of bruises, broken ribs, or other injuries may be the best initial guide to the force of the injury. With deep penetrating injuries of the upper abdomen, the probability of a pancreatic injury must be considered.

Symptoms immediately after the injury may be minor, such as only mild abdominal pain. With observation over a period of time, symptoms and signs of upper abdominal pain radiating into the back, deep abdominal discomfort, abdominal tenderness, a tender abdominal mass, or hypotension generally develop and increase in severity.

A serum or urinary amylase determination should be obtained in all patients with significant abdominal injuries, especially blunt injuries of the upper abdomen. Serum amylase levels are usually mildly elevated (300 to 500 Somogyi units) if pancreatic injury exists. In addition, paracentesis, four-quadrant abdominal taps, or peritoneal lavage and studies of the lavage fluid for the presence of elevated amylase levels, blood, or bile will help in establishing the diagnosis of pancreatic injury. If serum or peritoneal amylase levels are equivocal, the study should be repeated in 12 to 24 hr. Serial levels may be helpful. Blood hemoglobin or hematocrit levels may be useful, especially if there is intra-abdominal bleeding. Plain abdominal roentgenograms may be of value if a hazy distortion indicates the presence of intra-abdominal fluid or if a mass seems to be displacing the other organs. An upper gastrointestinal roentgenographic study of the stomach and duodenum using a water-soluble dye, Gastrograffin, may be helpful in identifying distortion of the duodenal C-loop or a duodenal injury.

All patients suspected of having a pancreatic injury should be operated upon for exploration of the pancreas.

Treatment

At operative exploration in patients with abdominal injuries, a quick inspection and superficial exploration of the pancreas can be achieved by opening the lesser peritoneal cavity through the gastrohepatic ligament above the stomach. However, if one suspects a pancreatic injury, the entire pancreas should be carefully inspected and palpated by (1) performing a Kocher maneuver, opening the retroperitoneum along the lateral border of the duodenum and mobilizing the duodenum and head of the pancreas medially to the midline, and (2) opening through the gastrocolic omentum into the lesser peritoneal cavity to expose the entire body and tail of the pancreas. Any evidence of injury to the pancreas, such as a retroperitoneal hematoma in the vicinity of the pancreas, should be thoroughly explored. The body and tail of the pancreas can be mobilized and explored by incising through the avascular plane below (caudad) the pancreas and mobilizing the gland cephalad, or by mobilizing the spleen and distal pancreas medially to inspect both ventral and dorsal sides of the gland. All organs or blood vessels in the vicinity of the pancreas should also be explored, carefully inspected, and palpated. It is frequently necessary to divide the ligament of Treitz and take down the third part of the duodenum, if there is a pancreatic injury in this vicinity, to look carefully for an accompanying retroperitoneal duodenal injury.

If a pancreatic injury is found, after the extent of the injuries to the pancreas and other structures has been determined, careful hemostasis is the next essential step. Hemorrhage, as noted above, is the major cause of death in patients who have suffered injury to the pancreas. Careful debridement of injured or devitalized pancreatic tissue should be done and suture ligation control of bleeding from the injured pancreas accomplished. Suture ligature, using figure-of-eight sutures, is the most effective method of controlling bleeding from small vessels in the pancreas. Silver clips, large and small, carefully applied may also be extremely effective.

A careful search for pancreatic duct injury and leakage of pancreatic juice is next in importance. With severe or massive crushing injuries, ductal injury at multiple sites can be assumed, even though a major duct injury may not be visualized. With a penetrating injury, such as a stab wound or gunshot wound, a careful search for a major duct injury should be made. With a transected pancreas, such as in a central gland injury over the spine, the divided major pancreatic duct can frequently be easily seen.

Management of Injuries of the Head of the Pancreas. Injuries of the head of the pancreas are the most difficult to manage and are potentially the most lethal. When the injury is not severe and there is no apparent injury to the duodenum, common bile duct, portal vein, or gastroduodenal artery, simple suture repair of the pancreas and any evident pancreatic duct injury, and sump suction drainage of the area may be adequate. Adding sphincteroplasty or catheterization of the pancreatic duct for duct drainage in this setting has not proved to be of any additional advantage.[3,4,6,10,12] If a more serious or massive injury of the head of the pancreas is found, various options should be considered, depending on the type and severity of the injury: (1) debridement and Roux-Y jejunal segment coverage of the area of injury (Figure 11-1); (2) distal gastrectomy and Billroth II gastrojejunostomy with closure of the duodenal stump (diverticulization of the injury), T-tube duodenostomy, and sump suction or Roux-Y jejunal coverage of the area of injured pancreas (Figure 11-2); or (3) pancreatoduodenectomy, removing the injured head of the pancreas and duodenum.[1,13] The magni-

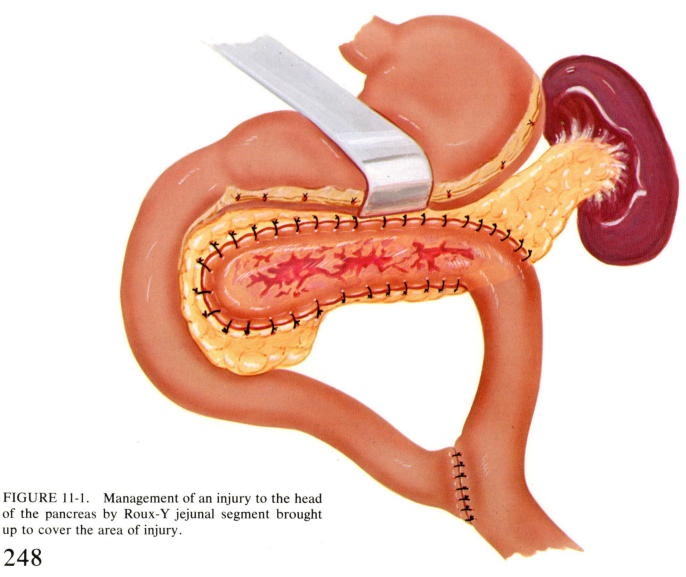

FIGURE 11-1. Management of an injury to the head of the pancreas by Roux-Y jejunal segment brought up to cover the area of injury.

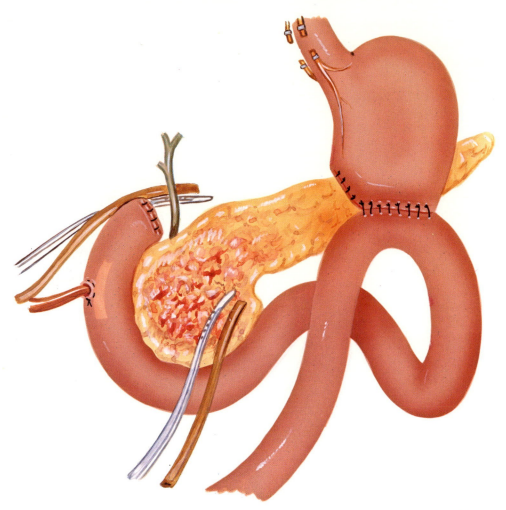

FIGURE 11-2.   More severe injury of the head of the pancreas treated by diverticulization of the injury.

tude of the operative procedure and probable mortality rate of these three options is, obviously, on an ascending scale. Pancreatoduodenectomy should be reserved for massive combined injuries of the head of the pancreas and duodenum; the mortality rate associated with the Whipple procedure in this setting is 20% to 30%.[1,2,6,13] Post-operative, liberal drainage of the remaining pancreas and right upper quadrant is essential, whichever procedure is performed.

Management of Injuries to the Midpancreas.   Most injuries of the middle portion of the pancreas are transection injuries of the gland as it crosses over the spine. These injuries may be handled in three general ways: (1) An attempt may be made to repair the injury if transection of the pancreas is not complete. This may entail anything from simple suturing of the pancreatic capsule alone to identifying the pancreatic duct and attempting to repair it over a catheter splint or small T-tube. The area of the pancreatic injury should be drained liberally after repair. (2) When the injury is more severe, an attempt to repair the injury using a Roux-Y jejunal segment may be made, covering the area of injury with the opened intestinal segment and preserving the distal pancreas. (3) Finally, if the injury is severe or extensive, one may debride the area of injury and resect the distal pancreas. A Roux-Y jejunal segment may be used for internal drainage of the divided proximal pancreas. In the past, some authors have suggested implanting the end of the divided pancreas into the stomach.[7] I have had no experience with this method of repair and would not advise it.

Management of Injuries to the Distal Pancreas. Injuries to the body and tail of the pancreas, to the left of the superior mesenteric vessels, should almost always be treated by resection of the distal pancreas and spleen. Only occasional, minor injuries should be repaired or drained without resection. If the entire injury is resected back to normal pancreas, the divided end of the gland can be closed with interrupted silk suture; an effort is made to identify the pancreatic duct and ligate it separately. If the area of transection of the gland is not in normal pancreas, then it is wise to drain the divided distal pancreas into a Roux-Y jejunal segment. The left upper quadrant and subdiaphragmatic area should be drained unless hemostasis and control of pancreatic leakage is unusually secure.

References

1. Owens, M. P., and Wolfman, E. F., Jr.: Pancreatic trauma. Management and presentation of a new technic. *Surgery, 73,* 881, 1973.
2. Sturim, H. S.: The surgical management of pancreatic injuries. *Surg. Gynecol. Obstet., 122,* 133, 1966.
3. Doubilet, H., and Mulholland, J. H.: Some observations on the treatment of trauma to the pancreas. *Am. J. Surg., 105,* 741, 1963.
4. Martin, L. W., Henderson, B. M., and Welsh, N.: Disruption of the head of the pancreas caused by blunt trauma in children: a report of two cases treated with primary repair of the pancreatic duct. *Surgery, 63,* 697, 1968.
5. Barnett, W. O., Hardy, J. D., and Yelverton, R. L.: Pancreatic trauma: review of 23 cases. *Ann. Surg., 163,* 892, 1966.
6. Northrup, W. F., III, and Simmons, R. L.: Pancreatic trauma: a review. *Surgery, 71,* 27, 1972.
7. Thompson, R. J., and Hinshaw, D. B.: Pancreatic trauma: review of 87 cases. *Ann. Surg., 163,* 1, 1966.
8. Werschky, L. R., and Jordan, G. L., Jr.: Surgical management of traumatic injuries to the pancreas. *Am. J. Surg., 116,* 768, 1968.
9. Carpenter, J. C., and Crandell, W. B.: Common bile duct and major pancreatic duct injuries during operations on the stomach. *Ann. Surg., 148,* 66, 1958.
10. Heitsch, R. C., Knutson, C. O., Fulton, R. L., et al.: Delineation of critical factors in the treatment of pancreatic trauma. *Surgery, 80,* 523, 1976.
11. Sturim, H. S.: Surgical management of traumatic transection of the pancreas: review of nine cases and literature review. *Ann. Surg., 163,* 399, 1966.
12. Doubilet, H., and Mulholland, J. H.: Surgical management of injury to the pancreas. *Ann. Surg., 150,* 854, 1959.
13. Salyer, K., and McClelland, R.: Pancreatoduodenectomy for trauma. *Arch. Surg., 95,* 636, 1967.

Operative Technics

12

Pancreatic Exploration

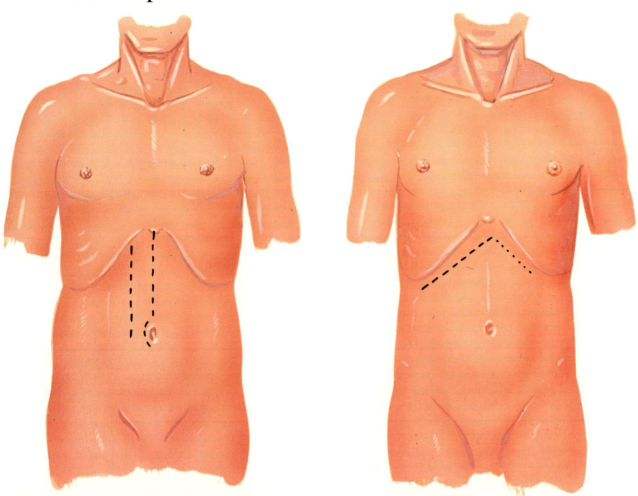

FIGURE 12-1.   The incisions I prefer for exploration of the pancreas: a midline upper abdominal incision or right paramedian incision for a thin patient with a narrow costal angle; or a right subcostal or bilateral subcostal incision for an obese patient with a wide costal angle.

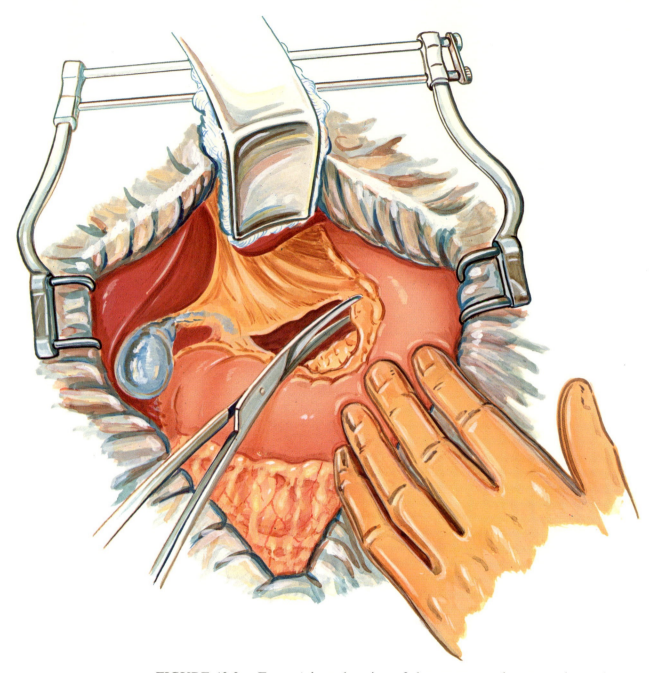

FIGURE 12-2.   For *quick* exploration of the pancreas, the stomach can be retracted inferiorly and the gastrohepatic ligament can be divided in an avascular
area, entering the lesser peritoneal cavity. The pancreas is seen under the stomach
and operative exploration with visualization and palpation of about 80% of the
gland can be obtained. This is an ideal way to assess the pancreas quickly when
the main thrust of the operative procedure is an operation on another organ system. This exposure of the pancreas is not adequate for *complete* evaluation of the
entire pancreas as a portion of the head and uncinate process are not clearly visible.

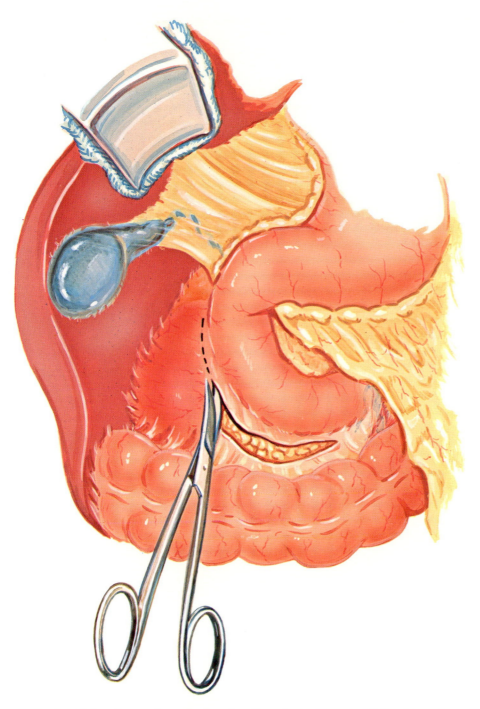

FIGURE 12-3.   To explore the head and uncinate process of the pancreas, a generous Kocher maneuver should be performed. The peritoneum lateral to the duodenum is sharply incised using a scissors; the duodenum is retracted medially by the surgeon's assistant. The surgeon can pick up the retroperitoneal tissues with a forceps and continue to dissect sharply the posterior wall of the duodenum and pancreas away from the inferior vena cava and other retroperitoneal structures.

253

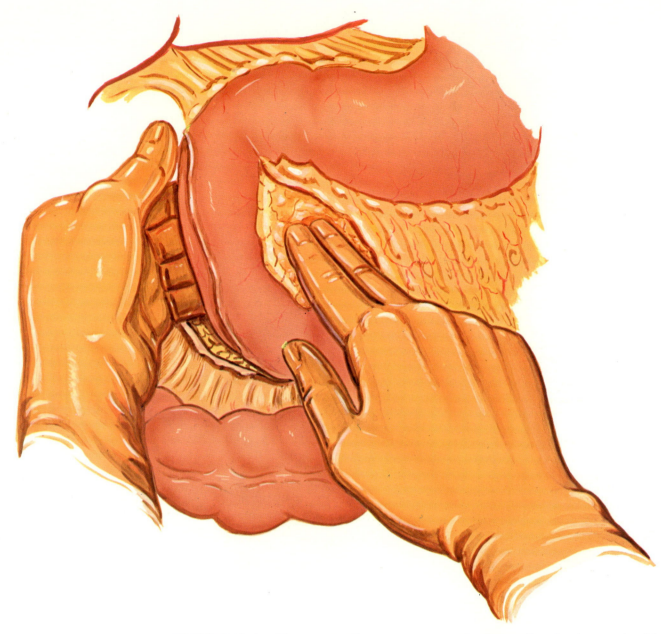

FIGURE 12-4.   The gastrocolic omentum over the descending duodenum should be excised and reflected medially so that the entire sweep of the second part of the duodenum and the head of the pancreas are adequately exposed. After the duodenum has been adequately mobilized from its retroperitoneal position to the midline, the surgeon can pass his left hand behind the head of the pancreas and, with his right hand, bimanually palpate and inspect the entire head of the pancreas and uncinate process. By mobilization of the duodenum medially, the posterior surface of the head of the pancreas can be visualized.

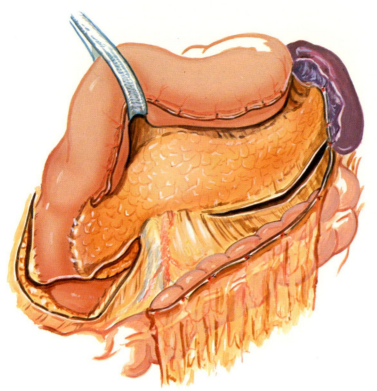

FIGURE 12-5. To explore the remainder of the pancreas, its neck, body, and tail, the gastrohepatic omentum should be divided below the gastroepiploic vessels. The stomach is mobilized up and the transverse colon with attached omentum down. The pancreas is fully exposed, from its head to the tail of the gland. By incision along the lower border of the pancreas lateral to the superior mesenteric artery and vein, the avascular plane behind the pancreas is entered.

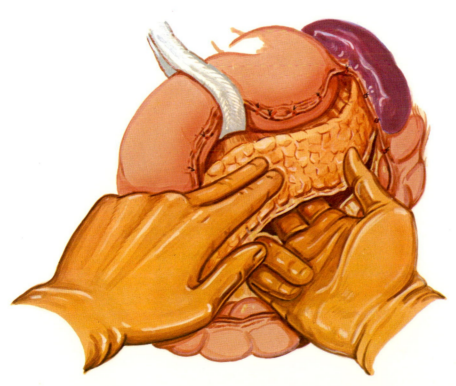

FIGURE 12-6. This avascular dissection plane is entered behind the pancreas and the distal gland is mobilized superiorly; the surgeon can then pass his right hand behind the body and tail of the pancreas and bimanually palpate this area. It is only by completely mobilizing the head, body, and tail of the pancreas, working through the gastrocolic omentum, that the surgeon can completely inspect and palpate the entire gland for thorough operative evaluation.

255

Operative Pancreatography

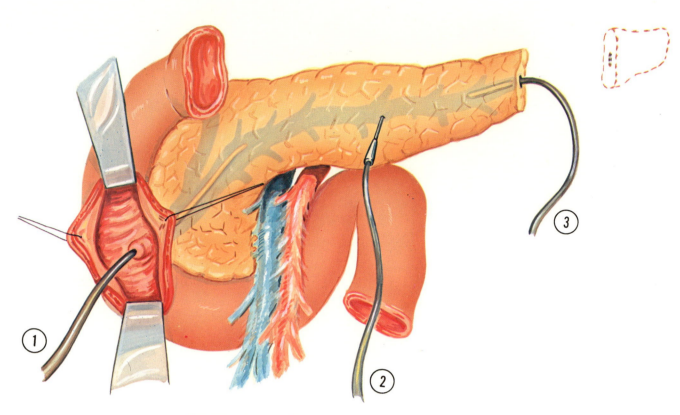

FIGURE 12-7. Three techniques of operative pancreatography are available: (1) Transduodenal catheterization of the pancreatic duct and retrograde pancreatography, (2) midduct needle injection pancreatography, and (3) catheterization of the distal pancreatic duct and prograde pancreatography.

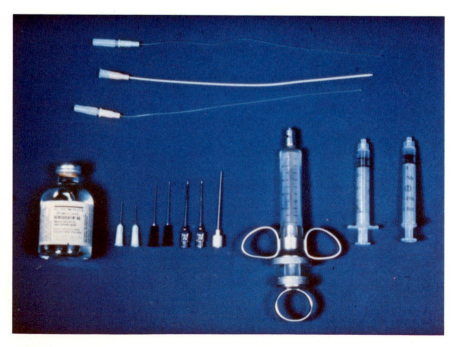

FIGURE 12-8. The instruments I use for operative pancreatography include 2-ml and 10-ml syringes, a series of 18- to 21-gauge needles, a series of 14- to 18-gauge polyethylene tubing (Intracath) with syringe attachment, and a bottle of Renografin-60 dye.

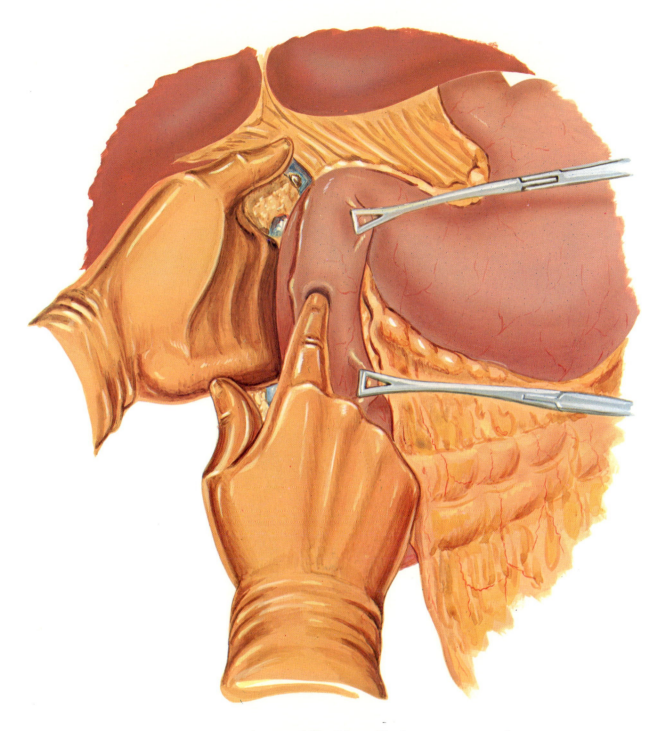

FIGURE 12-9.   The duodenum has been mobilized by a Kocher maneuver and the surgeon palpates for the papilla of Vater, usually felt along the medial wall of the duodenum as a firm projection. If the papilla of Vater cannot be palpated, its general location can be estimated by an operative cholangiogram. If necessary, the common bile duct can be opened above the duodenum and a small probe or catheter can be passed down the distal duct into the papilla of Vater for palpation.

257

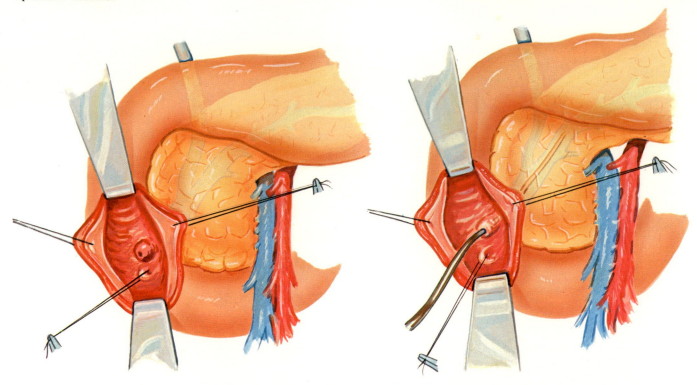

FIGURE 12-10.   A longitudinal duodenotomy is performed over the area of the papilla of Vater. Two small laparotomy gauze packs are placed in the proximal and distal limbs of the duodenum to prevent duodenal juice from obscuring the operative field. Two small right angle retractors are placed over these packs. A 3-0 silk suture is passed through the medial wall of the duodenum, below the papilla of Vater, to bring the medial wall forward. A small polyethylene catheter can usually be passed into the papilla of Vater and directly into the pancreatic duct. If there is difficulty in passing this catheter, a small sphincteroplasty can be performed. After the pancreatic duct has been catheterized, pancreatic juice is aspirated and approximately 1.5 to 2.0 ml of Renografin-60 dye is instilled for an operative pancreatogram. It is essential not to overfill the pancreatic duct system on the first instillation as this may induce pancreatitis. Two roentgenograms are taken. After these roentgenograms have been viewed, if the pancreatic duct is quite large or incompletely demonstrated, an additional 2.0 to 5.0 ml may be instilled for another roentgenographic study.

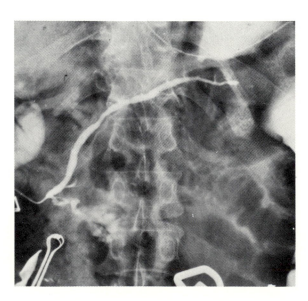

FIGURE 12-11.   Operative pancreatogram of a normal pancreatic duct.

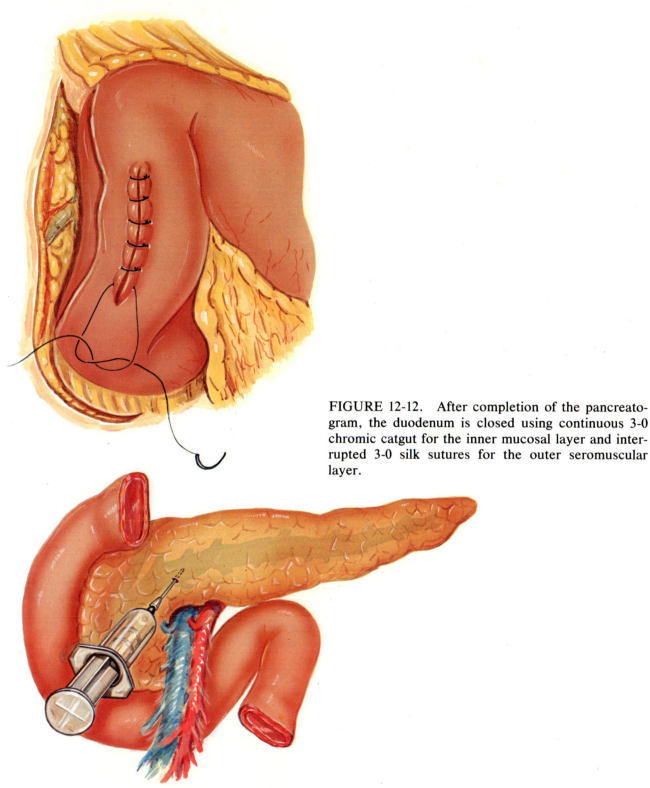

FIGURE 12-12. After completion of the pancreatogram, the duodenum is closed using continuous 3-0 chromic catgut for the inner mucosal layer and interrupted 3-0 silk sutures for the outer seromuscular layer.

FIGURE 12-13. If the surgeon does not wish to open the duodenum, or if there is extensive induration in the head of the pancreas, a midduct pancreatogram may be obtained. The pancreas should be exposed throughout its length. An obstructed and distended pancreatic duct may be palpated on the ventral surface of the gland. A 2-ml syringe attached to a 21-gauge needle is introduced into the mid-pancreatic duct, pancreatic juice is aspirated, and 1.5 to 2.0 ml of dye is instilled for an operative pancreatogram.

259

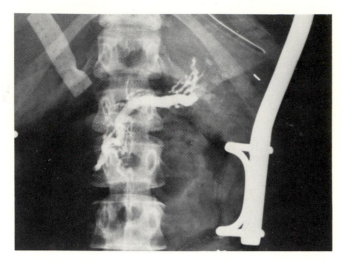 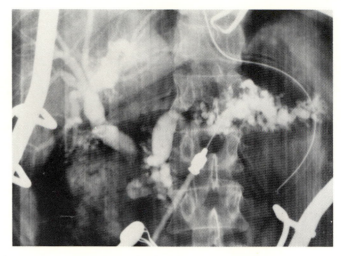

FIGURE 12-14. Operative pancreatograms obtained by midduct pancreatography.

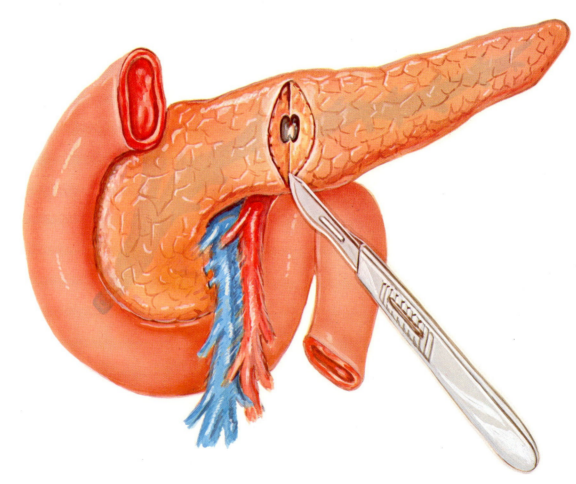

FIGURE 12-15. If the pancreatic duct cannot be palpated on the ventral surface of the pancreas, careful transverse sectioning of the pancreas may be performed to locate the duct. When the pancreatic duct is found, it can be cannulated and an operative pancreatogram can be performed.

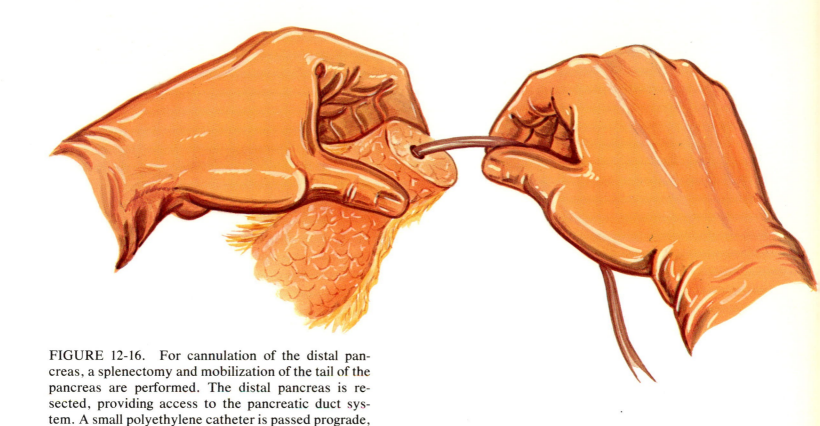

FIGURE 12-16. For cannulation of the distal pancreas, a splenectomy and mobilization of the tail of the pancreas are performed. The distal pancreas is resected, providing access to the pancreatic duct system. A small polyethylene catheter is passed prograde, from the tail toward the midpancreas, and 2 ml of dye is instilled for an operative pancreatogram.

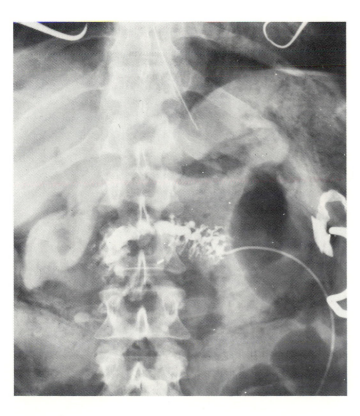

FIGURE 12-17. Operative pancreatogram showing this method of pancreatography.

261

Duodenojejunostomy for Annular Pancreas

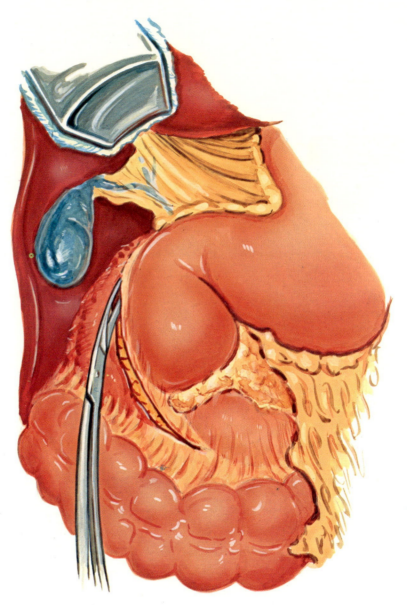

FIGURE 12-18.   The lateral peritoneal reflection over the duodenum is incised and a Kocher maneuver performed on a patient with an annular pancreas and a dilated proximal duodenum and stomach.

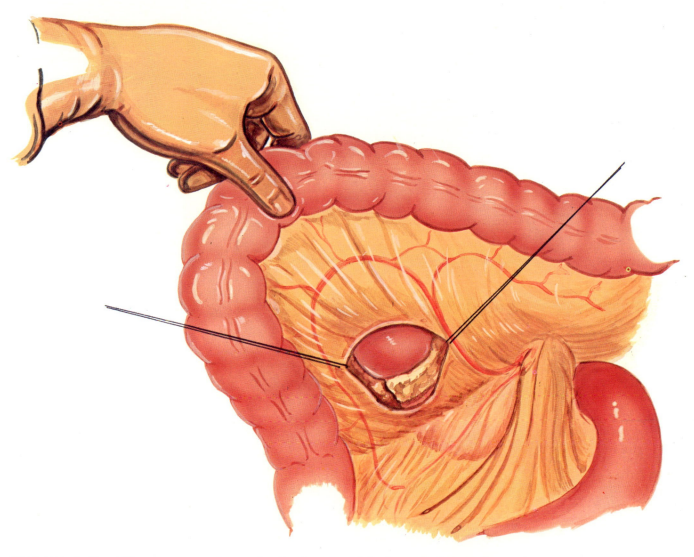

FIGURE 12-19.   The transverse mesocolon in the area of the hepatic flexure is elevated and a window is cut in the mesocolon to expose the proximal duodenum.

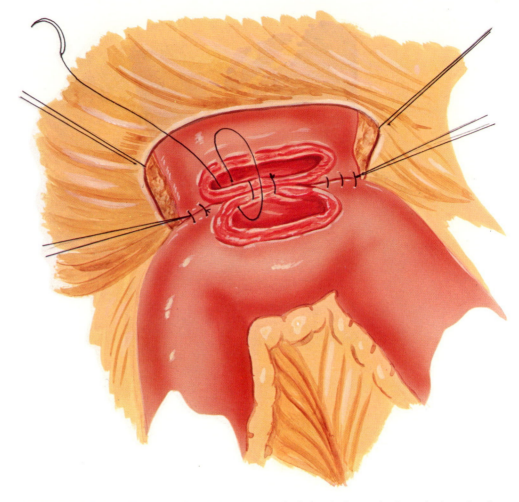

FIGURE 12-20. The proximal duodenum is joined through the window in the transverse mesocolon, side to side, to the first portion of the jejunum. The anastomosis is made immediately proximal to the annular pancreas in two layers, with interrupted 3-0 silk sutures to the posterior row, and a continuous 3-0 chromic catgut suture to the inner, mucosal layer.

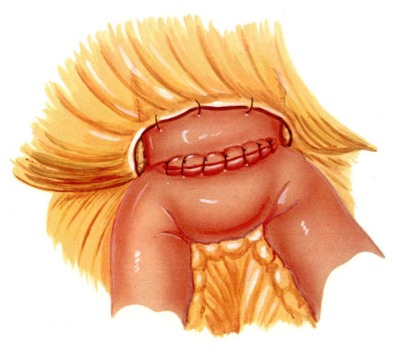

FIGURE 12-21. The anastomosis has been completed. Although duodenojejunostomy is preferred for bypassing an annular pancreas obstructing the duodenum, alternative methods include duodenoduodenostomy and gastrojejunostomy.

264

Drainage and Debridement of Pancreatic Necrosis or Abscess

During an operative procedure performed for acute, severe pancreatitis (hemorrhagic, necrotizing pancreatitis) the surgeon should (1) explore the abdomen to confirm the diagnosis of pancreatitis, (2) debride and drain any areas of necrosis, infected pancreatic tissue, or pancreatic juice collections, (3) drain the biliary system by cholecystostomy if there is evidence of bile duct obstruction, and (4) leave suction catheters in the peritoneal cavity for post-operative peritoneal drainage and lavage.

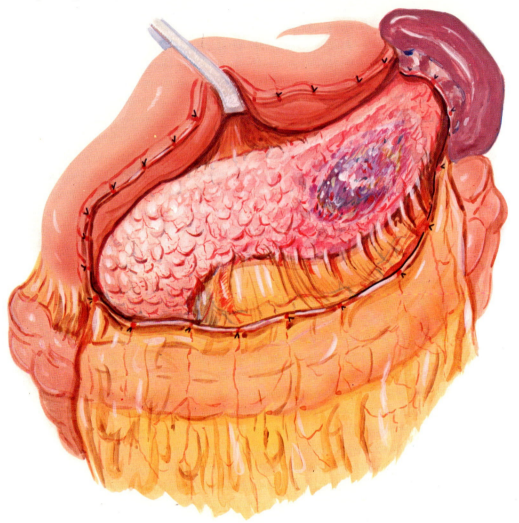

FIGURE 12-22.   Operative exposure of the pancreas is obtained by opening the gastrocolic omentum; an area of necrosis in the distal pancreas is shown.

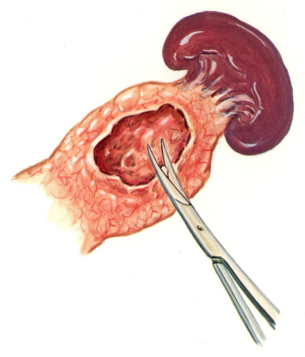

FIGURE 12-23. The area of pancreatic necrosis is debrided and collections of trapped pancreatic juice and areas of fat necrosis adjacent to the pancreas are drained.

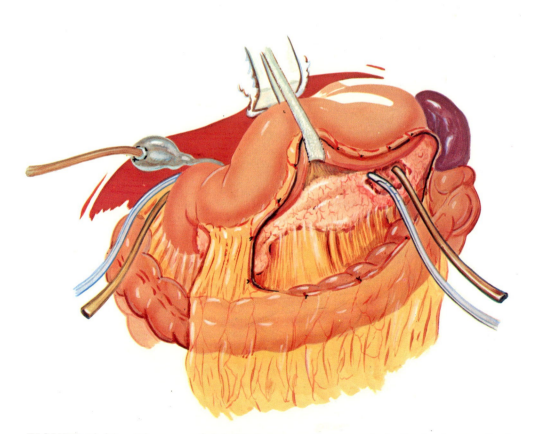

FIGURE 12-24. The area of debrided pancreatic necrosis in the body or tail of the pancreas is shown with drains and catheters placed into the lesser peritoneal cavity, a cholecystostomy tube in the gallbladder, and drains and catheters in the right subhepatic space. Additional drains or suction catheters may be placed in the lower abdomen or under the left diaphragm as needed. By means of sump suction catheters, approximately 1000 to 2000 ml of saline or Ringer's lactate solutions will be lavaged through the peritoneal cavity each 8 hr post-operatively for 2 to 3 days.

Sphincteroplasty and Pancreatic Duct Exploration

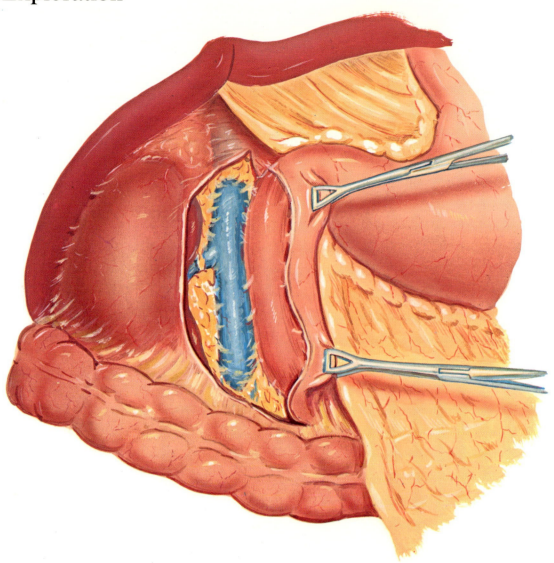

FIGURE 12-25.   The duodenum is mobilized from its retroperitoneal position by incising the lateral peritoneal reflection; the dissection should be carried beyond the vena cava to the lumbar spine to mobilize the duodenum into the incision.

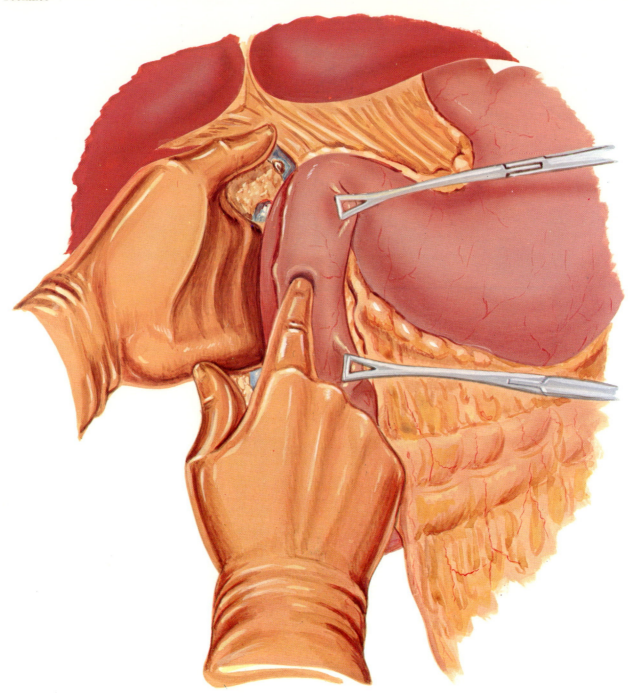

FIGURE 12-26.   The surgeon's left hand is placed behind the duodenum and the right hand palpates the papilla of Vater.

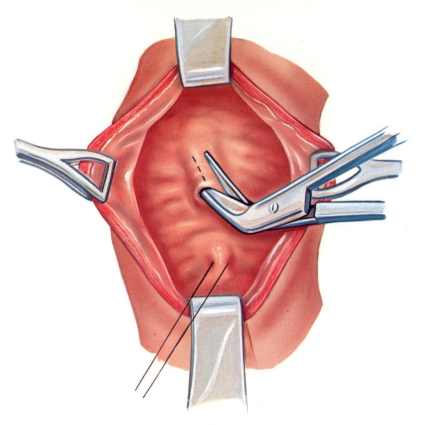

FIGURE 12-27. The duodenum is opened by longitudinal duodenostomy directly over the sphincter. Small laparotomy gauze pads are placed in the ascending and descending duodenum to occlude duodenal flow. A 3-0 silk suture is placed below the papilla of Vater in the medial wall of the duodenum to bring it forward. Pott's angled vascular scissors are used to cut the choledochal sphincter in the 11 o'clock position. This incision is carried superiorly for approximately 2.0 to 2.5 cm.

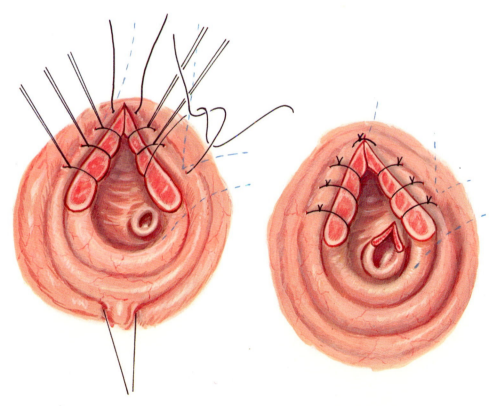

FIGURE 12-28.   The mucosa of the duodenum and distal bile duct are approximated with interrupted 4-0 chromic catgut sutures. It is important to place a suture at the apex of this incision, where the incision might carry through the posterior wall of the duodenum. The pancreatic duct orifice is also opened and the thickened septum between the orifice of the pancreatic duct and common bile duct is incised. A biopsy specimen of this thickened septum may be submitted to the pathologist.

269

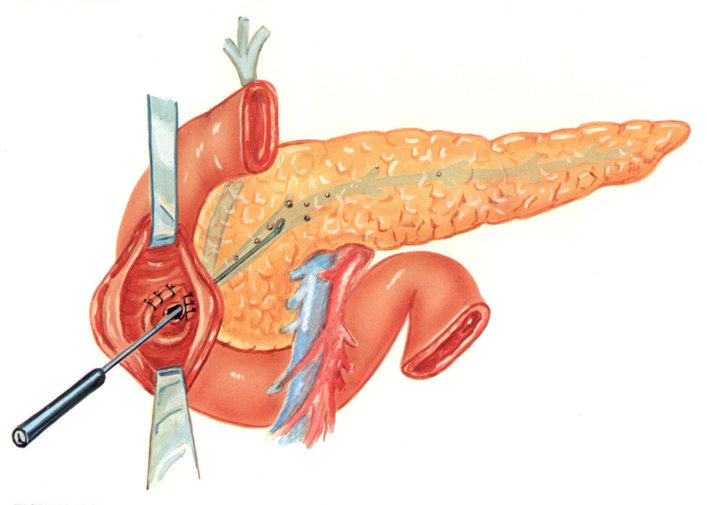

FIGURE 12-29. Instruments may be passed up the pancreatic duct retrograde to remove stones or calcific deposits occluding the pancreatic duct system.

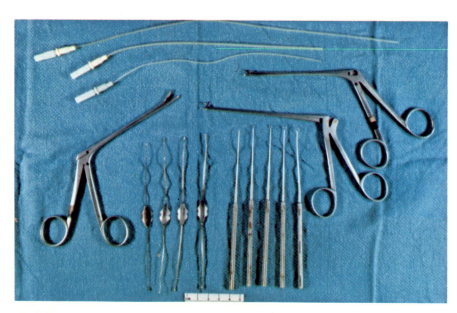

FIGURE 12-30. The instruments I use for exploration and debridement of the pancreatic duct include an assortment of small wire loops, curettes, small polyethylene catheters (Intracath), and fine rongeurs to crush and grasp stones.

270

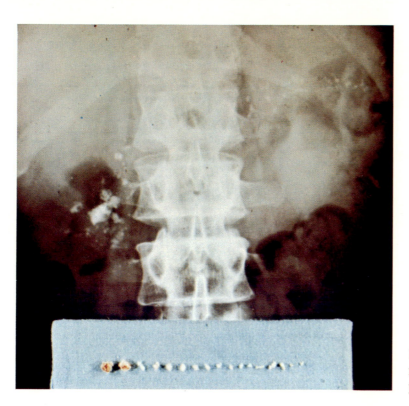

FIGURE 12-31. Stones and calculi removed during exploration of the pancreatic duct system.

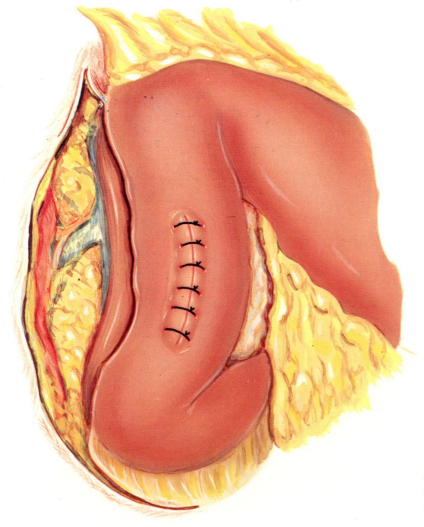

FIGURE 12-32. The duodenotomy incision is closed longitudinally in two layers with continuous 3-0 chromic catgut sutures to the mucosa and interrupted 3-0 silk sutures to the seromuscular layer.

271

Longitudinal Pancreatojejunostomy (Modified Puestow Procedure)

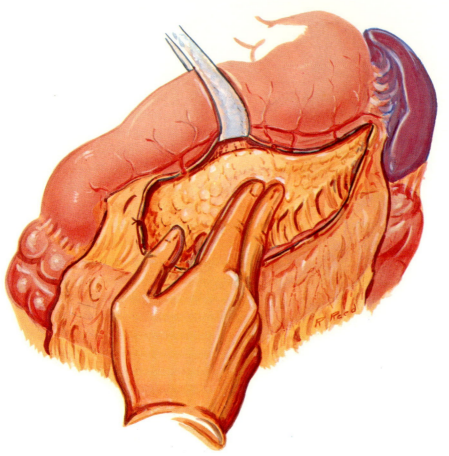

FIGURE 12-33. The pancreas has been exposed by dividing the gastrocolic omentum, protecting the gastroepiploic vessels along the greater curvature of the stomach. The surgeon's right hand is palpating the ventral surface of the pancreas to identify a dilated pancreatic duct.

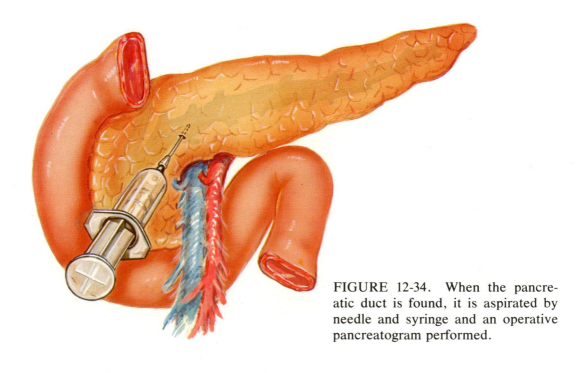

FIGURE 12-34. When the pancreatic duct is found, it is aspirated by needle and syringe and an operative pancreatogram performed.

272

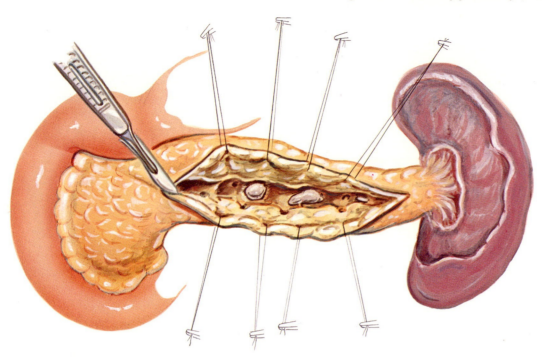

FIGURE 12-35.   The pancreatic duct is opened longitudinally through the ventral surface of the pancreas. Interrupted 3-0 silk sutures are used for hemostasis and traction. Calcium bicarbonate stones are often found in the pancreatic duct system and in secondary and tertiary duct orifices. All calcareous material should be removed, not only from the main duct but also from obstructed secondary and tertiary ducts. The longitudinal opening of the pancreatic duct system is carried almost to the duodenum in order to debride and open all obstructed pancreatic ducts.

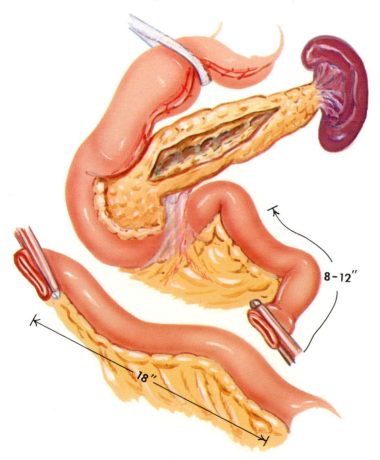

FIGURE 12-36.   A Roux-Y jejunal segment is then fashioned approximately 8 to 12 inches distal to the ligament of Treitz. The defunctionalized segment of jejunum should be about 18 inches long.

273

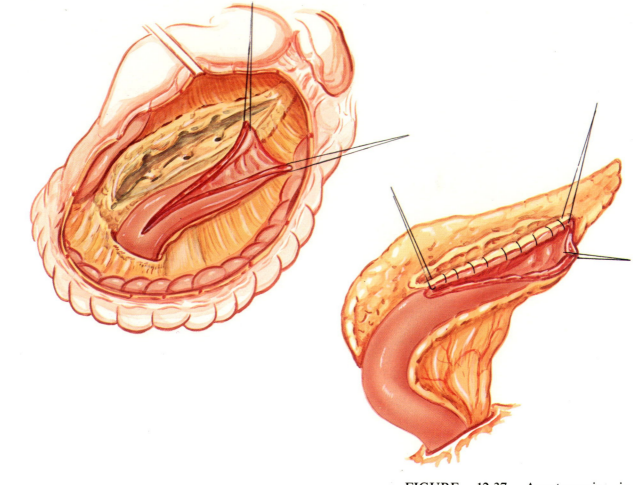

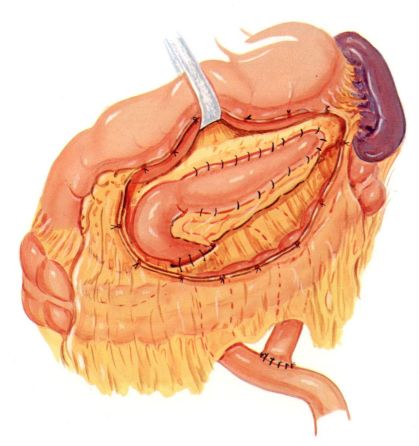

FIGURE 12-37. Anastomosis in progress. The Roux-Y jejunal segment is brought up under the colon through an opening in the transverse mesocolon to place it alongside the opened pancreas. The jejunal segment is opened along its antimesenteric border and a posterior row of interrupted 3-0 silk sutures is used to approximate the jejunum and pancreas. A second row of interrupted 3-0 synthetic absorbable or silk sutures is then placed to unite pancreatic duct mucosa with jejunal mucosa.

FIGURE 12-38. The anastomosis has been completed with two layers anteriorly; the jejunal segment covers the opened pancreatic ducts. The proximal divided jejunum is then rejoined end to side into the Roux-Y jejunal limb. The jejunum is fixed to the transverse mesocolon with loosely placed silk sutures. The anastomosis should be drained with a Penrose drain.

Subtotal Pancreatectomy and Pancreatojejunostomy

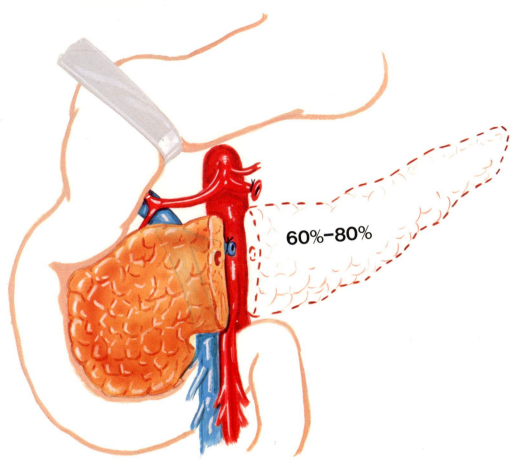

FIGURE 12-39.   When the most severe area of chronic pancreatitis is in the body or tail of the pancreas, a subtotal pancreatectomy should be performed. Usually there is enough disease in the head of the pancreas with some pancreatic duct obstruction to require retrograde drainage for this remaining segment of the pancreas. In most patients, resection of the body and tail of the pancreas to the superior mesenteric vessels or beyond will remove approximately 60% to 80% of the pancreas.

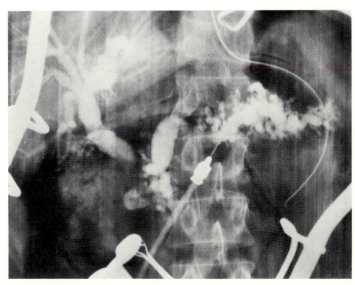

FIGURE 12-40.   Operative pancreatogram in a patient with a distended pancreatic duct in the head of the pancreas, resulting from obstruction at the ampulla of Vater, and a severely diseased duct system in the distal pancreas. Resection of the distal pancreas and drainage of the proximal remaining segment was performed in this patient.

275

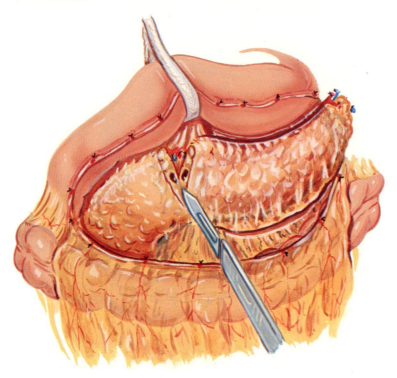

FIGURE 12-41.   The pancreas is exposed through the gastrocolic omentum, preserving the gastroepiploic vessels along the greater curvature of the stomach. The stomach is elevated superiorly, and the colon is retracted inferiorly. The spleen and tail of the pancreas are mobilized out of their bed and a splenectomy is performed. The distal pancreas is elevated by blunt dissection through the avascular plane behind the pancreas, and the splenic vessels are thereby mobilized with the gland. An incision along the inferior border of the pancreas provides access and entry to this retroperitoneal plane. The dissection is carried to the superior mesenteric vessels. At this point, the splenic vessels are ligated and the pancreas is transected; the distal pancreas is submitted to the pathologist. In transecting the pancreas, great care must be taken that the underlying superior mesenteric artery and vein are not damaged.

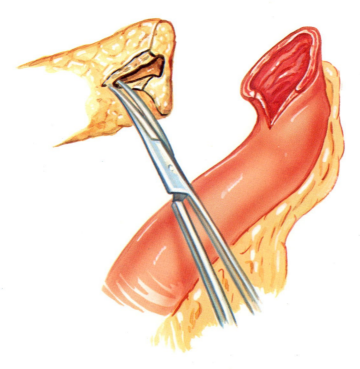

FIGURE 12-42. The remaining proximal segment of the gland is anastomosed to a Roux-Y jejunal segment brought up under the transverse colon. The pancreatic duct is opened longitudinally toward the duodenum to widely open the remaining pancreatic ducts for adequate drainage. The Roux-Y jejunal segment is opened by means of an incision along its antimesenteric border to overlap the opened pancreas.

276

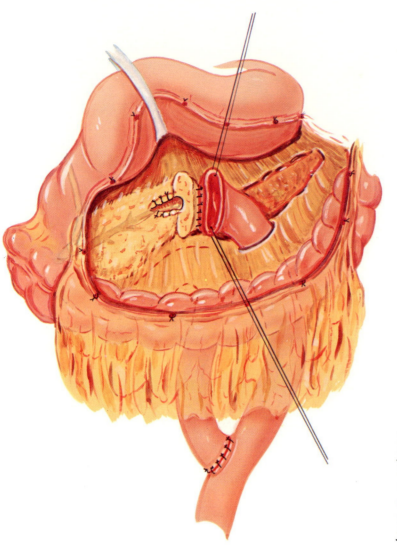

FIGURE 12-43. The opened jejunum is joined to the pancreas in two layers. Interrupted 3-0 silk sutures are used for the posterior row and interrupted 3-0 synthetic absorbable sutures are used to approximate the jejunal and pancreatic duct mucosa.

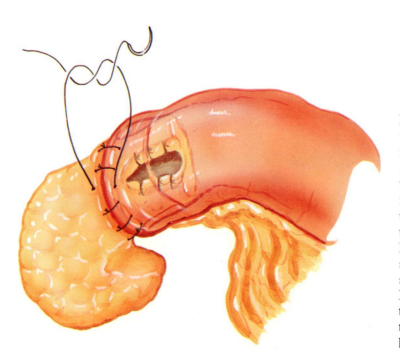

FIGURE 12-44. The two-layer anastomosis has been completed. The last interrupted 3-0 silk suture unites the seromuscular layer of the jejunum to the tough capsule of the chronically inflamed pancreas. It is always wise to drain the pancreatic anastomosis. If the anastomosis appears to be secure, Penrose drainage is adequate. If the surgeon is at all concerned about the security of the anastomosis, then both Penrose drains and sump suction tubes should be placed near the anastomosis to drain any pancreatic juice leakage.

Radical Subtotal Pancreatectomy

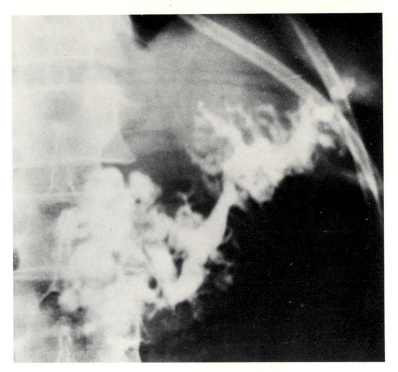

FIGURE 12-45. Operative pancreatogram of extremely severe chronic pancreatitis involving the entire pancreas. Subtotal pancreatectomy should be performed in this and the following situations: when previous duct drainage operations have failed or recurrent disease has occurred; or when the entire pancreas is fibrotic and calcified without evidence of ductal obstruction or distention (so that duct drainage operations would not be of value). I have never removed what I considered to be 95% of the pancreas, as described by Child and associates. On several occasions, I have performed a subtotal pancreatectomy of up to 85% of the pancreas.

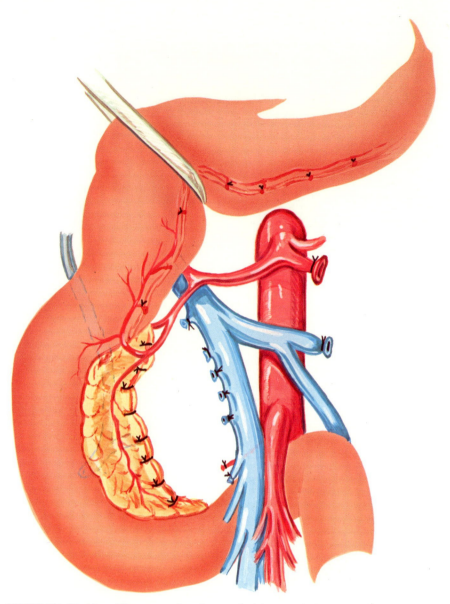

FIGURE 12-46. The resection is carried beyond the superior mesenteric vein; branch veins are ligated to the remaining rim of pancreas around the C-loop of the duodenum. It is important to protect the superior and inferior pancreatocoduodenal arteries from the gastroduodenal and to protect the common bile duct. It may be wise to open the common bile duct and place a metal probe in the distal bile duct to aid in its identification. The remaining rim of pancreatic tissue may be sutured closed without drainage by a Roux-Y jejunal segment. It is important to identify and to ligate the main pancreatic duct separately. After completion of the operative procedure, one must be assured that the blood supply to the duodenum and remaining pancreas is intact. I believe this operative procedure is preferable and has a lower operative mortality than a pancreatoduodenal resection (Whipple operation) for chronic pancreatitis. The Whipple operation also sacrifices, unnecessarily I believe, the antrum of the stomach, duodenum, and distal bile duct, all of which are preserved by subtotal pancreatectomy. However, if more severe pancreatitis is in the head of the pancreas and the distal pancreas is less involved (an infrequent occurrence), then a pancreatoduodenal resection may be advisable. After subtotal pancreatectomy, drainage of the remaining pancreas is necessary. I place two sets of drains, one to the edge of the resected pancreas through the left upper quadrant of the abdomen and another into the right subhepatic space through the right upper abdomen.

Cystogastrostomy

Pseudocysts of the pancreas may be most effectively drained into the stomach when the anterior wall of the pseudocyst is adherent to the posterior wall of the stomach.

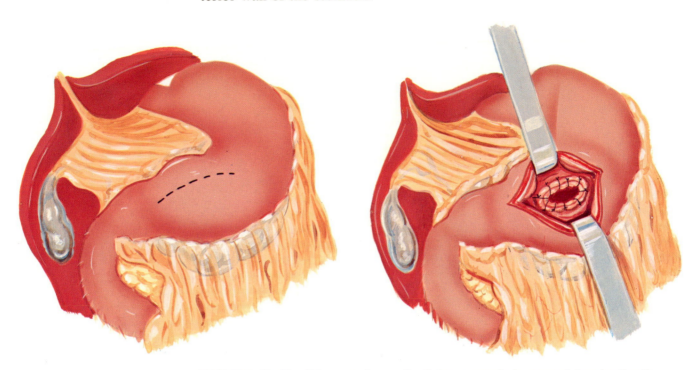

FIGURE 12-47.   The anterior wall of the stomach is opened longitudinally, as indicated by the dotted line. Once the stomach is opened, a pseudocystogram may be obtained by needling through the posterior wall of the stomach into the pseudocyst cavity. The fluid from the pseudocyst is submitted for culture, cytological, study, and amylase levels. After aspiration of 15 to 30 ml of cyst fluid, approximately 15 to 30 ml of Renografin-60 dye is instilled into the cyst cavity. A pseudocystogram is obtained to show the position of the pseudocyst in relationship to the stomach, whether it is unilocular or multilocular, and to aid the surgeon in deciding on dependent drainage. If it appears appropriate to proceed with a cystogastrostomy, a longitudinal incision is made through the combined posterior wall of the stomach–anterior wall of the pseudocyst, entering the cyst cavity. A segment of the pseudocyst wall should be excised for biopsy. The cystogastrostomy opening should be at least 3 to 4 cm for effective drainage. I suture the cystogastrostomy opening with interrupted 3-0 synthetic absorbable sutures to control bleeding from the cut edge of the stomach, to approximate the gastric mucosa to the cyst lining, and to prevent early closure of the opening. In exploring the cavity of the pseudocyst, any loose or necrotic pancreatic tissue or debris is excised. After completion of the cystogastrostomy, the stomach is closed with a continuous 3-0 chromic catgut suture to the mucosa and a second layer of interrupted 3-0 silk sutures to the seromuscular wall. Drainage of the abdominal cavity is rarely necessary.

Cystojejunostomy

When a pseudocyst is located below the stomach or through the transverse mesocolon such that the anterior wall of the cyst and the posterior wall of the stomach are not in close approximation, or when cystogastrostomy would not provide dependent drainage of the pseudocyst, it is more effective to drain the pseudocyst by means of a Roux-Y jejunal segment.

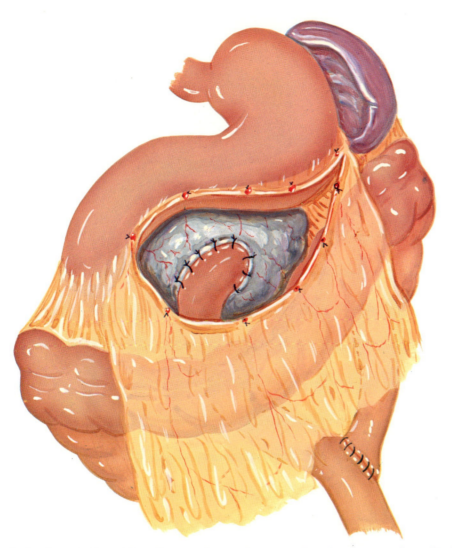

FIGURE 12-48.   After the pseudocyst is exposed and an appropriate site for dependent drainage is selected, a large needle is inserted into the cyst, 15 to 30 ml of cyst fluid is aspirated, and 15 to 30 ml of Renografin-60 dye is instilled into the cavity for a pseudocystogram. The most dependent area of the pseudocyst on the area of needle aspiration is selected for the point of drainage. A Roux-Y jejunal segment is constructed and brought up to the pseudocyst; the Roux-Y segment is passed under the transverse colon or, occasionally, over the transverse colon, as depicted. An opening is made in the wall of the pseudocyst and a segment of the wall is again submitted for biopsy. A cystojejunostomy anastomosis is made in two layers using interrupted 3-0 silk sutures to the outer row and interrupted 3-0 synthetic absorbable sutures for the inner layer. The anastomosis should be at least 3 to 4 cm. After construction of this anastomosis, drainage of the abdomen is usually not necessary.

Cystoduodenostomy

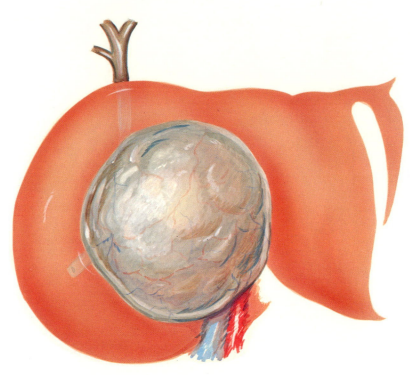

FIGURE 12-49. When a pseudocyst is in the head of the pancreas, stretching the C-loop of the duodenum, the cyst may be effectively drained into the duodenum. Cystoduodenostomy is slightly more hazardous than cystogastrostomy or cystojejunostomy.

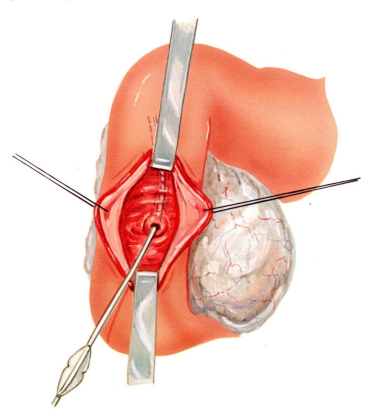

FIGURE 12-50. Adequate mobilization of the descending duodenum is performed and a longitudinal duodenotomy employed to open the duodenum. The papilla of Vater should be identified and a small metal probe passed up the distal bile duct to determine its location.

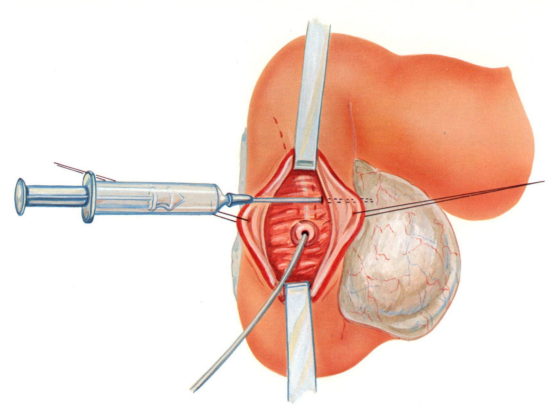

FIGURE 12-51.   Needle aspiration of the pseudocyst is performed to identify the size and location of the pseudocyst and a pseudocystogram is performed.

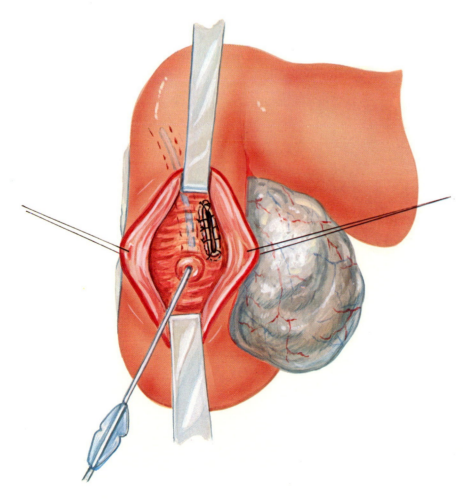

FIGURE 12-52. A cystoduodenostomy is created that opens through the medial wall of the duodenum into the cyst cavity to create a 3 to 4 cm opening. A portion of the cyst wall is submitted for biopsy. This opening must be placed to avoid injury to the distal bile duct, identified by a metal probe in the duct. Interrupted 3-0 synthetic absorbable sutures are used to suture this opening, both to provide hemostasis and to prevent early closure. After completion of the cystoduodenostomy, the probe is removed from the distal bile duct and the duodenotomy incision is closed longitudinally in two layers, with continuous 3-0 chromic catgut to the inner layer and interrupted 3-0 silk sutures to the outer, seromuscular layer. Drainage of the abdomen is not usually necessary.

283

Pancreatoduodenal Resection (Whipple Procedure)

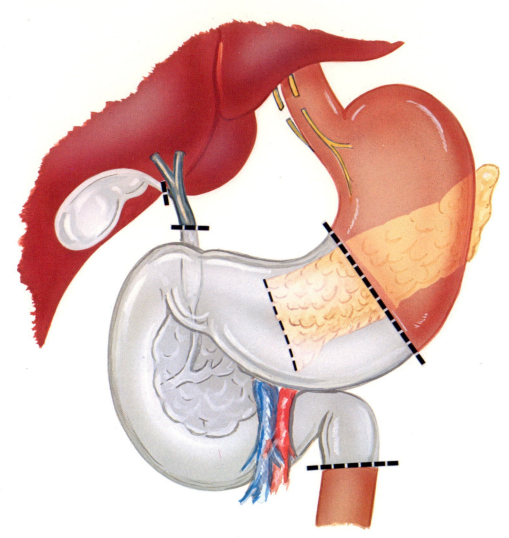

FIGURE 12-53. The extent of a pancreatoduodenal resection (Whipple operation). The specimen resected includes the antrum of the stomach, distal bile duct, duodenum, and head and uncinate process of the pancreas. In addition, a cholecystectomy and vagotomy are performed. The vagotomy decreases gastric acidity and aids in preventing post-operative stomal ulceration. The cholecystectomy is performed because the gallbladder is rendered non-functional by resection of the distal bile duct; if it remained, it would act as a diverticulum of the biliary system and a potential nidus for stone formation. Although some surgeons have preserved the gallbladder and used it for cholecystojejunostomy reconstruction of the biliary system, I prefer to remove it.

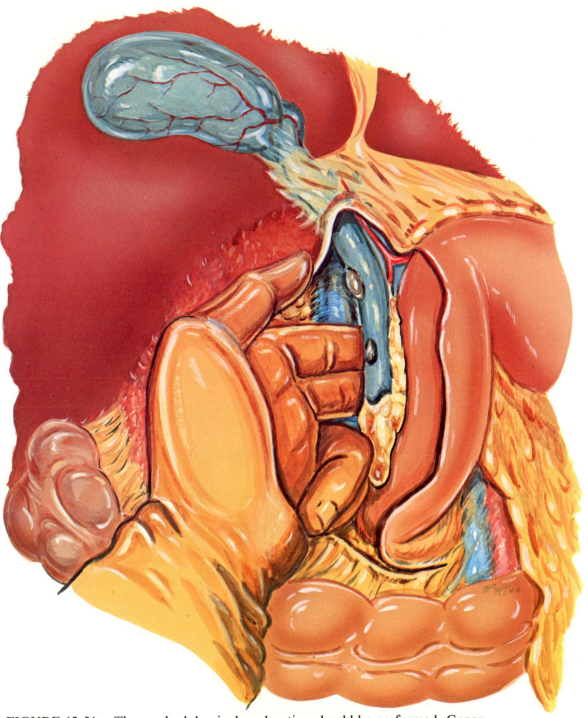

FIGURE 12-54. Thorough abdominal exploration should be performed. Generous mobilization of the duodenum and head of the pancreas from their retroperitoneal position should be performed; this dissection should be carried medial to the vena cava to the level of the spine or aorta. This exposes the posterior aspect of the duodenum, pancreas, and distal common bile duct. Any lymph nodes found in this area should be excised for biopsy. At this time, the abdominal cavity should be examined for metastases. Close attention should be given to potential metastases in the lymph node groups draining the pancreas—the paraduodenal, common bile duct, hepatic, celiac, and superior mesenteric lymph nodes. Biopsies should be performed on any suspicious nodes. In addition, biopsy should be done of any suspicious areas or possible metastases in the liver.

285

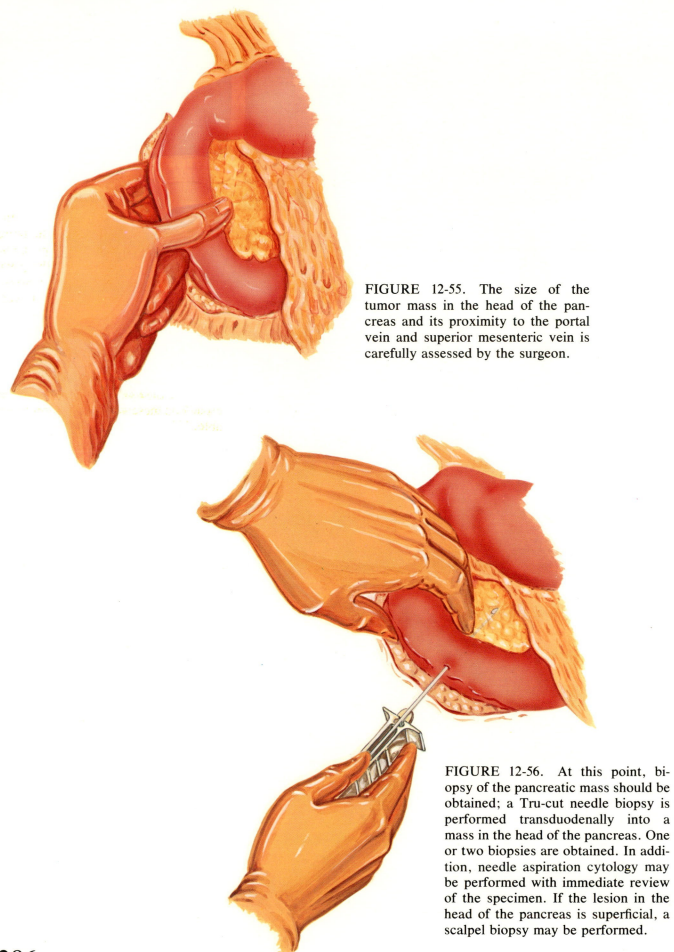

FIGURE 12-55. The size of the tumor mass in the head of the pancreas and its proximity to the portal vein and superior mesenteric vein is carefully assessed by the surgeon.

FIGURE 12-56. At this point, biopsy of the pancreatic mass should be obtained; a Tru-cut needle biopsy is performed transduodenally into a mass in the head of the pancreas. One or two biopsies are obtained. In addition, needle aspiration cytology may be performed with immediate review of the specimen. If the lesion in the head of the pancreas is superficial, a scalpel biopsy may be performed.

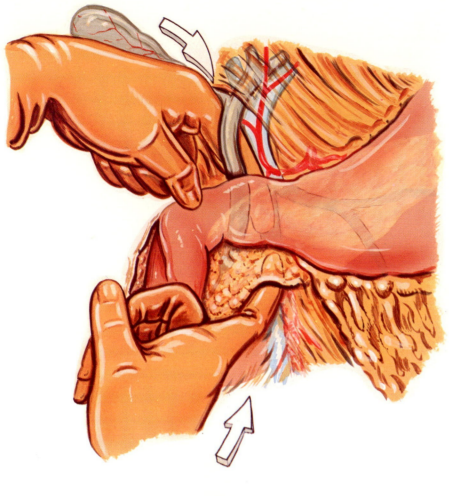

FIGURE 12-57. After biopsy is obtained, if the lesion appears resectable by virtue of no distant metastases, the dissection is carried along the third part of the duodenum to expose the superior mesenteric vein at the point where it crosses the duodenum and enters under the neck of the pancreas. By bimanual palpation along the superior mesenteric vein from below and the portal vein from above, the size and extent of the tumor mass and its proximity to these vessels are evaluated. If the lesion is so large as to encroach on these vessels, it is unresectable. If it is small enough to be safely removed from these vessels and there are no distant metastases, it is potentially resectable.

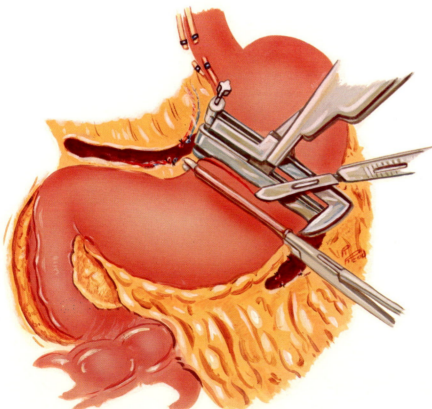

FIGURE 12-58. After it has been determined that the tumor mass in the head of the pancreas is potentially resectable, a vagotomy is performed and the antrum of the stomach is divided. A TA-90 automatic stapler is placed across the distal stomach at the site selected and the stomach is stapled closed. a noncrushing clamp is placed below the stapler and the stomach is divided.

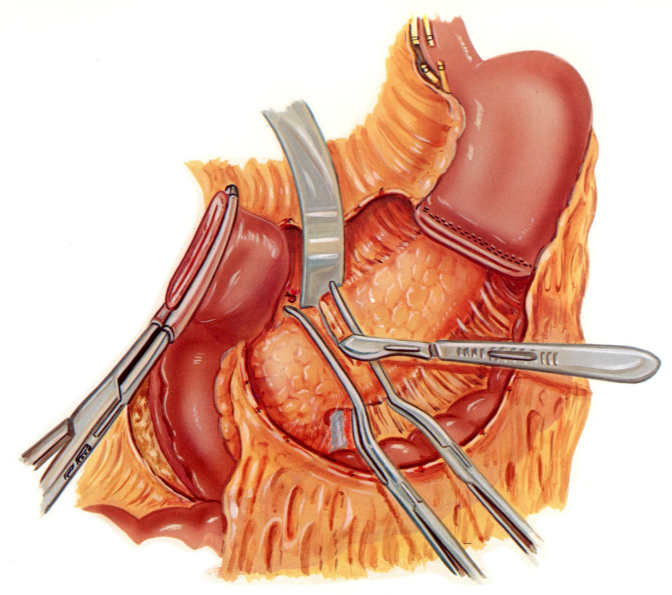

FIGURE 12-59.   The antrum of the stomach and its adjacent omentum is reflected to the right and inferiorly; the gastroduodenal artery is identified, ligated,
and divided; and by blunt finger dissection on top of the superior mesenteric and
portal veins, the neck of the pancreas is gently elevated from these vessels. It is
rare to have a branch vein on the ventral surface of these vessels to the pancreas;
an avascular space can almost always be found in this area. Two noncrushing,
Glassman clamps are placed across the neck of the pancreas and the pancreas is
carefully divided between clamps. These clamps control bleeding from the divided
pancreas.

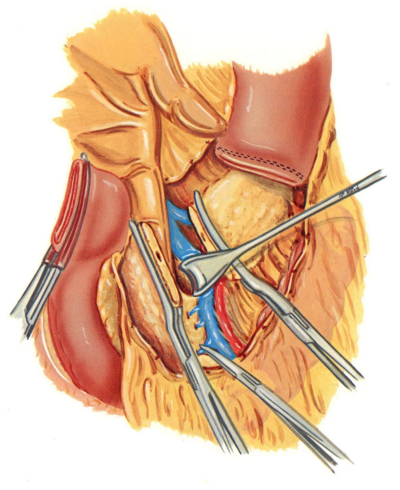

FIGURE 12-60. The head of the pancreas and uncinate process are carefully freed by sharp and blunt dissection from the superior mesenteric vein and its branches, and the individual branches are carefully identified, ligated, and divided. This is most safely performed by the surgeon placing his left hand behind the head of the pancreas, and an assistant retracting the superior mesenteric vein with a small vein retractor or a Kittner dissector.

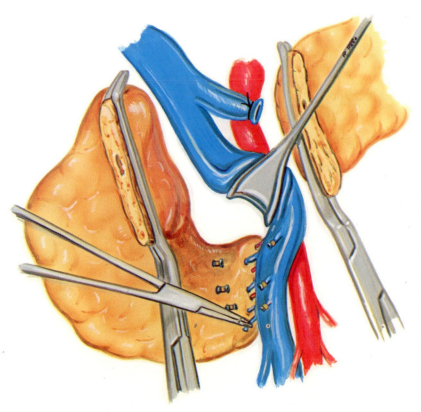

FIGURE 12-61. Ligation of the several delicate branches of the superior mesenteric vein may be performed by silk sutures or silver clips. The disadvantage of clips is that they may later be rubbed off with bleeding. An effort is made to remove the entire pancreas and uncinate process from the superior mesenteric vein. However, in some patients, when the uncinate process passes well behind the superior mesenteric vein, it may be transected and a portion of the tip may be left in place. This has caused no problems.

289

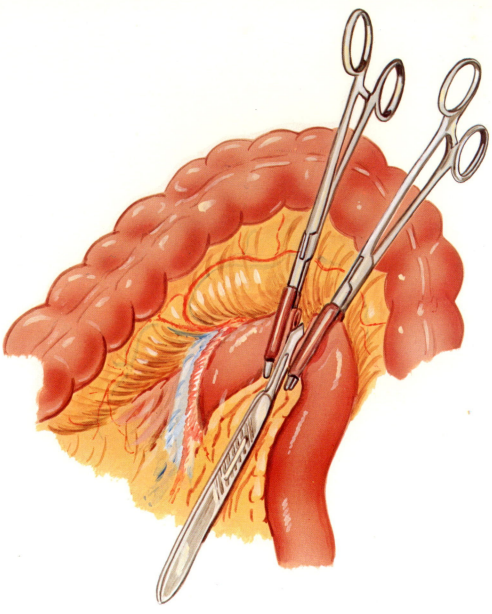

FIGURE 12-62.   Attention is turned to the duodenojejunal junction at the ligament of Treitz. The duodenum is mobilized as dissection of the pancreas from the superior mesenteric vessels proceeds. At the point where the entire blood supply to the duodenum has been divided with ligation of the inferior pancreatoduodenal arcade, the duodenum is completely mobilized and freed. A non-crushing clamp is then placed across the duodenojejunal junction and it is divided. The specimen is removed and given to the pathologist.

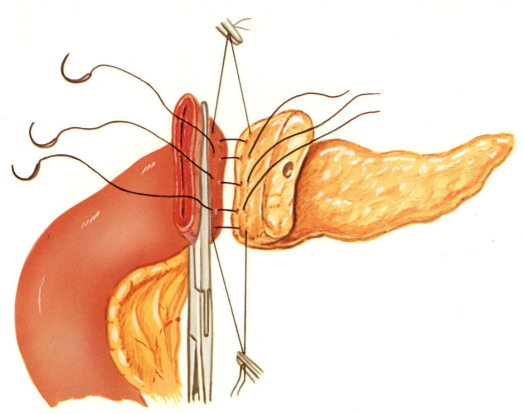

FIGURE 12-63. Technic of pancreatojejunostomy. The jejunum is then brought under the superior mesenteric vessels into the subhepatic space. I prefer to reconstruct by means of an end-to-end pancreatojejunostomy. However, if the end of the jejunum cannot be brought up to the end of the pancreas, the end of the jejunum may be closed and the end of the pancreas anastomosed into the lateral wall of the jejunum, with the entire head of the pancreas stuffed into the jejunum. An external row of interrupted 3-0 silk sutures is placed. A second row of interrupted 3-0 synthetic absorbable sutures is placed to suture the jejunal mucosa to the cut margin of the pancreas; the pancreatic duct is thus sutured open to the jejunal mucosa. In many instances, as a splint for the pancreatojejunal anastomosis, I place a polyethylene catheter into the pancreatic duct extending several inches into the jejunum. The entire cut end of the pancreas is placed inside the jejunum, whether the anastomosis is performed end to end or end to side.

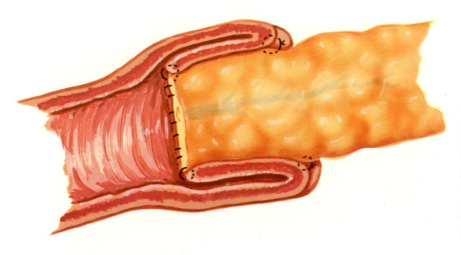

FIGURE 12-64. The construction of a pancreatojejunal anastomosis. The entire end of the pancreas is stuffed into the end of the jejunum with a two-layer anastomosis; the intussuscepted jejunum is wrapped around the end of the pancreas to prevent leakage. The technic of this anastomosis is critical; every effort must be made to prevent leakage of pancreatic juice.

291

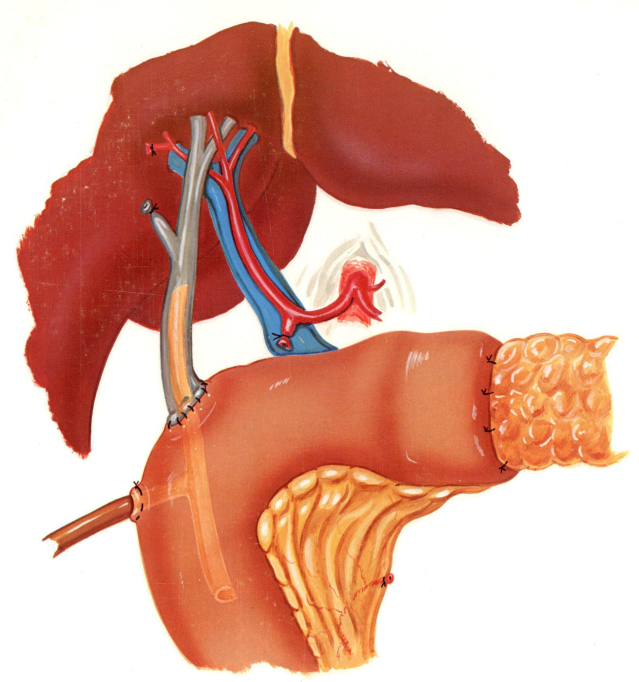

FIGURE 12-65.   After completion of the pancreatojejunal anastomosis, a choledochojejunal anastomosis is created end to side. I frequently splint this anastomosis with a large T-tube brought out through the wall of the jejunum. However, in many patients with a large, dilated common bile duct, splinting of the anastomosis is not necessary. A two-layer anastomosis is performed with interrupted 3-0 chromic catgut sutures to the inner row and interrupted 3-0 silk sutures to the outer. If a T-tube is brought out through the wall of the jejunum, a purse-string suture of 2-0 chromic catgut encircles the exit point.

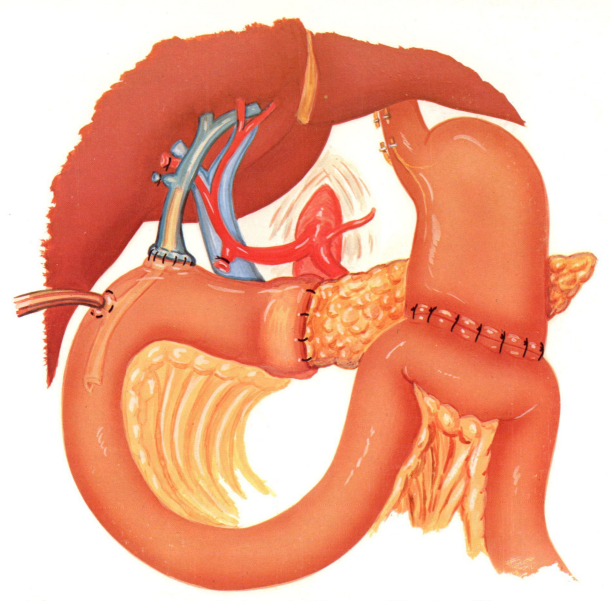

FIGURE 12-66.   The reconstruction is completed by a gastrojejunostomy. This is performed, antecolic and end to side, by dividing the stapled transected end of the stomach along the greater curvature for a distance of 4 to 6 cm. A two-layer gastrojejunostomy is created using a continuous 3-0 chromic catgut suture to the inner row and interrupted 3-0 silk sutures to the outer row. After a Whipple operation, sump suction tubes and Penrose drains should be placed to the pancreatojejunal anastomosis and to the right subhepatic space for post-operative drainage. The sump suction tubes are usually left for 3 or 4 days and then removed. The Penrose drains may be left slightly longer, up to 6 or 7 days. Most patients do not become diabetic nor do they need pancreatic enzyme supplements after pancreatoduodenal resection. However, all patients must be carefully monitored for evidence of pancreatic exocrine or endocrine insufficiency. If supplemental pancreatic enzymes are needed in the diet because of post-operative steatorrhea or weight loss, I prefer Viokase or Cotazyme tablets with meals. A bland, high-protein, low-fat diet is prescribed after patients resume eating.

293

Total Pancreatectomy

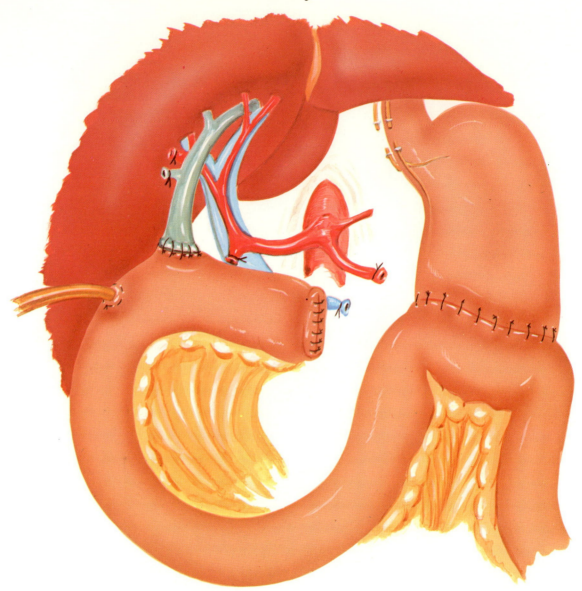

FIGURE 12-67.   If total pancreatectomy is performed, a pancreatoduodenal resection is the mechanism of removal of the head and uncinate process of the pancreas. Following completion of the pancreatoduodenal resection, the end of the jejunum is closed and an end-to-side choledochojejunostomy and gastrojejunostomy are made as previously described. The distal pancreas is then resection by either of two methods. The dissection may be carried from right to left; the cut edges of the pancreas are elevated and mobilized from the superior mesenteric vessels, and the splenic artery and vein are divided as they enter the distal pancreas. Once the splenic vessels are divided, an avascular plane behind the distal pancreas is entered and the distal pancreas and spleen are then excised. An alternative method is to remove the spleen and mobilize the tail of the pancreas from left to right; the dissection is carried to the superior mesenteric vessels and the splenic artery and vein are divided as the last step of the procedure.

Local Resection of Ampullary Tumor

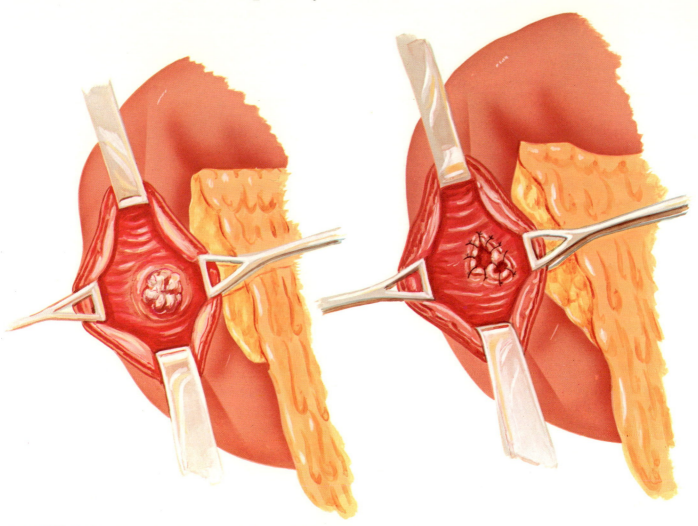

FIGURE 12-68.   Occasionally, especially in elderly patients, a polypoid carcinoma or villous adenoma with carcinoma-in-situ may be locally excised. The descending duodenum is mobilized by a Kocher maneuver and longitudinal duodenotomy is performed. The localized, polypoid tumor mass of the ampulla of Vater
can be seen in the left drawing. The distal bile duct should be opened by a sphincterotomy. If a stalk can be identified, the tumor is simply excised locally by division through the stalk of the tumor mass. A segment of the adjacent wall of the
duodenum is excised with the polypoid tumor and its stalk, opening widely into
the distal common bile duct and pancreatic duct. After excision of the tumor, a
careful reconstruction of the mucosa of the common bile duct and pancreatic duct
to the duodenal mucosa is accomplished, as seen on the right. The longitudinal
duodenotomy is then closed in two layers in the usual fashion.

Palliative Procedures
for Carcinoma of the Pancreas

Biliary Bypass: Cholecystojejunostomy

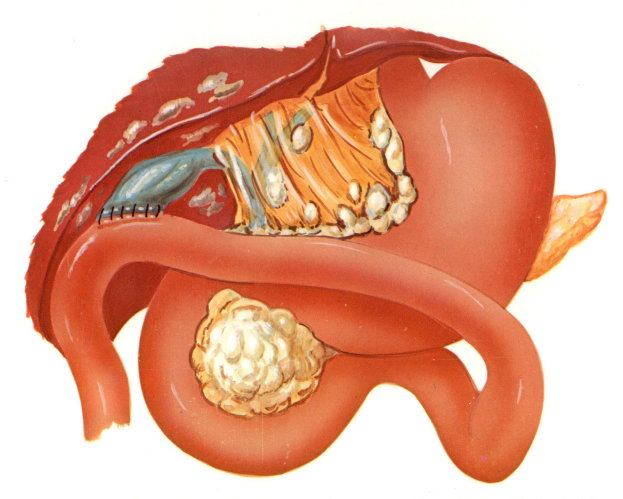

FIGURE 12-69. When an extensive, unresectable carcinoma of the head of the pancreas is found, palliation of the obstructed biliary system may be obtained by a cholecystojejunostomy. If this technic of biliary drainage is used, the surgeon must be certain that the tumor mass does not encroach on the cystic duct–hepatic duct junction. An operative cholangiogram through the gallbladder should be obtained. If the cystic duct is widely patent and joins the common hepatic duct well above the area of obstruction, a cholecystojejunostomy may be performed. The fundus of the gallbladder is joined to the side of the first portion of the jejunum, anterior to the colon, creating a two layer anastomosis, with interrupted 3-0 chromic catgut to the inner row and interrupted 3-0 silk sutures to the outer row.

Biliary Bypass: Choledochoduodenostomy

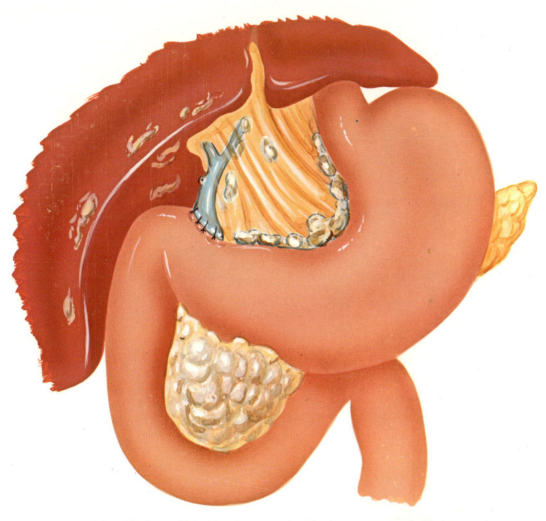

FIGURE 12-70.   If the gallbladder has previously been removed, if the cystic duct is not widely patent, or if it joins the common hepatic duct too close to the area of tumor obstruction for effective drainage of the biliary system, a choledochoduodenostomy should be performed. The first part of the duodenum is mobilized and joined side to side to the dilated common bile duct, creating a 2.5 to 3 cm anastomosis. A two-layer anastomosis is performed with interrupted 3-0 silk sutures to the outer layer and interrupted 3-0 chromic catgut sutures to the inner layer. It is rarely necessary to splint this anastomosis with a T-tube.

Gastrojejunostomy

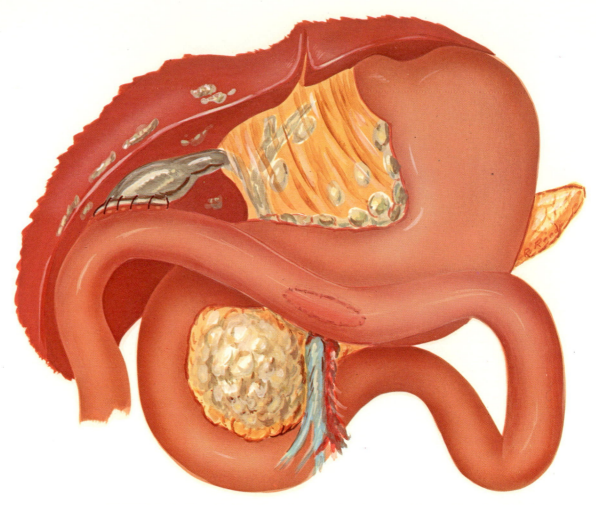

FIGURE 12-71.   If there is evidence of existing or impending duodenal obstruction because of the size of the tumor mass, a complementary gastrojejunostomy should also be constructed. The gastrojejunostomy should be performed in the most dependent portion of the antrum of the stomach, anterior to the colon, near the pylorus.

Bilateral Splanchnic Resection

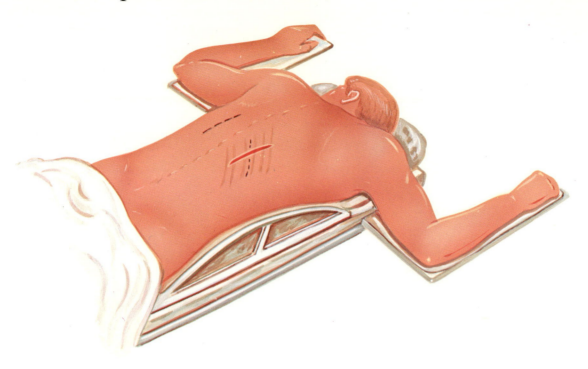

FIGURE 12-72.   When a carcinoma of the body and tail of the pancreas is found and is unresectable, as is the usual case, attention must be paid to relieving the patient's pain. After the diagnosis is established by abdominal exploration and biopsy and any necessary palliative procedures (biliary bypass and/or gastrojejunostomy) have been performed, the abdomen is closed. Under the same anesthesia, we turn the patient onto the abdomen, exposing the back. A neurosurgeon then performs a bilateral splanchnic resection through two longitudinal paraspinous incisions.

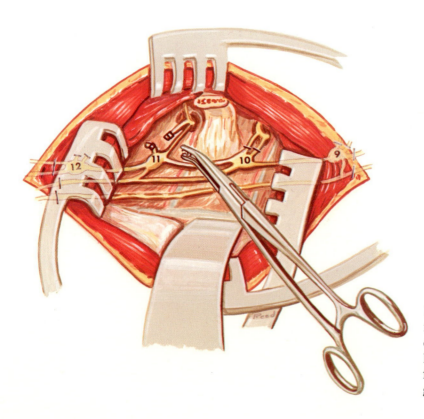

FIGURE 12-73.   Complete splanchnic resection is performed on each side, dividing and excising the greater, lesser, and least splanchnic nerves from the 9th through the 12th thoracic ganglia.

299

Index

Index